SOFT TISSUE TUMORS

Edited by **Fethi Derbel**

Soft Tissue Tumors
Edited by Fethi Derbel

Published by InTech
Janeza Trdine 9, 51000 Rijeka, Croatia

Publishing Process Manager Marija Radja

Technical Editor Teodora Smiljanic

Cover Designer InTech Design Team

Additional hard copies can be obtained from orders@intechopen.com

Soft Tissue Tumors, Edited by Fethi Derbel
p. cm.
ISBN 978-953-307-862-5

For EU product safety concerns:
IN TECH d.o.o., Prolaz Marije Krucifikse Kozulić 3, 51000 Rijeka, Croatia,
info@intechopen.com or visit our website at intechopen.com.

Meet the editor

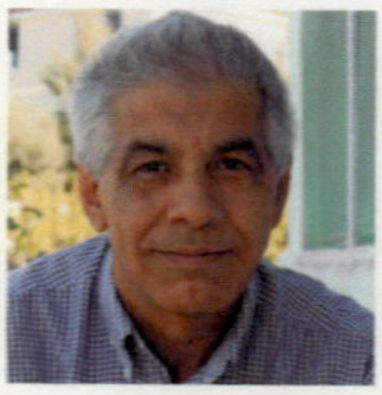

Professor Fethi Derbel was born in 1960, in Tunisia. He received his medical degree from the Sousse Faculty of Medicine at Sousse, Tunisia. He completed his surgical residency in General Surgery at University Hospital Farhat Hached of Sousse and was a member of Unit of Liver Transplantaion in the University of Rennes, France. He is presently working in the department of surgery in Sahloul Hospital, Sousse. His hospital activities are mostly concerned with laparoscopic, colorectal,pancreatic, hepato-biliary and gastric surgery. He is a professor at the school of Medicine in Djibouti, past member of the medical committee in the University Hospital Sahloul, Sousse,Member of the National College of Surgeons in Tunisia. He has published many articles in journals and collaborates intensively with InTech Open Access Publisher as an editor.

Contents

Preface

Soft tissue tumors include a heterogeneous group of diagnostic entities, most of them benign in nature and behavior. Malignant entities, soft tissue sarcomas, are rare tumors that account for 1% of all malignancies. These are predominantly tumors of adults, but 15% arise in children and adolescents. The wide biological diversity of soft tissue tumors, combined with their high incidence and potential morbidity and mortality represent challenges to contemporary researches, both at the level of basic and clinical science. Determining whether a soft tissue mass is benign or malignant is vital for appropriate management.

This book is the result of collaboration between several authors, experts in their fields; they have tried to convey to the reader the complexity of soft tissue tumors and the diversity in the diagnosis and management of these tumors.

In this book, entitled Soft Tissue Tumors, we have highlighted many of the significant advances in the diagnosis and treatment of soft tissue tumors; we tried to offer a comprehensive overview of this wide field, from basic mechanisms underlying soft tissue tumors to current advances and future directions in the prevention, early detection and management of these neoplasms.

The presented textbook is subdivided into five sections termed: Fundamental Aspects of Soft Tissue Tumors, Diagnosis and Investigations,Types and Classification of Soft Tissue Tumors, Treatment of Soft Tissue Tumors, Prognosis of Soft Tissue Tumors.

Although this book does not cover all aspects related to soft tissue tumors, it is intended for at least two kinds of readers : residents of intermediate and advanced courses in medicine; oncologist, pathologist, surgeon, radiologists and all doctors whatever their specialty.

As editor in chief of this textbook, I would like to acknowledge the efforts made by all of the contributing authors and the entire editorial team in the publishing of this book especially Mrs Marija Radja for her very precious collaboration. Their dedication to the publication of the most contemporary and comprehensive scientific data has this excellent work as a result. I would like to dedicate this textbook to all my colleagues surgeons, pathologist, oncologist and radiologist at Sahloul Hospital, the past and actual deans of our university Professor Mohsen Jeddi, Sahloul Essoussi, Abdelkrim Zbidi, Nejib Mrizak and Ali Mtiraoui for their encouragement, and Professor Moncef Mokni pathologist in the department of pathology at Farhat Hached Hospital in Sousse.

I would like to express a special dedication to our first dean and professor of pathology who had dedicated a lot of his scientific efforts to the soft tissue tumors. His name is Professor Chedly Bouzakkoura. He passed away last year.

I also dedicate this book especially to Professor Ridha Ben Hadj Hamida, and Professor Rached Letaief, surgeons at the department of surgery in Sousse. A special dedication to Professor Gharbi Slaheddine and Hamadi Farhat, the first surgeons at Sousse University who died a few years ago.

You have taught me, since my first steps as resident, not only to manage different types of digestive malignancies using the highest quality surgical and medical care but as well instilled in me a sense of responsibility to improve as a person and as a clinician.

Fethi Derbel
Professor of General and Digestive Surgery
University Hospital Sahloul
Sousse
Tunisia

Part 1

Fundamental Aspects of Soft Tissue Tumors

1

Considerations for Treatment Development in Rhabdomyosarcoma: *In Vitro* Assessment of Novel DNA Binding Drugs

Steven J. Wolf[1,3], Laurence P.G. Wakelin[2] and Daniel R. Catchpoole[1,3]
[1]*The Biospecimens Research Group and Tumour Bank, Children's Cancer Research Unit, The Kids Research Institute, The Children's Hospital at Westmead, Westmead, NSW,*
[2]*The School of Medical Science, The Faculty of Medicine, The University of New South Wales, Sydney, NSW,*
[3]*Faculty of Medicine, The University of Sydney, NSW, Australia*

1. Introduction

Rhabdomyosarcoma (RMS) is the most common soft tissue sarcoma in children and is believed to originate from mesenchymal cells that resemble undifferentiated striated muscle cells (Wexler and Helman, 1997). It is a relatively rare tumour type with approximately 350 patients below the age of 20 diagnosed each year in the USA (Gurney et al, 1999). Incidence in Australia is also low with only 31 RMS cases out of the total 1,003 childhood cancers diagnosed between 2001 and 2005 in the state of NSW (Tracey et al 2007). Histological staining of tumour samples led to the classification of two distinct forms of tumour types: embryonal (ERMS) and alveolar (ARMS). ERMS is the most common histologically diagnosed variant of the disease and is associated with an earlier onset, most commonly around the age of 2 to 5 years (Qualman et al, 1998). Diagnosis of ERMS is made when the cells fit the criteria of appearing as stroma-rich spindle cells which are not densely packed and show no alveolar pattern of growth which characterises ARMS. Variant forms of ERMS, including botryoid and spindle cell types, have been described as being histologically similar to standard ERMS (Wexler and Helman, 1997).

Treatment of rhabdomyosarcoma employs a multimodal approach that utilizes surgical, radiological and chemotherapeutic protocols. Unlike in the treatment of adult sarcomas, surgical removal of the tumour mass in paediatric RMS patients is usually only attempted if complete resection can be guaranteed without causing cosmetic or developmental damage to the child. For this reason chemotherapy is the frontline option in the treatment of paediatric RMS both as a means of local tumour mass control and for the prevention of residual and micrometastatic disease (Stevens, 2005). Over 70% of patients with non-metastatic RMS will respond well to chemotherapy and reach a 5 year event free survival milestone. Patients with metastatic or stage IV ERMS however, and those with ARMS who generally present at diagnosis with an advanced metastatic form of the cancer, continue to face a poor prognosis as a result of diminished tumour response to the current chemotherapy options. Currently, less than 30% of patients with metastatic disease survive

without relapse and despite this drastic difference in tumour response, chemotherapy protocols continue to utilize the same compounds regardless of tumour subtype, progression or stage (Wexler and Helman, 1997).
Without agents to target specific molecular pathways and proteins of RMS, such as the PAX3-FKHR chimeric protein, chemotherapy protocols continue to utilize general cytotoxic compounds that rely on the rapid proliferation of tumour cells for selectivity and optimal efficacy. Most of these agents bind to DNA and disrupt key molecular processes involved in DNA transcription and replication. Treatment usually involves the vinca alkaloid vincristine, the transcription inhibitor actinomycin D and the alkylating prodrug cyclophosphamide (Breitfeld et al, 2005). Several other general cytotoxic agents, including the topoisomerase poisons etoposide, doxorubicin, epirubicin, topotecan and irinotecan as well as the alkylating agents ifosfamide and carboplatin have also been used in alternative treatment protocols and large scale clinical trials (Table 1). Many agents included in RMS clinical trials and standard treatment protocols can be broadly classified as general cytotoxic agents, a large proportion, including etoposide, doxorubicin and topotecan, specifically target and poison the function of the topoisomerase enzymes, whilst actinomycin D is a transcription inhibitor that has been successful in the treatment of a wide variety of tumours, including RMS.

2. DNA binding agents underpin RMS therapy – a review of clinical trials

Prior to the 1970s the prognosis for RMS patients was extremely poor regardless of tumour subtype. The earliest large scale collaboration to be established was the Intergroup Rhabdomyosarcoma Study Group (IRSG), a joint effort between US and Canadian researchers. Five trials were carried out by this group between 1972 and 2000 at which point the group merged into the Children's Oncology Group (COG) under which more recent trials have been carried out. Patients enrolled in IRSG or COG clinical trials were grouped based on various prognostic factors before an appropriate treatment schedule was assigned. The second collaboration to be established was the European based group 'International Society for Paediatric Oncology' (SIOP) which launched several large cohort trials in 1975, 1984, 1989 and 1995 from which many findings were reported. A selection of key findings from IRSG, COG and SIOP clinical trials are presented in summarized form in Table 1. With 5 year event-free survival rates (EFS) reaching 70%, patients with gross residual tumour were believed to have benefited the most in early studies. It was clear however, that patients with stage III or IV RMS required more intense chemotherapy than those in stage I and II and it was concluded that despite the successes of the VAC combinational therapies, introducing additional agents, such as topoisomerase I poisons, would help subdue the onset of local and distant failures. The prognosis for patients with non-metastatic RMS continued to improve after the fourth and fifth IRSG studies were completed, yet despite years of large cohort clinical trials and the subsequent retrospective analysis of data, response rates in patients with metastatic ERMS and ARMS remained considerably low. This has been attributed to many factors including combination chemotherapy leading to additive and overlapping adverse side effects which limit the dosages used as well as intrinsic or acquired drug resistance mechanisms.

3. Therapeutic advancement in RMS requires new agents

It is clear from this review of the chemotherapeutic treatment options available for RMS that novel agents are desperately required to improve the prognosis for patients with metastatic

Study	RMS Classification	Protocol Tested	Results	References
IRSG Study I	Group I	VAC + R	No benefit from additional R	Maurer et al, 1988
	Group II	VC + R + A	No benefit from additional A	
	Group III + IV	VAC + R + D	No benefit from additional D	
IRSG Study II	Group III	Intense repetitive pulse VAC + radiation or VDC + radiation	Improvement over IRSG 1: (SR) increased -50% to 66% (CRR) increased - 56% to 73%.	Maurer et al, 1993
	Groups I - IV	VDC	No improvement vs. VAC. Fatal side effects	
	Groups I – II	VA + C	No improvement from additional C	
	Groups I – II	Repetitive pulse VAC	Improvement over IRSG 1	
IRSG Study IV	Groups I – II	VAC, with either VAI or VIE	3yr EFS: 75% VAC, 77% VAI, 77% VIE Overall EFS of 83%. Surgery + VAI + VIE was equally effective as VAC only	Crist et al, 2001
IRSG Study IV	Intermediate risk ERMS	3yr FFS improved due to doubling of alkylating agent dosage compared to the treatment protocol used in IRSG study III. Cyclophosphamide or ifosfamide had same effect.		Baker et al, 2000
	High Risk / Stage IV	VAI or VIE every 3 wks / 12 wks + VAC every 3 wks for 36 wks.	63% OR (12 weeks)	Sandler et al, 2001
SIOP MMT89	Group III, Stage III	Novel treatment which combined 6 drugs (IVA) + (CbEV) + (IVE).	60% OS (5yr) versus 42% OS (5yr) MMT84	Stevens et al, 2005
Independent Phase I	Recurring solid tumours	varying doses of Cb + fixed doses of I + E	33% OR (4% increased)	Marina et al, 1993
Indepe-ndent Phase I/II	Refractory STS sarcomas	ICbE	32% CR 63% OR	Kung et al, 1995
CCG Study I	27 RMS patients in a total cohort of	ICbE	78% 1yCR, 33% 2yCR, 66% OR ERMS ARMS	Van Winkle et al, 2005

Study	RMS Classification	Protocol Tested	Results	References
	97 STS patients		82% 1 yr OS 40% 1 yr OS 46% 2 yr OS 20% 2 yr OS	
SIOP MMT89	Untreated Stage IV RMS	Single Course C, Epi + V	53% Total OR ERMS ARMS 46% OR 58% OR	Frascella et al, 1996
IRSG V	Stage IV RMS	T or T + VAC	46% Total OR ERMS ARMS 28% OR 65% OR	Pappo et al, 2001
Independent Trial	Intermediate risk RMS	VDC + EI at 3 week intervals over a total 10 cycle course.	91% OS 85% EFS	Arndt et al, 1998

Table 1. Results from Selected RMS clinical trials involving general cytotoxic compounds. A=actinomycin D, C=cyclophosphamide, D=Doxorubicin, E=etoposide, Epi=Epirubicin, I=ifosfamide, R=radiotherapy, V=vincristine, Cb=Carboplatin; CR=Complete Response, CRR=Complete Response Rate, EFS=Event Free Survival, OR=Overall Response, OS=Overall Survival, SR=Survival Rate.

or stage IV ERMS and ARMS. To date, the only genetic abnormality consistently associated with ARMS is the t(2:13)/t(1:13) translocations that produce the oncogenic PAX3/7-FKHR chimeric proteins. One day these may be targeted by small molecules or genetic based therapies, however, the immediate future of RMS treatment remains highly dependant on general cytotoxic agents. Unfortunately, all of the available general cytotoxic agents are associated with adverse side effects that place severe limitations on the concentrations of drug that can be administered to children with the disease. To minimize these side effects each agent is used in low doses both in combination with other general cytotoxic agents and over an extended period of time. Such treatment protocols rarely guarantee full recovery and often promote the development of drug resistance mechanisms within the cancer cells that manifest themselves either during initial rounds of therapy, or more commonly, following tumour relapse.

Optimization of existing chemotherapy protocols, and the introduction of established cytotoxic agents into RMS clinical trial, has resulted in improved response rates for ERMS patients in recent decades. Despite this, ARMS and metastatic ERMS, are still associated with a poor prognosis (Breitfeld and Meyer, 2005). With such a high dependency on general cytotoxic agents for the treatment of RMS, novel compounds with improved efficacy and fewer side effects must be developed. Efforts to improve the outcome in poor prognosis patient groups focus largely on trials involving new combinations of existing clinically-active compounds. Some of the most commonly used agents in RMS protocols exploit the fragility of DNA transcription, and chromosome integrity, by physically interfering with these processes and structures. For example, actinomycin D inhibits transcription by intercalating into DNA and impeding the progression of DNA-dependant RNA polymerases. Etoposide, along with the anthracyclines, camptothecin and its analogues, trap topoisomerases in their DNA cleavable complexes, resulting in the accumulation of DNA double strand breaks, fragmented chromosomes, and cell death at mitosis (Pommier Y,

2006). Given the apparent importance of these biochemical targets in RMS therapy, here, we have investigated the efficacy of a number of novel DNA binding transcription inhibitors and topoisomerase poisons in 5 RMS cell lines that represent both ERMS (RD and JR1) and ARMS (RH30, RH3 and RH4) tumour subtypes. We have also compared their activity with that of the established transcription inhibitors actinomycin D, chromomycin, and nogalamycin, and the topoisomerase poisons etoposide, amsacrine, doxorubicin, mitoxantrone, and topotecan. Each new agent has been designed with altered DNA association/dissociation kinetics, improved tumour penetration compared to the established agents and with this in mind, their efficacy and vulnerability to common mechanisms of resistance are examined.

3.1 Novel DNA binding cytotoxic agents

With a range of novel cytotoxic compounds available to us through colleagues at the University of New South Wales and the Auckland Cancer Society Research Centre, we aimed to assess the efficacy of selected agents from various classes in an in vitro RMS cell line model that best represented both subtypes of the disease. In doing so it was our intention to identify agents with the potential to expand treatment options for RMS patients and further improve the efficacy of chemotherapy protocols that utilize general cytotoxic agents. Each of the novel compounds assessed in this study contain tricyclic carboxamide moieties that act as DNA intercalating chromophores and have previously been shown to be cytotoxic in leukaemia and/or solid tumour cell lines (Wakelin et al, 2003; Baguley et al, 1995; Atwell et al, 1984).

One group of novel transcription inhibitors (Figure 1A) contain dual intercalating chromophores that are joined via their 9-amino groups by linker chains of various structures and contain N,N-dimethylaminoethyl (DMAE) active side chains. These agents bind to DNA in a bisintercalating threading fashion inspired by the binding mechanism of nogalamycin (Wakelin et al, 2003). In this design the carboxamide sidechains spear the DNA helix and make bonding interactions with guanine bases in the major groove to promote transcription inhibition by enhancing DNA residence time without increasing binding affinity. This is a desirable characteristic for activity in solid tumours where tumour penetration correlates inversely with DNA binding affinity (Wakelin et al, 2003). Differences in these compounds are found in their linker chains with flexibility, charge and length all varying. With the linker chains laying in the minor groove of the DNA helix they play a crucial role in the overall activity of the compound by placing a physical block in the path of DNA tracking enzymes (Wakelin et al, 2003).

The second class of transcription inhibitors (Figure 1B,C) contain representatives of phenazine-1-carboxamide dimers bridged via their side chains with alkylamino linkers of various structures (Spicer et al, 2000). Within this class, the clinical candidate MLN944/XR5944 bisintercalates with its linker in the DNA major groove making hydrogen bonding interactions to guanines in a sequence specific manner. This compound possesses a unique mechanism of action, including the inhibition of transcription factor binding to DNA, which ultimately leads to the inhibition of transcription (Byers et al, 2005). The bis(phenazine-1-carboxamides) studied are of two structural types: SN26356 (MLN944/XR5944) and SN26700 are 9-methylphenazines joined via a dicationic -(CH2)2NH(CH2)NH(CH2)2- linker, and differ in that SN26700 has the amines substituted with a methyl group (Figure 1B). SN26871 has an N-methylated monocationic -(CH2)3N(Me)(CH2)3- linker and an 8,9-benzphenazine chromophore (Figure 1C). ¶

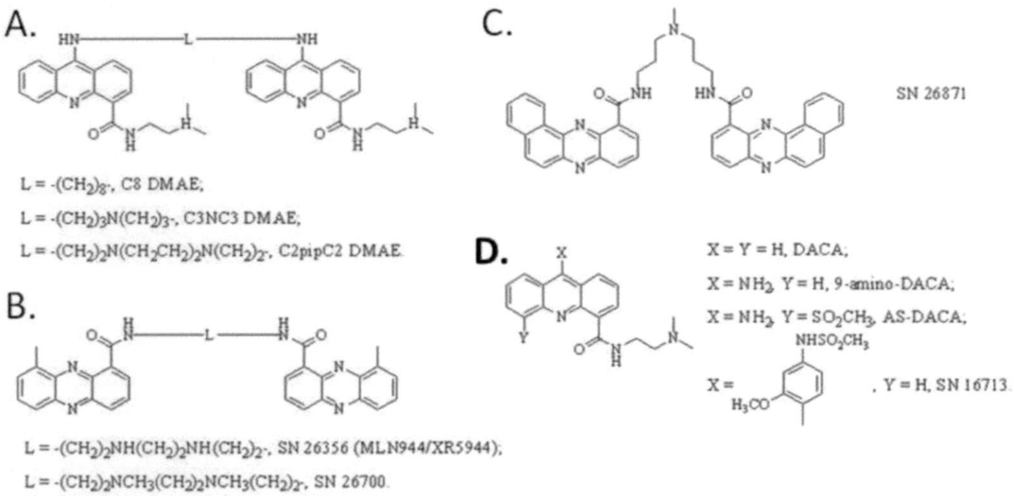

Fig. 1. *Molecular structure* of **(A)** novel transcription inhibitors Bis(9-aminoacridinecarboxamides), C8 DMAE, C3NC3 DMAE and C2pipC2 DMAE, **(B-C)** novel transcription inhibitors Bis(phenazine-1-carboxamides), 26356 (MLN944/XR5944), 26700 and 26871 **(D)** novel topoisomerase poisoning, monointercalating acridine-4-carboxamides, DACA, 9-amino-DACA, AS-DACA and SN16713.

A third class of novel compounds, also structurally based around the acridine-4-carboxamide intercalating chromophore, have previously been identified as topoisomerase poisons (Finlay et al., 1996) and act as monointercalating agents that feature electron-withdrawing moieties in place of a single active side chain (Figure 1D). N-[2-(dimethyl)aminoethyl]-acridine-4-carboxamide (DACA), a dual topoisomerase I/II poison and the parent compound from this class of agents, was unsuccessfully taken into phase II clinical trial in patients with non-small cell lung carcinoma, advanced ovarian cancer, recurrent glioblastoma and advanced colorectal cancer (Twelves et al, 2002; Caponigro et al, 2002). 9-amino derivatives of DACA, however, have greater cytotoxic and dose potencies, and modifications in the 5-position, such as the methyl sulphone group in AS-DACA, promote solid tumour activity (Atwell et al, 1987). In contrast to DACA, 9-amino-DACA and AS-DACA appear to be more specific poisons for topoisomerase II (Bridewell et al, 2001) with AS-DACA, a less lipophillic derivative (Haldane et al,1999) also known to have a wide spectrum of activity in solid tumours (Atwell et al,1987).

4. Screening novel agents indicates differential response

A panel of 5 RMS cell lines were selected for in vitro assessment of cytotoxicity of novel and established transcription inhibitors and topoisomerase poisons. RD and JR1 were selected to represent the ERMS subtype whilst RH30, RH3 and RH4 were selected to represent the ARMS subtype. We assessed the cytotoxicity of a range of novel and established transcription inhibitors and topoisomerase poisons against 5 established RMS cell lines. MTT cell viability assays were used to determine cell survival after a 72 hour exposure to each compound. Published IC_{50} values (Wolf et al, 2009) are plotted as 'Δ Plots' which graphically represent the differences in efficacy of each drug in each cell line relative to the median (m) IC_{50} of all drugs in all cell lines (Figure 2).

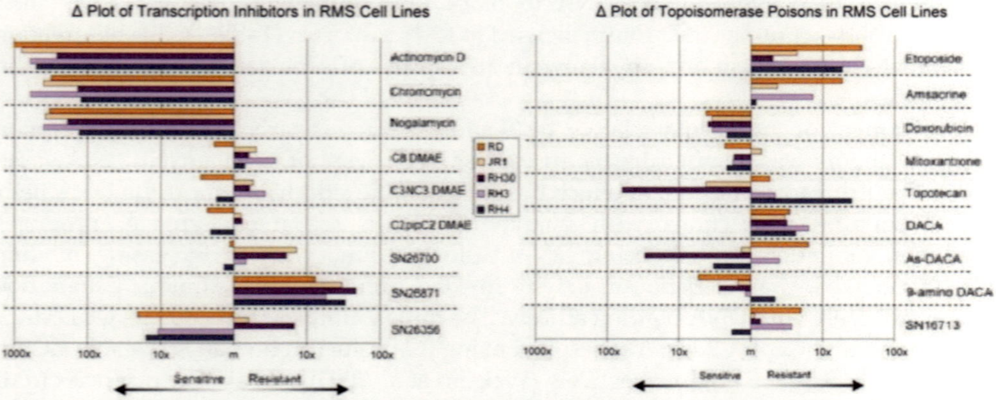

Fig. 2. *Δ plots showing variations in drug potency in 5 RMS cell lines.* IC_{50}s are plotted as a log_{10} measure of sensitivity or resistance against the median (m) IC_{50} of all agents across all cell lines (m = 600 nM). This measure of potency, taken as a whole across all RMS cell lines, serves to highlight the relative differences in drug efficacy. (Wolf, 2009)

Our findings enable classification of these agents into 3 classes; those that are potent in all 5 cell lines; those that show differential responses across the panel; and those that require higher concentrations to be toxic in all cell lines. The first class includes the naturally occurring transcription inhibitors actinomycin D, chromomycin and nogalamycin, which are the most potent amongst the agents studied, the topoisomerase II poisons doxorubicin and mitoxantrone, and the experimental acridine-4-carboxamide topoisomerase II poison 9-amino-DACA. Class two includes the bis(phenazine-1-carboxamide) SN 26356, otherwise known as MLN944/XR5944, identified as a transcription inhibitor and topoisomerase I poison, the topoisomerase I poison topotecan, and the acridine-4-carboxamide topoisomerase poison AS-DACA. AS-DACA and topotecan have the same spectrum of cytotoxic activity, which is complementary to that of SN 26356. Agents such as those described in group 2 may offer alternative treatment options for RMS tumours unresponsive to the traditional chemotherapy protocols.

4.1 Cytotoxicity of novel and established transcription inhibitors in RMS cells

The antitumour antibiotics actinomycin D, chromomycin and nogalamycin are amongst the classical template inhibitors of transcription, each binding to DNA reversibly, but dissociating slowly so as to present a long-lived block to the passage of RNA polymerases. Actinomycin D is a monofunctional intercalating agent which places bulky cyclic peptides in the DNA minor groove, chromomycin is a minor groove binding agent (Yang et al, 1999) and nogalamycin is a monofunctional threading agent which intercalates with its nogalose sugar lying in the minor groove and its bicyclic amino sugar spearing the duplex making hydrogen bonding interactions with guanines in the major groove (Li and Krueger, 1991). All are known to bind selectively to GC-rich sequences and block RNA polymerase progression by placing a bulky group in the DNA minor groove. Furthermore, all cause similar profound perturbation to transcription profiles (Zilhif et al, 2006). We have found that all three agents have indistinguishable activity in the 5 RMS cell lines and that they are the most potent agents studied, with activity in the nM range (Figure 2). Seemingly, the fine details of how they interact with DNA to block RNA polymerase do not affect their cytotoxicity. With actinomycin D routinely used in RMS protocols (Table 1), this observation suggests that chromomycin and nogalamycin are worthy of consideration for inclusion in clinical studies.

The development of the bisintercalating bis(9-aminoacridine-4-carboxamide) transcription template inhibitors was inspired by the threading mechanism of nogalamycin (Wakelin et al, 2003). Their threading design, in which the carboxamide sidechains spear the DNA helix to make bonding interactions with guanine bases in the major groove, promotes transcription inhibition by enhancing DNA residence time without increasing binding affinity, a desirable characteristic for activity in solid tumours where tumour penetration correlates inversely with DNA binding affinity. The three examples studied here, C8 DMAE, C3NC3 DMAE and C2pipC2 DMAE, despite having IC_{50} values in human leukaemia CCRF-CEM cells of 35, 50 and 63 nM respectively (Wakelin et al, 2003), and similar potencies (nM) in a range of human cancer cell lines (Wakelin unpublished), are found to be about 4 to 40 times less potent in the rhabdomyosarcoma cells, which is some 100 to 1000 times less active than the naturally occurring transcription inhibitors. RD is the only RMS cell line that could be considered sensitive and is the only one in which all three threading dimers produced IC_{50}s marginally lower than m (Figure 2). The origins of the intrinsic resistance of the RMS cell lines to these agents are unclear.

This generalized resistance to the bisacridines also extends to the bis(phenazinecarboxamide) dimers, with one important exception. These compounds were designed as bisintercalating topoisomerase I and II poisons (Spicer et al, 2000), but their actual mechanism of action is complex and appears to involve both transcription inhibition, along with topoisomerase I poisoning (Byers et al, 2005). The three compounds studied here are potently cytotoxic in mouse leukemia P388, mouse Lewis lung and Jurkat human leukemia cells (Gamage et al, 2001). The toxicity of SN26700 and SN26871 however, is diminished some 35 to 2200 times in the RMS panel, with their IC_{50}s clustering around m or greatly exceeding it (Figure 2). The exceptional response is found with SN26356 which was used in clinical trial as MLN944/XR5944 (Verborg et al, 2007). Its potent activity in previous studies is maintained in the RD, RH3 and RH4 cell lines, with an average IC_{50} of about 40 nM. The origins of this selectivity are unknown, but our findings point to the importance of considering SN26356 as a possible clinical trial candidate in RMS.

4.2 Cytotoxicity of novel and established topoisomerase poisons in RMS cells

The trapping of topoisomerases in a cleavable complex with DNA is a well established mechanism of action of many DNA binding drugs (Li and Liu, 2001). Representative topoisomerase poisons, both established and novel, were examined in this study, and produced widely ranging results. For example, amongst the clinically used topoisomerase II poisons, etoposide and amsacrine were uniformly, poorly active across the RMS cell line panel, with IC_{50}s all greater than m, ranging from 600nM to 22mM (Figure 2). Such a finding sits oddly with the inclusion of etoposide in clinical RMS protocols (Van Winkle et al, 2005). In contrast, doxorubicin and mitoxantrone are uniformly active in the RMS cells with average IC_{50}s of about 200nM and 400nM respectively, a finding that supports their inclusion in clinical studies. The only clinical topoisomerase I poison studied, topotecan, produced a differential response with activity of 10nM and 140nM in RH30 and JR1 cells, but IC_{50}s of 1mM to 15mM in the remaining 3 RMS lines. Interestingly, this is the inverse selectivity of SN26356, which is inactive in RH30 and JR1, and raises the intriguing question of the potential clinical activity of their use in combination.

The novel topoisomerase poisons evaluated are structurally based on the acridine-4-carboxamide chromophore, the parent compound of which, DACA (Figure 1), has been identified as a dual topoisomerase I/II poison (Finlay et al., 1996). Despite its wide solid tumour activity and its clinical evaluation (Twelves et al, 2002; Caponigro et al, 2002; Haldane et al, 1993), it shows poor potency in all RMS cell lines with IC_{50}s about 2 to 4 mM. In contrast, its dicationic derivative, 9-amino-DACA, which binds to DNA 6-fold more tightly than DACA and is only weakly active as a topoisomerase I poison (Finlay et al., 1996), is 10 times more potent in all RMS cell lines, making its activity comparable to that of doxorubicin and mitoxantrone (Figure 2). Although the extra charge on the chromophore of 9-amino-DACA enhances cytotoxic potency and antileukaemic activity in mouse tumour models (Atwell et al, 1987), it diminishes solid tumour activity as a consequence of poor tumour penetration due to its elevated DNA affinity. Electron withdrawing substituents in the acridine 5-position lower the chromophore pK, and AS-DACA, bearing a 5-methylsulphone, has a neutral chromophore at physiological pH, binds DNA with an affinity between that of DACA and 9-amino-DACA, and is intermediate between these two agents with respect to topoisomerase selectivity (Finlay et al, 1996). These characteristics make it generally more cytotoxic than DACA, and endow it with widespread solid tumour activity (Atwell et al, 1987). In the RMS panel it returns a differential response, strongly reminiscent of topotecan, with JR1 and RH30 cells being sensitive, but the remaining three cell lines have IC_{50}s above 1mM (Figure 2). Lastly, within the acridinecarboxamide family, we examined the activity of SN16713, a monofunctional threading agent that superposes the structures of amsacrine and 9-amino-DACA, selectively poisons topoisomerase II which has an IC_{50} of 120nM in CCRF-CEM cells (Zihlif et al, 2006) and 7nM in Jurkat leukaemia (Finlay et al, 1996), is poorly active in RMS cells (Figure 2).

Several novel agents displayed comparable or improved efficacy over their established counterparts in our in vitro drug cytotoxicity study in RMS cell lines. Despite the resistance of some cell lines to these agents their overall efficacy necessitates further preclinical development for possible inclusion in RMS clinical trials. Of particular interest were the novel agents AS-DACA and 9-amino-DACA. 9-amino-DACA showed efficacy across all cell lines comparable to the established topoisomerase poisons flagging its potential as a candidate for future RMS clinical trials. By contrast AS-DACA produced a variable cytotoxic response across the cell line panel. Many factors may be responsible for this observed variation, in particular the 190x fold difference observed between two archetypal RMS cell lines, RD and RH30 (Wolf et al, 2011). The remainder of this discussion will explore our study of AS-DACA cytotoxicity in two RMS cell lines; RD and Rh30, along with AS-DACA-resistant cell line we derived from RH30, named Res30 (Wolf et al, 2011), as an illustration of the complexities of developing new treatment strategies for RMS.

5. Causes for differential drug cytotoxicity in RMS cells

Drug "resistance" is a phenomenon that impedes the efficacy of every compound used in the treatment of cancer at some stage. Mechanisms governing cellular resistance to chemotherapy may be intrinsic, however in most cases they are acquired following repeated or extended exposure to chemotherapy. Although "acquired" drug resistance is a term that is used to describe the development of drug resistance within cells that were originally chemosensitive, it may in fact result from a clonal proliferation of a subpopulation of intrinsically resistant cells within the original tumour or cell culture. This has been noted to occur within RMS with resistant, differentiated cells making up the majority of tumour remaining after chemotherapy treatment (Klunder et al, 2003). The complexity and number of mechanisms that contribute to drug resistant phenotypes makes identifying and circumventing the source of the problem a challenge for researchers and clinicians alike. Some well established mechanisms of resistance include alterations in drug target levels and function, enhanced drug efflux via membrane bound transport proteins and drug sequestration/altered intracellular drug distribution. Further, it must be assumed that drug resistance mechanisms, intrinsic only to certain RMS cell types, act in a manner dependent on the subtle structural differences which exist between the DNA-binding compounds used. Given the importance of in vitro studies in pre-clinical drug investigations, it is worthwhile investigating commonly used RMS cell lines to identify the subtle biological mechanisms which are intrinsic to them and produce these selective drug resistance phenotypes. Consequently, in the remaining sections of this review, the impact of different mechanisms of resistance will be explored, with a specific focus on the differential response of AS-DACA in RD and RH30 as a paradigm of this complexity.

5.1 'Classical' drug resistance involving transport proteins

One of the most described mechanisms of drug resistance in RMS cell lines, is ATP-Binding Cassette (ABC) transport protein mediated drug efflux. ABC transport proteins span the plasma membranes of almost all cells and are responsible for active transport of many compounds, including a number of agents used in cancer therapy (Klein et al, 1999). In total 49 human genes have been described that encode various ABC transport pumps (Chang, 2007). Whilst each protein is structurally and functionally distinct, all members of the ABC transport protein family share three conserved sequence motifs within nucleotide binding domains and are common to many proteins that bind ATP (Leslie et al, 1999). For many years it was believed that the MDR1 gene, also known as ABCB1, which encodes P-glycoprotein (P-gp), was the prime contributor to drug efflux (Leslie et al, 1999). Subsequent studies however led to the identification of several related proteins which have also been linked to the multidrug resistance phenotype and include multidrug resistance-associated proteins MRP1 to MRP5 and Breast Cancer Related Protein (BCRP) (Komdeur et al 2003).

5.1.1 Multidrug Resistance-Associated Protein 1 (MRP1)

MRP1 (ABCC1) is a 170kDa protein (190kDa in its glycosylated form), that belongs to the ABC family of membrane bound transport proteins. MRP1 is comprised of 17 transmembrane segments that are grouped into three transmembrane domains (TMDs), two cytoplasmic linker regions and two cytoplasmic nucleotide binding domains. This structure is common to most members of ABCC subfamily. Although the cytoplasmic linker region, which lies between TMD0 and TMD1, has been shown to be vital for drug transport, loss of TMD0 does not greatly affect drug transport (Chang, 2007). MRP1 is understood to transport a greater number of substrates than P-gp, despite being an anion transporter. The anthracycline antibiotics, vinca alkaloids, folate based antimetabolites, antiandrogens, organic anions and heavy metals are just some of the known substrates for MRP1 (Munoz et al, 2007). This phenomenon has been attributed to the presence of glutathione (GSH) with several studies indicating that without physiological concentrations of GSH present, MRP1 has no ability to transport unmodified anti-cancer drugs. Hence it is considered that MRP1 may co-transport GSH together with anticancer drugs, or GSH may bind to MRP1 and enhance the transport of hydrophobic molecules (Chang, 2007).

MRP1 is overexpressed in many tumours including RMS and other soft tissue sarcomas. In 2005 a study that assessed the expression levels of various ABC transport proteins detected MRP1 in 43% of the surgically resected STS samples examined and found that its expression correlated to a larger tumour size and age of the patient (>20 years) (Oda et al, 2005). Similarly, an earlier study reported MRP1 expression in 11 out of 13 paraffin-embedded primary tumour RMS samples before chemotherapy. In follow up assessments it was found that a metastasis of a tumour which had previously not expressed the protein did so after chemotherapy, and showed increased expression in three other primary tumour samples also following chemotherapy. All other samples however showed equal or decreased levels of expression following drug exposure (Klunder et al, 2003). In a separate study of 29 paediatric and 16 adult RMS cases it reported that MRP1 was expressed in 56% of cases however this expression did not contribute to the poorer response to therapy in older RMS patients (Komdeur et al, 2003).

5.1.2 P-Glycoprotein (P-gp)

P-gp is a 170 kDa protein that predominantly transports cationic or uncharged molecules and is known to efflux many of the compounds used in RMS therapy including the anthracycline antibiotics, actinomycin D, etoposide and the vinca alkaloid vincristine (Larsen et al, 2000). The extent to which P-gp contributes to the poor drug response associated with metastatic RMS has seen much debate with many studies presenting conflicting evidence on the matter. In 2003 a study that screened P-gp levels in 13 pairs of paraffin-embedded RMS samples from patients before and after treatment could not identify any consistent pattern of change in the expression levels of the protein. Of the 13 samples tested, 4 cases saw a decrease in expression of P-gp, 5 cases showed no change and only 4 cases showed an increase in expression post treatment (Klunder et al, 2003). Similarly, in 1996 it was reported that high P-gp expression was not correlated to poor drug response in RMS patients following therapy (Kuttesch et al, 1996). This study, which used immunohistochemistry to detect and measure P-gp levels from 71 patients that had been treated between 1969 and 1991 found no association between the expression levels at diagnosis and patient outcome following treatment. Instead it was suggested that multidrug resistance is a consequence of combining agents from several drug classes that subsequently induce a range of resistance mechanisms within a single population of cells. Another separate study found that despite a poorer prognosis in older RMS patients, age at diagnosis has no effect on expression levels of the protein (Komdeur et al, 2003). Whilst these studies suggested P-gp contributed little to the poor drug response associated with metastatic RMS, several papers had previously presented a strong relationship between patient prognosis and P-gp expression level. One such example correlated P-gp levels with relapse in 30 biopsy samples from RMS and STS patients, and found that of the 9 patients with detectable P-gp levels, all relapsed. Of the 21 patients without detectable P-gp levels, only 1 patient relapsed (Chan et al, 1990).

5.1.3 MRP1 transport of AS-DACA in RMS cells

The monointercalating acridine-4-carboxamide compounds used in this study are vulnerable to transport via these efflux pumps. AS-DACA is a substrate for P-gp whilst DACA, the parent compound from this class, is not (Haldane et al, 1999). Using western blot analysis the influence of AS-DACA on the expression levels of MRP1 was investigated in both resistant and sensitive cell lines. Western blot analysis of MRP1 expression levels showed substantial change in RD and RH30 cells following a 16 hour exposure to double the IC_{50} of AS-DACA for each cell line (Figure 3A). This protein was also expressed in Res-30

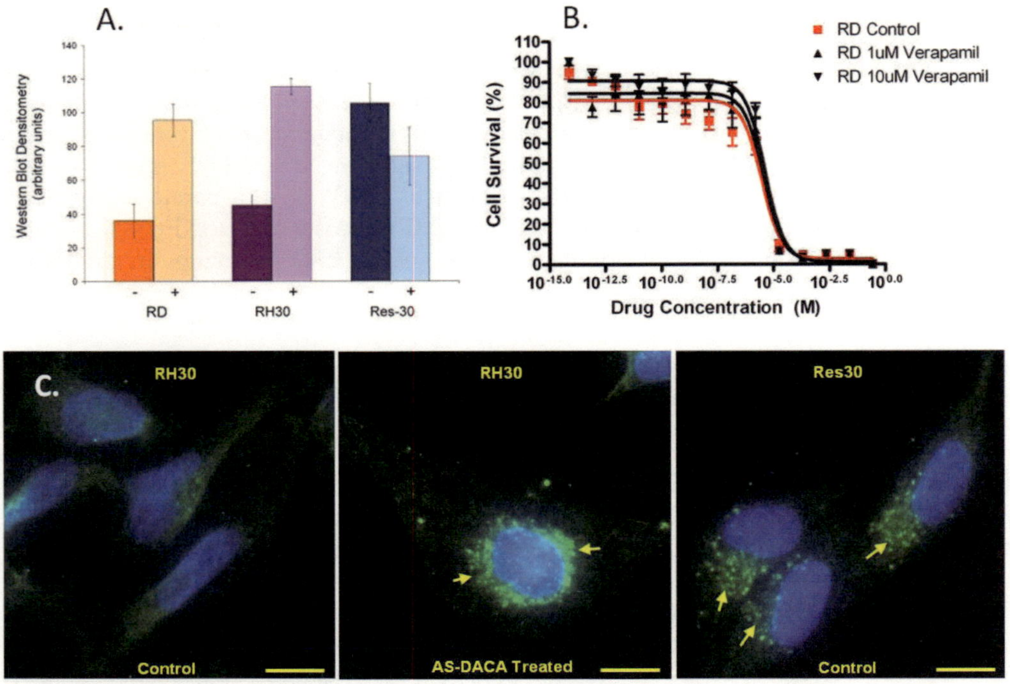

Fig. 3. *The influence of MRP1 expression on AS-DACA activity in RMS cells.* **(A)** Expression levels of MRP1 (170kDa) were determined by western blot before (-) and after (+) exposure to AS-DACA ($2xIC_{50}$ for 16 hours). Densitometry was performed on triplicate blots with band intensity normalized for both background noise and total protein loading differences as determined by Ponceau S staining. **(B)** The influence (R)-verapamil has on AS-DACA efficacy was established using MTT cell viability assays. RD and Res-30 cells were treated with 1μM and 10μM of verapamil whilst being exposed to various concentrations of AS-DACA for 72 hours. Error bars represent the SEM of three independent experiments in each case. **(C)** Intracellular localization of MRP1 in RH30 cells before and after AS-DACA exposure as determined by immunofluorescence microscopy. MRP1 appears green. Highlighted with yellow arrows is a bright staining vesicular structure in the perinuclear region following exposure to AS-DACA. All cells are co-stained with the nuclear stain DAPI (blue) and displayed as merged artificially coloured monochromatic images. Untreated Res30 show the same structures indicating it has acquired this feature during selection. Scale bars = 10μm.

cells without an additional exposure to AS-DACA. Exposure to the MRP1 inhibitor (R)-verapamil at concentrations of 1 and 10 mM failed to alter AS-DACA-induced cytotoxicity (Figure 3B), indicating the differential toxicity of AS-DACA in the RMS cells is not simply explained by understanding classical drug resistance involving MRP1 (Wolf et al 2011). So whilst the higher levels of the ABC transport protein MRP1 following treatment with AS-DACA was detected, typical of a 'classical' multidrug resistance phenotype in RMS cells, this treatment-induced increased expression of MRP1 in cell lines does not explain the differential in sensitivity to AS-DACA induced cell death. Firstly, both RD and RH30 cell lines demonstrated an equivalent increase in MRP1 expression (Figure 3A). The absence of any effects of the MRP1 inhibitor verapamil (Figure 3B), indicate that despite the changes in protein levels, impedance of MRP1 activity did not alter AS-DACA toxicity in any RMS cells.

Interestingly, MRP1 protein was shown to localize to vesicular membranes in all three cell lines (Wolf et al, 2011) this being most prominent in cells directly after exposure to AS-DACA (Figure 3C). Active mechanisms that drive sequestration of weakly basic compounds into vesicles of the membrane trafficking system are not uncommon. Several of the ABC transport pumps have been implicated in such mechanisms and alternative pathways involving the trans-golgi network (TGN), lung-resistance-related protein 1 and major vault proteins have been proposed to modify intracellular drug distributions by altering transport between the nucleus, endosomal vesicles, lysosomes and the cytoplasm. Rajagopal *et al* (2003) used HeLa cells to demonstrate MRP1, P-gp and BCRP were localized to membranes of intracellular vesicles that they contributed to drug resistance phenotypes via sequestration-based mechanisms at these sites. With this growing evidence suggesting that various ABC transport proteins, including MRP1, are localized to vesicles of the membrane trafficking system where they actively transport drug from the cytoplasm into lysosomes (Rajagopal et al, 2003) these experiments further implicated MRP1 with drug sequestration, rather than drug efflux from the cell. It is clear that understanding this impact is vital for the future development of AS-DACA and other members of the class of monointercalating acridine-4-carboxamides and hence, deserves further attention in future studies.

5.2 Alterations in drug target: Reduced topoisomerase levels

The consequence of trapping topoisomerase enzymes in cleavable complexes with DNA is an accumulation of double strand breaks in the DNA helix. There is strong evidence that AS-DACA induced cell death results from an accumulation of double stranded DNA breaks following the trapping of topoisomerase II in a cleavable complex with DNA (Bridewell et al, 2001). Hence, we determined that the expression level of each topoisomerase isoform was a contributing factor in the variation of RMS cell response to AS-DACA exposure. We first establish the level of DNA damage induced by the compound correlated with the degree of sensitivity or resistance exhibited by each cell line. Using an enzyme linked immunosorbent assay (ELISA) for phosphorylated histone 2A (γH2AX) (Burma et al, 2001), DNA damage was assessed in both sensitive and resistant cell lines following low dose exposures equivalent to the IC_{50} in RH30 cells (20nM) of AS-DACA over a time course of 48 hours. The results are displayed in Wolf et al 2011. DNA damage was substantially reduced in Res-30 cells when compared to the parental RH30 cell line even after 48 hours exposure to the drug. Whilst DNA damage was evident after just 1 hour in the sensitive RH30 cells, it does not appear until 24 hours later in the resistant Res-30 cells. Interestingly, DNA damage is detected in RD cells after just 4 hours despite the drug exposure being approximately 450 times lower than its IC_{50} in this cell line. After 48 hours the level of DNA damage has reached 40% of what would be reached when the cells are exposed to their IC_{50} dose for the same length of time. In Res-30 cells only 10% of the DNA damage induced with a 4μM dose of AS-DACA was observed after a 48 hour exposure to 20nM of AS-DACA. From these findings it is clear that the level of DNA damage induced in each cell line correlates to the IC_{50} of AS-DACA in each cell line. Not surprisingly, the levels of DNA damage increase as the time of exposure to AS-DACA increases and this is most obvious in the sensitive cell line RH30.

The immediate interpretation of this result is that AS-DACA is being prevented from intercalating with the DNA and forming cleavable complexes. With DNA damage having been confirmed as a primary consequence of AS-DACA exposure (Wolf et al, 2011), it was essential to assess the relationship between the expression levels of each topoisomerase isoform and the levels of DNA damage induced in each cell line following exposure to the drug. Since the trapping of topoisomerase in its cleavable complex with DNA is the primary mechanism by which AS-DACA induces DNA damage (Finlay et al, 1996), we hypothesized that the differences in response between the RD and RH30 cell lines to AS-DACA was due, in part, to intrinsic differences in the levels of the primary drug target, topoisomerases. Mechanisms are known to reduce the efficacy of topoisomerase poisons through decreased expression of the target enzyme, topoisomerase. It is well established, for example, that the topoisomerase I enzyme is reduced following cell exposure to the topoisomerase I poison camptothecin and the subsequent activation of the ubiquitin/26S proteasome pathway. As described in Desai et al 1997, topoisomerase I-ubiquitin conjugates were discovered to form within minutes of camptothecin treatment in Chinese hamster ovary (CHO) cells decreasing levels of topoisomerase I by up to 80%, 2 hours after treatment. The expected reduction of topoisomerase I following camptothecin treatment was reversed using the 26S proteosome inhibitors MG-132 and lactacystin demonstrating that the ubiquitin/26S pathway was involved in the camptothecin induced down regulation of topoisomerase I (Desai et al, 1997). This correlation was further highlighted using a panel of breast cancer cell lines that had previously been shown to exhibit a high variability in their response to the drug, which was shown to result from the down regulation of topoisomerase I (Li and Liu, 2001).

This phenomenon is not exclusive to the topoisomerase I isoform however with published data suggesting that both topoisomerase IIα and topoisomerase IIβ may also be down regulated following exposure to various topoisomerase II poisons. One study highlighted that in a panel of cell lines representing various tumour types, both isoforms of topoisomerase II were degraded following activation of a proteasome pathway that specifically targeted the enzyme when it was trapped to DNA in complex with etoposide (Fan et al, 2008). The down regulation of topoisomerase IIα as a means to circumvent drug cytotoxicity is however controversial as this enzyme has previously been shown to be essential for cell survival with topoisomerase IIβ unable to compensate in its absence (Austin et al, 1998). On the other hand it has been shown that topoisomerase IIα is overexpressed in several tumour types (Murphy et al, 2007) and hence may permit a down regulation of the enzyme to a level that does not compromise cell viability yet limits the efficacy of topoisomerase IIα poisons.

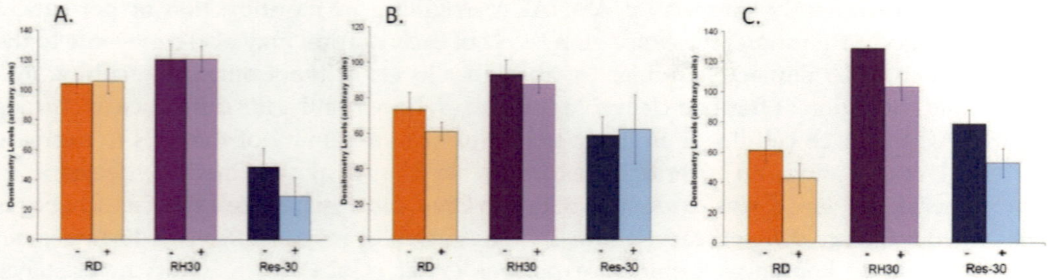

Fig. 4. (A) Topoisomerase I (90kDa), (B) Topoisomerase IIa (175kDa) and (C) Topoisomerase IIβ (180kDa) levels were determined by western blot before (-) and after (+) exposure to AS-DACA (2x IC_{50} for 16 hours). Densitometry was performed on triplicate blots with band intensity normalized for both background noise and total protein loading differences as determined by Ponceau S staining. Error bars represent the SEM of intensity for each band in three independent experiments.

As topoisomerase levels are known to be reduced in many cell lines in response to topoisomerase poison exposure, we explored using western blotting whether one or more isoforms of the enzyme were altered in our RMS cell lines following AS-DACA exposure. The expression levels of each topoisomerase isoform were assessed in both treated and untreated cells following an overnight exposure to AS-DACA (16 hours) at a concentration double the IC_{50} for each individual cell line. From this analysis of topoisomerase I and II western blots (Figure 4), it was evident that the basal levels of each isoform varied in the cell lines assessed. Basal levels of topoisomerase I appeared marginally higher in the RH30 cell line compared to RD and were substantially reduced in Res-30 cells - to at least 50% of the level observed in the parental RH30 cell line. Levels of topoisomerase I were unaffected by a 16 hour exposure to AS-DACA in both RD and RH30 cell lines whilst a modest reduction was observed in the Res-30 cell line. No change in topoisomerase IIα levels were observed following an overnight exposure to AS-DACA in any cell line, however RH30 cells again appeared to possess modestly higher basal levels of this protein compared to both RD and Res-30 cells. Although Res-30 cells possessed the least amount of this protein, its expression was similar to that observed in the RD cells. Topoisomerase IIβ was the only isoform to be reduced, albeit modestly, in each cell line following overnight exposures to AS-DACA. Again RH30 appeared to possess an increased basal expression of this enzyme in comparison to both RD and Res-30 cell lines and unlike the former two isoforms, the expression of topoisomerase IIβ was at least double that of RD.

Upon examination of the expression levels of each topoisomerase isoform in RD and RH30 cells (Figure 4) (Wolf et al, 2009), it became clear that intrinsic differences in their basal levels were present as hypothesized. As all isoforms are clearly expressed in RD, and DNA damage is induced with even small concentrations of drug (Wolf et al, 2011), it is unlikely that the levels of each isoform exclusively promote the resistant phenotype, although it may be a contributing factor. In comparison, the modest overexpression of topoisomerase I and topoisomerase IIα isoforms as well as the substantial overexpression of topoisomerase IIβ in RH30 cells may promote an enhanced drug efficacy. A higher expression of the target enzyme could translate to an increased frequency in the formation of cleavable complexes which are subsequently trapped by AS-DACA, resulting in the induction of permanent DNA damage. Furthermore, the expression levels of each isoform may also contribute to the rate at which DNA damage is induced with higher levels of topoisomerase resulting in a more rapid formation of trapped cleavable complexes. Importantly, the difference in efficacy of AS-DACA in each cell line is unlikely to be linked to an ability of the cells to decrease protein levels during an overnight exposure to the drug. A modest decrease in topoisomerase IIβ levels was evident in both sensitive and resistant cell lines and hence is unlikely to influence drug efficacy(Figure 4). The AS-DACA resistant Res-30 which was not cross resistant to known topoisomerase poisons (Wolf et al 2011) suggests a resistance mechanism peculiar to AS-DACA. The absence of double strand breaks in the Res-30 line (Wolf et al, 2011) indicates extensive impedance of the agent from its primary cytotoxic target.

5.3 Drug sequestration through the endosomal pathways

It was not long after the discovery of the lysosome by Nobel laureate Christian de Duve in the 1960's that a mechanism of drug sequestration involving acidic vesicles had been proposed (Kaufmann and Krise, 2007). In early studies of lysosomal sequestration correlation was drawn between the pKa of compounds and their ability to "induce vacuolization" (Yang et al, 1965). It was well known that weak acids and bases are capable of readily diffusing lipid bilayer membranes providing pH gradients exist on either side of the membrane partition.

The membrane trafficking system, illustrated in Figure 5A, is responsible for the transport and processing of proteins, cellular waste and foreign materials. It is comprised of several vesicle types that traffic along the cytoskeletal network of microtubules to various locations throughout the cell. Some of these vesicles include lysosomes, late stage endosomes (LSE), early endosomes (EE), multi-vesicular bodies (MVB) and macropinosomes. Each vesicle differs not only in their function but also in their intravesicular pH and in the receptors they express. Early endosomes, which originate from clathrin coated pits (CCP) in the cell's plasma membrane, are an integral component in the endocytic uptake of extracellular material (Saraste et al, 2007). These vesicles, with an approximate pH of 6.2, express SNARE proteins, the GTPases Rab4 and Rab5 and the early endosome antigen 1 (EEA1) protein. During the fusion of vesicles and formation of late stage endosomes, the vesicle pH drops to around 5.5 which not only aids in the degradation of intravesicular material but promotes recycling of the various membrane bound proteins back to the plasma membrane in recycling vesicles (Luzio et al 2001). Late stage endosomes, which express the membrane bound proteins Rab7, Lysosome Associated Membrane Protein-1 (LAMP-1) and mannose-6-phosphate receptor, receive and process material from both early endosomes and the TGN (Luzio et al 2001). The TGN is the end point in many endocytic pathways, internalizing a range of extracellular materials which are destined for endosomes or lysosomes And are trafficked in transport vesicles through a process regulated by the mannose-6-phosphate receptor. Material contained within the late stage endosomes is generally destined for degradation and when this cannot be achieved by the endosomes themselves, fusion of the vesicles with lysosomes will take place. Lysosomes, which continue to express the membrane bound protein LAMP1, may have a pH as low as 4.7 and contain acid hydrolases that degrade cellular waste including proteins and lipids (Luzio et al 2001).

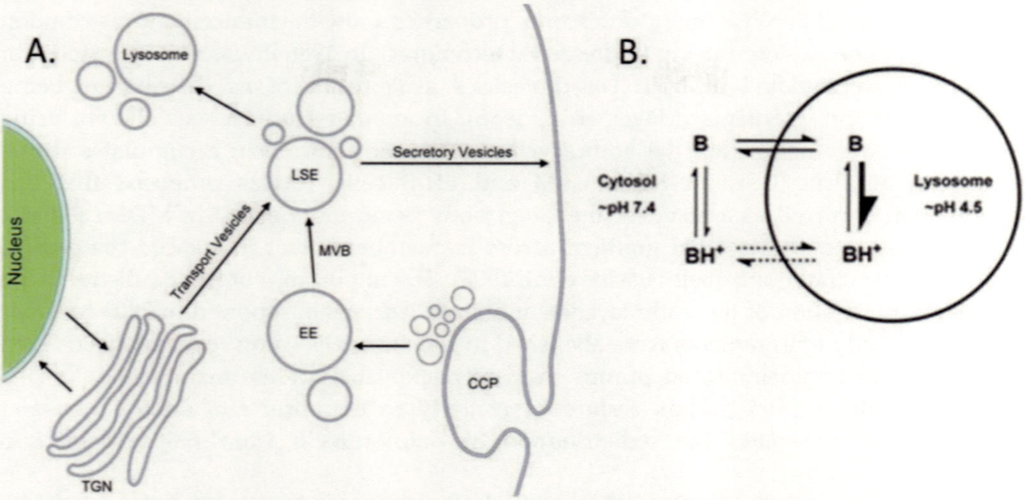

Fig. 5. **(A)** *Schematic Diagram of the Membrane Trafficking System*. This system is responsible for the distribution and processing of various proteins, lipids, foreign material and cellular waste. In this diagram CCP stands for Clathrin Coated Pit, EE for early endosome, LSE for Late Stage Endosome and MVB for multi-vesicular body, TGN for trans-golgi-network. **(B)** *Partitioning Theory* - Schematic diagram of the pH partition that is believed to be the predominant driving force in the sequestration of weakly basic in lysosomes. In the neutral conditions of the cytosol, compounds with pKa's near neutral will exist mainly in the free base form, maintaining its membrane permeability. In the lower pH of the lysosomes weak bases will exist predominately in the ionized or protonated form rendering the molecule impermeable to lipid bilayers. This figure has been reproduced from Kaufmann et al, 2007.

Classically, vesicle sequestration of the anthracycline antibiotics appears to be dictated by the "partitioning theory". The partitioning theory (Figure 5B) of drug sequestration, which was proposed not long after the discovery of the lysosome in the 1960's, is still believed to contribute significantly to drug resistance. This basic biochemical property formed the foundation of the partitioning theory of drug sequestration that was described by Christian de Duve is still accepted today (De Duve et al, 1974). The partitioning theory is based upon the principle that weak acids and bases are capable of readily diffusing lipid bilayer membranes down pH gradients, rendering these compounds able to accumulate in acidic vesicles due to protonation by free H+ ions present in the vesicular lumen. Such ionization renders the drug impermeable to the membrane and accumulation will continue whilst vesicular H^+ ion concentrations are maintained. So long as H^+ ion concentrations are maintained by V-type H^+-ATPase vacuolar proton pumps, drug accumulation will continue (Kaufmann and Krise, 2007). It has also recently been noted that this theory may be extended to explain the rapid drug efflux that occurs from tumour cells growing in hypoxic conditions. This occurs as a result of acidification of the extracellular space from anaerobic glycolysis and the subsequent exaggeration of the cytosol-extracellular fluid pH gradient (Chen et al, 2006).

Without an ability to view the intracellular distribution of weakly basic compounds, this sequestration may go completely unnoticed. As a research tool, the anthracycline antibiotics are commonly used because their fluorescence properties allow the intracellular distribution of the drugs to be explored using fluorescence techniques. In 1986 it was first reported that doxorubicin accumulated in lipid based vesicles as a result of its distribution being determined by pH gradients (Mayer et al, 1986). In another study it was shown, using microspectrofluorometry, that the anthracycline antibiotic pirarubicin accumulates in the Golgi body of drug resistant K562, CEM and LR73 cells. It was proposed that this accumulation occurred as a result of the Golgi body being more acidic in MDR cells and hence possessing a stronger pH gradient across its membrane that influenced the passive diffusion of the compound (Belhoussine et al, 1998). The importance of pH gradients in the vesicular sequestration of the anthracycline antibiotics was again reported in 2003 by Ouar et al. In this study pH gradients were abolished in resistant cells using concanamycin A, an inhibitor of the vacuolar proton pumps that are responsible for the maintenance of pH. Inhibition of the proton pumps restored sensitivity to daunorubicin, doxorubicin and epirubicin and prevented the redistribution of daunorubicin from the nucleus into lysosomes.

Although vesicular sequestration of weakly basic compounds is still believed to be facilitated by passive diffusion down pH gradients, several recent studies have indicated that other mechanisms may influence this process. In 2007 it was shown that knockdown of the major vault protein (MVP) using siRNA disrupted lysosomal uptake of not only doxorubicin, but also the intracellular pH probe LysoSensor and the lysosomal specific antigen LAMP1. This study indicated that MVP was integral in redistributing the drug away from the nucleus to the lysosomes (Herlevsen et al, 2007). In another study, cells were exposed to various weak bases before lysosomes were isolated and their contents quantified using high performance liquid chromotography. It was found that the lysosomes sequestered 3 to 15 times the volume of compound that would be expected if passive diffusion was the only mechanism facilitating this process. Hence this study also arrived at the conclusion that alternative mechanisms were active in the lysosomal sequestration of weakly basic compounds (Duvvuri and Krise, 2005).

Despite strong evidence implicating acidic vesicles of the membrane trafficking system in the sequestration of weakly basic compounds in in vitro settings, there is poor understanding of the influence this mechanism plays in the overall efficacy of compounds in a clinical setting. It was recently reported that disruption of vesicular sequestration following cellular exposure to the proton pump inhibitor omeprazole increases not only the potency of doxorubicin but also its penetration through an in vitro multicell layer culture (Lee and Tannock, 2006). This article hypothesized that it is in the effective treatment of solid tumours that vesicular sequestration of anti-cancer drugs may be truly relevant. As an effective treatment is dependant on the compound's ability to penetrate the tumour mass, in situations where drug is captured in the outer layers of a tumour, penetration is limited and treatment will be rendered ineffective. Furthermore, it is important to note that other agents used in the clinic in combination with weakly basic compounds may inadvertently promote their vesicular sequestration. In 2007 it was revealed that vincristine treatment produced not only a larger number of acidic vesicles retained in the cell but also the presence of unusually large lysosomal compartments. It was believed that this occurs following destabilization of the microtubule network, which is required to direct and maintain the movement of the lysosomes, endosomes and autophagosomes (Groth-Pedersen et al, 2007).

5.3.1 AS-DACA fluorescence allows monitoring of its distribution in RMS cells

AS-DACA is a unique compound that has dynamic fluorescence properties. These had never been characterized nor had they been exploited for experimental purposes. Clearly, such a property provides an invaluable tool in the assessment of intracellular drug distribution and for this reason an experimental protocol was optimized that allowed the visualization of the drug in our RMS cell lines. Initial examination of the intracellular distribution of AS-DACA revealed that it was being localized to areas other than the nucleus, but also that each compound fluoresced different colours depending on the area to which they had localized. This latter finding was unexpected as all other established cytotoxic agents that are associated with fluorescence, emit only single colours, in all intracellular situations. The findings presented in Figures 6 highlight that AS-DACA emits different colours when excited at a single wavelength. This suggests that depending on the microenvironment to which the compounds had localized, a change in drug structure may alter the emission wavelength.

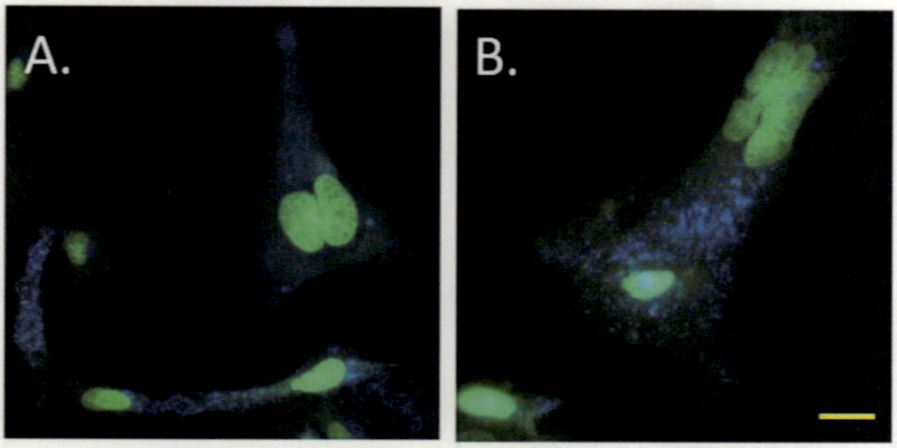

Fig. 6. *Images of the intracellular distribution of AS-DACA* in (A) RD and (B) RH30 cells. Images were captured using digital colour photography after a 4 hour exposure to 2μM of the drug. The agent was excited between 330nm - 385nm. Images were captured at 600x magnification. Scale Bar = 10mm (Wolf et al, 2011 for experimental details)

As we had hypothesized that AS-DACA would be vulnerable to protonation in low pH environments such as those found in vesicles of the membrane trafficking system, we reasoned that this shift in colour emission may correlate directly with the pH of the microenvironment in which the drugs had localized. Furthermore, AS-DACA is known to be lipophilic (Haldane et al, 1999) and thus vulnerable to sequestration in acidic vesicles. AS-DACA not only retains the ability to passively diffuse membranes but also contains a site in its structure that may be protonated at a lower pH making it subject to the partitioning theory. These factors together make the drug vulnerable to such a mechanism of sequestration. To determine if this hypothesis was correct, the influence of pH on the fluorescence properties of each compound was assessed. A luminescence spectrophotometer was used to measure the entire spectrum of emission from both compounds following excitation at 262nm in a range of solutions of differing pH. The results presented by Wolf et al 2011 clearly highlight that pH influences AS-DACA's fluorescence profile substantially. Although green emission does not appear to change greatly, blue emission, particularly at around 440nm, decreases significantly as pH rises, indicates that between pH 6.2 and pH 6.8, the intensity of blue fluorescence becomes lower than the intensity of green fluorescence. Above pH 6.6 the intensity of green fluorescence is stronger than that of blue (Wolf et al 2011).

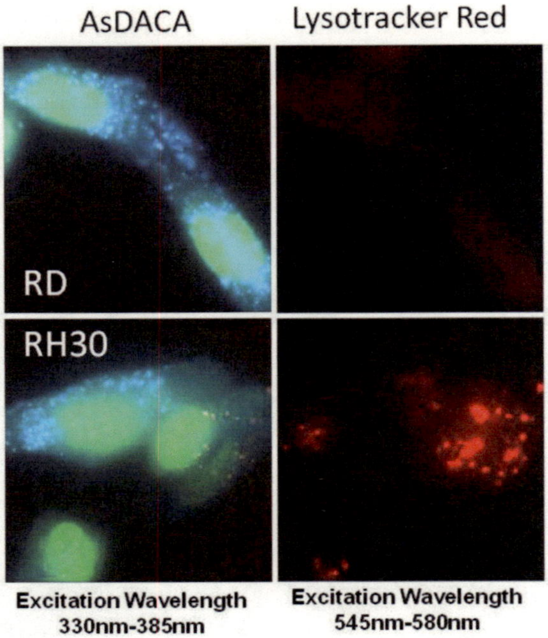

Fig. 7. *Intracellular Distribution of AS-DACA and LysoTracker™ Red in RD and RH30 Cells.* RD and RH30 cells were exposed to 2μM of AS-DACA for 4 hours and 100nM of LysoTracker™ Red for 45 minutes before being viewed on an epifluorescent microscope. Images were captured at 600x magnification. Scale bars represent 10μm.

In defining the influence pH has on the fluorescent properties of AS-DACA, it was shown that the compound fluoresced blue in the pH range below ~6.2. This provided evidence that the membrane trafficking system plays a role in AS-DACA's intracellular distribution. However, as this was only correlative, a more direct approach was taken to assess this potential link. Figure 7 highlights that following simultaneous short incubation with AS-DACA and LysoTracker™ Red, an intracellular probe that stains vesicles of low pH, RH30 cells consistently failed to stain with LysoTracker™ Red yet showed a strong sequestration of AS-DACA. In the RD cell line, whilst LysoTracker™ Red was observed within acidic vesicles co-localization was rare with most cells displaying vesicular accumulation of LysoTracker™ Red or AS-DACA individually. In rare instances however co-localization of AS-DACA and LysoTracker™ Red was observed in RD cells. Careful deconvolution of images following epifluorescence microscopy indicated that in RD cells exposed to LysoTracker™ Red, simultaneously with AS-DACA, some incomplete co-localization was observed, and limited to only a proportion of cellular vesicles (Wolf et al, 2011).

5.3.2 Determining which vesicles sequester AS-DACA

With all the evidence thus far suggesting that the observed sequestration of AS-DACA was a specific redistribution mechanism involving acidic vesicles of the membrane trafficking system, it became important to establish which vesicles were involved, and to determine how this redistribution of AS-DACA was taking place. As each intracellular vesicle functions as part of a larger network. Early endosomes traffic material to late stage endosomes which in turn traffic material to lysosomes. AS-DACA was shown to fluoresce blue when in environments below pH 6.2 (Figure 7), this confirmed that sequestration of the drug was occurring in acidic vesicles. However, this did not provide any insight into which vesicle types were responsible. To help determine which vesicles were involved in AS-DACA's sequestration, expression levels of markers specific for the various vesicle types were assessed using Western blot analysis (Figure 8). Sensitive (RH30) and resistant (RD and Res-30) cells were exposed to double the IC_{50} of AS-DACA overnight and the expression levels of early endosome antigen 1 (EEA1), Rab5, LAMP1 and Rab7 were assessed. As detailed above, the two former markers are localized to the membranes of early endosomes whilst the latter two are found on late stage endosomes and lysosomes. We suspected that in order to assist in the drug's redistribution away from the nucleus, an increase in vesicle number may occur in resistant cells following drug exposure. This would be reflected by an increase in the expression levels of the marker proteins localized to the vesicle involved.

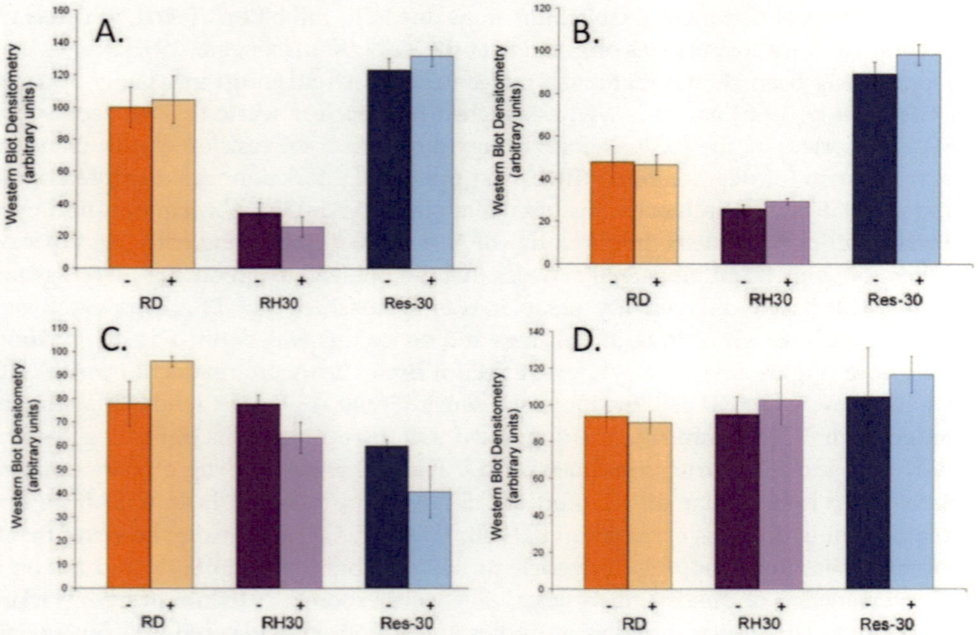

Fig. 8. *Expression levels of (A) EEA1, (B) Rab5, (C) LAMP-1 and (D) Rab7 in RMS cells.* Cells were processed by western blot for each protein before (-) and after (+) exposure to AS-DACA (2x IC_{50} for 16 hours). Densitometry was performed on triplicate blots with band intensity normalized for both background noise and total protein loading differences as determined by Ponceau S staining. Error bars represent the SEM of intensity for each band in three independent experiments.

Shown in Figure 8A, expression of EEA1, a marker of early endosomes, was not altered in any cell line following a 16 hour exposure to double the IC_{50} of AS-DACA. Expression of the protein was however, substantially higher in the resistant RD and Res-30 cell lines and the clear increase observed in Res-30 cells relative to RH30 cells was independent of an additional overnight treatment of drug. Similarly, Rab5 which is also associated with early endosomes, showed no change in expression level in any cell line following a 16 hour exposure to AS-DACA (Figure 8B). A marked increase however was again observed in Res-30 cells relative to RH30 which supported the overexpression of EEA1 in Res-30 cells. LAMP-1, which is associated with both lysosomes and late stage endosomes, showed minimal change in expression levels in all cell lines following a 16 hour exposure to AS-DACA (Figure 8C) This was supported by the expression levels of Rab7, a protein associated with late stage endosomes, which also showed minimal change in expression levels in all cell lines following a 16 hour exposure to AS-DACA (Figure 8D). This opposed our original hypothesis and implicated early endosomes, or unidentified transport vesicles with similar markers, in the sequestration and redistribution of AS-DACA.

5.3.3 Disrupting the membrane trafficking system: Influence of Brefeldin A

To further assess the hypothesis that AS-DACA is selectively redistributed away from the nucleus into vesicles of the membrane trafficking system, drug efficacy and intracellular distribution were assessed in resistant cell lines following pretreatment with Brefeldin A (BFA). BFA, a potent disrupter of Golgi, functions due to its inhibition of Arf1, which is vital for formation of transport vesicles originating at the TGN (Klausner et al, 1992).

It has previously been shown that small molecules may be taken up into Golgi apparatus (Belhoussine et al, 1998) and it is well established that nuclear waste is often removed via the ER and sorted in the TGN before being transported to vesicles of the membrane trafficking system for degradation. With this in mind Golgi function was disrupted by BFA in order to establish the influence this organelle plays in AS-DACA's sequestration by the membrane trafficking system. Importantly, BFA is known to be inherently cytotoxic and could therefore only be administered at doses that did not lead to a reduction in cell growth. Using an MTT based cell viability assay it was established that BFA was cytotoxic at concentrations above 15nM in both cell lines and hence this was defined as the maximum tolerated dose (Figure 9A). The cytotoxic effect of Brefeldin A pretreatment on AS-DACA efficacy in the resistant RD cell line increased sensitivity to AS-DACA modestly with a two fold reduction in IC_{50} (Figure 9B). This suggested that disruption of the trafficking system at the TGN may influence drug resistance of RD. These changes to drug efficacy appear to correlate to the intracellular distribution of AS-DACA in both cell lines with little to no vesicular accumulation was observed in RD cells (Figure 9 C,D). To ensure however that the BFA pretreatment impacted only on vesicle formation from the Golgi body and not on the integrity or function of preexisting vesicles, cells were exposed to 100nM of LysoTracker™ Red for 1 hour. This probe provides an indication of both vesicular pH and functionality after BFA exposure and it is clear (Figure 9 C,D) that BFA exposure does not alter the frequency, integrity or functionality of vesicles in the RD RMS cell line.

Following pretreatment of these cells with agents that disrupt various stages of the membrane trafficking pathway, such as brefeldin A, provides further evidence to suggest resistance to AS-DACA is determined by sequestration into the endosomal trafficking pathways. Together, these results highlight that AS-DACA is sequestered by acidic vesicles of the membrane trafficking system through a range of mechanisms. It appears that the TGN contributes to the redistribution of drug in RD cells whilst MRP1, or other membrane bound transport pumps, localize to vesicles in RH30 and Res-30 where they contribute to drug uptake into acidic vesicles. The results presented highlight not only that AS-DACA is vulnerable to sequestration in vesicles of the membrane trafficking system in RMS cell lines. Although the exact mechanisms that drive sequestration has not been fully defined, it appears that several pathways contribute to the removal of drug from the nucleus and subsequent accumulation in vesicles of low pH. Whether AS-DACA is merely redistributed away from the nucleus or whether it is effluxed from the cells remains unknown.

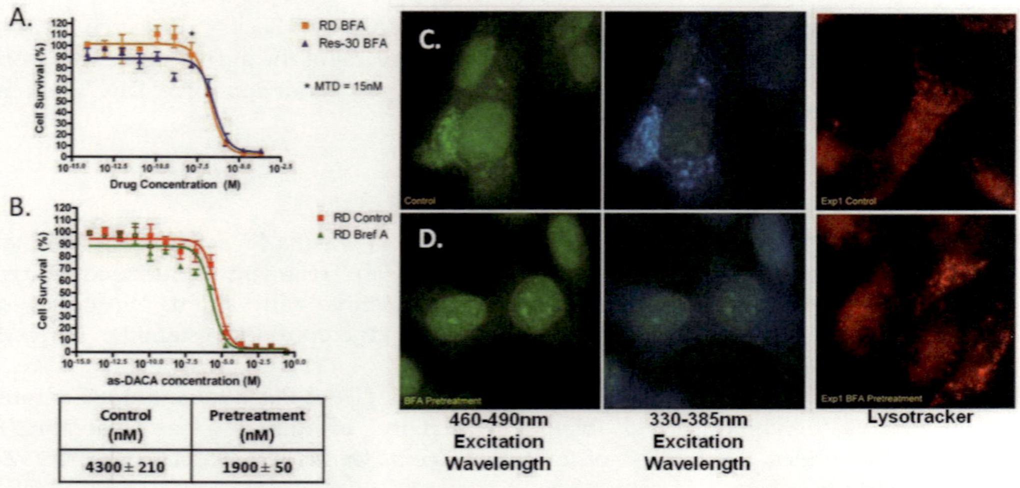

Control (nM)	Pretreatment (nM)
4300 ± 210	1900 ± 50

Fig. 9. *The influence BFA has on AS-DACA efficacy in RMS cells.* **(A)** MTT cell viability assay for BFA to determine maximum tolerated dose (MTD). **(B)** RD and Res-30 cells were pretreated for 16 hours with 15nM of BFA before being exposed to various concentrations of AS-DACA for 72 hours. A two fold difference in drug efficacy was seen in the RD cell line. **(C-D)** Images of AS-DACA distribution in RD cells with **(D)** and without **(C)** 16 hour exposure to 15nM of BFA and subsequent 4 hour exposure to 2μM of AS-DACA. For comparison, RD cells were pretreated with 15nM of BFA for 16 hours followed by 100nM of the acidicc vesicular probe LysoTracker™ Red for 1 hour. Images were captured using epifluorescence microscopy at 600x magnification with excitation of the probe between 545nm and 580nm.

6. Conclusion

With RMS being one of the most common paediatric solid tumours associated with poor drug response, this mechanism deserves further attention. Despite significant improvements in the treatment of non-metastatic ERMS in the past 30 years, patients with metastatic ERMS and ARMS continue to face a poor prognosis. This is due, in part, to a lack of response of the tumours to current the chemotherapy options. In this chapter, the cytotoxic effect of novel topoisomerase poisons and transcription inhibitors assessed in a panel of human RMS cell lines have been described. Findings were presented that reveal variable cell responses following exposure to a novel topoisomerase poison, AS-DACA. With this series of experimenst we have illustrated some of the cell biology which needs to be considered when exploring the therapeutic potential of new agents. Complexities include "non-classical" resistance mechanisms that are driven by the reduction of key target proteins (eg topoisomerases), drug sequestration mechanism which result in the accumulation of AS-DACA in acidic vesicles of the membrane trafficking system. This complex suite of cellular responses to general cytotoxics raises the consideration that such patient-specific differences in RMS tumours may lead to these agents contributing to personalised therapeutic strategies.

7. Acknowledgment

We thank Professor Bill Denny from the Auckland Cancer Society Research Centre, University of Auckland, New Zealand, for providing several of the agents used. This work was supported by funding from the Children's Oncology Foundation (SJW, DRC), and an Australian Postgraduate Research Award (SJW).

8. References

Arndt CAS, Nascimento AG, Schroeder G, Schomberg PJ, Neglia JP, Sencer SF, Silberman TL, Moertel CL, Tillisch JK, and Miser JS. (1998) Treatment of intermediate risk rhabdomyosarcoma and undifferentiated sarcoma with alternating cycles of vincristine/doxorubicin/cyclophosphamide and etoposide/ifosfamide. *European Journal of Cancer,* 34, 1224-1229

Atwell GJ, Cain BF, Baguley BC, Finlay GJ, Denny WA. (1984) Potential antitumor agents. Part 43. Synthesis and biological activity of dibasic 9-aminoacridine-4-carboxamides, a new class of antitumor agent. *Journal of Medicinal Chemistry,* 27: 1481-1485

Atwell GJ, Rewcastle GW, Baguley BC and Denny WA. (1987) Potential antitumour agents, 50, In vivo solid-tumour activity of derivatives of N-[2-(dimethylamino)ethyl]acridine-4-carboxamide. *Journal of Medicinal Chemistry* 30: 664-669

Austin CA, and Marsh KL (1998) Eukaryotic DNA topoisomerase IIβ. *Bioessays,* 20, 215-226

Baguley BC, Zhuang L and Marshall E. (1995) Experimental solid tumour activity of N-[2-(dimethylamino)ethyl]-acridine-4-carboxamide. *Cancer Chemotherapy and Pharmacology,* 36: 244-248

Baker KS, Anderson JR, Link MP, Grier HE, Qualman SJ, Maurer HM, Breneman JC, Wiener ES, and Crist WM. (2000) Benefit of intensified therapy for patients with local or regional embryonal rhabdomyosarcoma: Results from the Intergroup Rhabdomyosarcoma Study IV. *Journal of Clinical Oncology,* 18, 2427-2434

Belhoussine R, Morjani H, Millot JM, Sharonov S, and Manfait M. (1998) Confocal scanning microspectrofluorometry reveals specific anthracycline accumulation in cytoplasmic organelles of multidrug-resistant cancer cells. *Journal of Histochemistry and Cytochemistry,* 46, 1369-1376

Breitfeld PP, and Meyer WH. (2005) Rhabdomyosarcoma: new windows of opportunity. *The Oncologist* 10: 518-27

Bridewell DJ, Finlay GJ and Baguley BC. (2001) Topoisomerase I/II selectivity among derivatives of N-[2-(dimethylamino)ethyl]acridine-4-carboxamide (DACA). *Anticancer Drug Design* 16: 317-324

Burma S, Chen BP, Murphy M, Kurimasa A, and Chen DJ. (2001) ATM phosphorylates Histone H2AX in response to DNA double-strand breaks. *Journal of Biological Chemistry,* 276, 42462-42467

Byers SA, Schafer B, Sappal DS, Brown J, Price DH. (2005) The antiproliferative agent MLN944 preferentially inhibits transcription. *Molecular Cancer Therapeutics,* 4: 1260-1267

Caponigro F, Dittrich C, Sorensen JB, Schellens JH, Duffaud F, Paz Ares L, Lacombe D, de Balincourt C, Fumoleau P. (2002) Phase II study of XR 5000, an inhibitor of topoisomerases I and II, in advanced colorectal cancer. *European Journal of Cancer,* 38: 70-74.

Chang XB, (2007) A molecular understanding of ATP-dependent solute transport by multidrug resistance-associated protein MRP1. *Cancer Metastasis Reviews,* 26, 15-37

Chen V, and Rosania GR. (2006) The great multidrug-resistance paradox. *ACS Chemical Biology,* 1, 271-273

Crist WM, Anderson JR, Meza JL, Fryer C, Raney B, Ruymann FB, Breneman J, Qualman SJ, Wiener E, Wharam M, et al. (2001) Intergroup Rhabdomyosarcoma Study-IV: Results for patients with nonmetastatic disease. *Journal of Clinical Oncology,* 19, 3091-3102

De Duve C, De Barsy T, Poole B, Trouet A, Tulkens P and Van Hoof F. (1974) Commentary: Lysosomotropic agents. *Biochemical Pharmacology,* 23, 2495-2531

Desai SD, Liu LF, Vazquez-Abad D, and D'Arpa P. (1997) Ubiquitin-dependent destruction of topoisomerase I is stimulated by the antitumour drug camptothecin. *The Journal of Biological Chemistry.* 272, 24159-24164

Duvvuri M, and Krise JP. (2005) A novel assay reveals that weakly basic model compounds concentrate in lysosomes to an extent greater than pH-partitioning theory would predict. *Molecular Pharmaceutics,* 2, 440-448

Fan TR, Peng AL, Chen HC, Lo SC, Huang TH, and Li TK. (2008) Cellular processing pathways contribute to the activation of etoposide-induced DNA damage responses. *DNA Repair,* 7, 452-463

Finlay GJ, Riou JF, Baguley BC. (1996) From amsacrine to DACA (N-[2-(dimethylamino)ethyl]acridine-4-carboxamide): selectivity for topoisomerases I and II among acridine derivatives. *European Journal of Cancer,* 32A: 708-714

Frascella E, Pritchard-Jones K, Modak S, Mancini AF, Carli M, Pinkerton CR. (1996) Response of previously untreated metastatic rhabdomyosarcoma to combination chemotherapy with carboplatin, epirubicin and vincristine. *European Journal of Cancer,* 32A, 821-825

Gamage SA, Spicer JA, Finlay GJ, Stewart AJ, Charlton P, Baguley BC, and Denny WA. (2001) Diatonic Bis(9-methylphenazine-1-carboxamides): Relationships between biological activity and linker chain structure for a series of potent topoisomerase targeted anticancer drugs. *Journal of Medicinal Chemistry* 44: 1407-1415

Groth-Pedersen L, Ostenfeld MS, Hoyer-Hansen M, Nylandsted J and Jaattela M. (2007) Vincristine induces dramatic lysosomal changes and sensitizes cancer cells to lysosome-destabilizing siramesine. Cancer Research, 67, 2217-2225

Gurney JG, Young JL, Roffers SD, Smith MA and Bunin GR, (1999) Soft Tissue Sarcomas. *Cancer Incidence and Survival among Children and Adolescents: United States SEER Program 1975-1995,* (eds. Ries L.A.G, Smith M.A, Gurney J.G, Linet M, Tamra T, Young J.L, Bunin G.R)pp. 111-124 *National Cancer Institute, SEER Program.* Bethesda

Haldane A, Finlay GJ, Hay MP, Denny WA, Baguley B. (1999) Cellular uptake of N-[2-(dimethylamino)ethyl]acridine-4-carboxamide (DACA). *Anti-cancer Drug Design,* 14: 275-280

Herlevsen M, Oxford G, Owens CR, Conaway M and Theodorescu D. (2007) Depletion of major vault protein increases doxorubicin sensitivity and nuclear accumulation and disrupts its sequestration in lysosomes. *Molecular Cancer Therapeutics,* 6, 1804-1813

Kaufmann AM, and Krise JP. (2007) Lysosomal sequestration of amine-containing drugs: Analysis and therapeutic implications. *Journal of Pharmaceutical Sciences,* 96, 729-746

Klausner R, Donaldson JG, Lippincott-Schwartz J. (1992) Brefeldin A: insights into the control of membrane traffic and organelle structure. *Journal of Cell Biology,* 116, 1071-1080

Klein I, Sarkadi B, and Varadi A. (1999) An inventory of the human ABC proteins. *Biocimica et Biophysica Acta,* 1461, 237-262

Klunder JW, Komdeur R, Van Der Graaf WTA, De Bont EJSM, Hoekstra HJ, Van Den Berg E, and Molenaar WM. (2003) Expression of multidrug resistance-associated proteins in rhabdomyosarcomas before and after chemotherapy: The relationship between lung resistance-related protein (LRP) and differentiation. *Human Pathology,* 34, 150-155

Komdeur R, Klunder J, van der Graaf WTA, van den Berg E, de Bont ESJM, Hoekstra HJ, and Molenaar WM. (2003) Multidrug resistance proteins in rhabdomyosarcomas. *Cancer,* 97, 1999-2005

Kung FH, Desai SJ, Dickerman JD, Goorin AM, Harris MB, Inoue S, Krischer JP, Murphy SB, Pratt CB, Toledano S, et al (1995) Ifosfamide/carboplatin/etoposide (ICE) for recurrent malignant solid tumors of childhood: a Pediatric Oncology Group Phase I/II study. *Journal of Pediatric Hematology/Oncology,* 3, 265-269.

Lee CM, Tannock IF. (2006) Inhibition of endosomal sequestration of basic anticancer drugs: influence on cytotoxicity and tissue penetration. *British Journal of Cancer.* 94, 863-869

Leslie EM, Deeley RG, and Cole SPC. (2005) Multidrug resistance proteins: role of P-glycoprotein, MRP1, MRP2, and BCRP (ABCG2) in tissue defense. *Toxicology and Applied Pharmacology,* 204, 216-237

Li LH, and Krueger WC. (1991) The biochemical pharmacology of nogalamycin and its derivatives. *Pharmacology and Therapeutics,* 51: 239-255

Li TK, and Liu LF. (2001) Tumor cell death induced by topoisomerase-targeting drugs. *Annual Review of Pharmacology and Toxicology.* 41, 53-77

Luzio JP, Mullock BM, Pryor PR, Lindsay MR, James DE, and Piper RC. (2001) Relationship between endosomes and lysosomes. *Biochemical Society Transactions.* 29, 476-480

Marina NM, Rodman J, Shema SJ, Bowman LC, Douglass E, Furman W, Santana VM, Hudson M, Wilimas J, Meyer W, et al (1993) Phase I study of escalating targeted doses of carboplatin combined with ifosfamide and etoposide in children with relapsed solid tumors. *Journal of Clinical Oncology,* 11, 554-560

Maurer HM, Beltangady M, Gehan EA, Crist W, Hammond D, Hays DM, Heyn R, Lawrence W, Newton W, Ortega J, et al (1988) The Intergroup Rhabdomyosarcoma Study-I: A final report. *Cancer,* 61, 209-220

Maurer HM, Gehan EA, Beltangady M, Crist W, Dickman PS, Donaldson SS, Fryer C, Hammond D, Hays DM, Herrman J, et al (1993) The Intergroup Rhabdomyosarcoma Study-II. *Cancer,* 71, 1904-1922

Mayer LD, Bally MB and Cullis PR. (1986) Uptake of adriamycin into large unilamellar vesicles in response to a pH gradient. *Biochimica et Biophysica Acta,* 857, 123-126

Murphy AJ, Hughes CA, Barrett C, Magee H, Loftus B, O'Leary JJ, and Sheils O. (2007) Low-level TOP2A amplification in prostate cancer is associated with HER2 duplication, androgen resistance, and decreased survival. *Cancer Research,* 67, 2893-2898

Ouar Z, Bens M, Vignes C, Paulais M, Pringel C, Fleury J, Cluzeaud F, Lacave R and Vandewalle A. (2003) Inhibitors of vacuolar H+-ATPase impair the preferential accumulation of daunomycin in lysosomes and reverse the resistance to the anthracyclines in drug-resistant renal epithelial cells. *Biochemical Journal,* 370, 185-193

Pappo AS, Lyden E, Breneman J, Wiener E, Teot L, Meza J, Crist W and Vietti T. (2001) Up-front window trial of topotecan in previously untreated children and adolescents with metastatic rhabdomyosarcoma: An Intergroup Rhabdomyosarcoma. *Journal of Clinical Oncology,* 19: 213-219

Pommier Y. (2006) Topoisomerase I inhibitors: Camptothecins and beyond. *Nature Reviews,* 6, 789-802

Qualman SJ, Coffin Cheryl M, Newton WA, Hojo H, Triche TJ, Parham DM, and Crist WM. (1998) Intergroup Rhabdomyosarcoma Study: Update for pathologists. *Pediatric and Developmental Pathology,* 1: 550-561

Rajagopal A, and Simon SM, (2003) Subcellular localisation and activity of multidrug resistance proteins. *Molecular Biology of the Cell,* 14, 3389-3399.

Sandler E, Lyden E, Ruymann F, Maurer H, Wharam M, Parham D, Link M, Crist W. (2001) Efficacy of ifosfamide and doxorubicin given as a phase II "window" in children with newly diagnosed metastatic rhabdomyosarcoma: A Report from the Intergroup Rhabdomyosarcoma Study Group. *Medical and Pediatric Oncology,* 37: 442-448.

Saraste J, and Goud B. (2007) Functional symmetry of endomembranes. *Molecular Biology of the Cell,* 18, 1430-1436

Spicer JA, Gamage SA, Rewcastle GW, Finlay GJ, Bridewell DJA, Baguley BC, and Denny WA. (2000) Bis(phenazine-1-carboxamides): Structure-activity relationships for a new class of dual topoisomerase I/II-directed anticancer drugs. *Journal of Medicinal Chemistry,* 43: 1350-1358

Stevens MCG, Rey A, Bouvet N, Ellershaw C, Flamant F, Habrand JL, Marsden HB, Martelli H, Sanchez de Toledo J, Spicer RD, et al (2005) Treatment of nonmetastatic rhabdomyosarcoma in childhood and adolescence: Third study of the International Society of Paediatric Oncology – SIOP Malignant Mesenchymal Tumor 89. *Journal of Clinical Oncology,* 23, 2618-2628

Tracey E, Baker D, Chen W, Stavrou E, and Bishop J. (2007) Cancer in New South Wales: Incidence, Mortality and Prevalence, 2005. Sydney: Cancer Institute NSW

Twelves C, Campone M, Coudert B, Van den Bent M, de Jonge M, Dittrich C, Rampling R, Sorio R, Lacombe D, de Balincourt C, and Fumoleau P. (2002) Phase II study of XR5000 (DACA) administered as a 120-h infusion in patients with recurrent glioblastoma multiforme. *Annals of Oncology,* 13: 777-780

Van Winkle P, Angiolillo A, Krailo M, Cheung YK, Anderson B, Davenport V, Reaman G, Cairo MS. (2005) Ifosfamide, carboplatin, and etoposide (ICE) reinduction chemotherapy in a large cohort of children and adolescents with recurrent/refractory sarcoma. *Pediatric Blood and Cancer,* 44: 338-347

Verborg W, Thomas H, Bissett D, Waterfall J, Steiner J, Cooper M, and Rankin EM. (2007) First-into-man phase I and pharmacokinetic study of XR5944.14, a novel agent with a unique mechanism of action. *British Journal of Cancer*, 97: 844-850

Wakelin LPG, Bu X, Eleftheriou A, Parmar A, Hayek C, and Stewart B. (2003) Bisintercalating threading diacridines : Relationships between DNA binding, cytotoxicity, and cell cycle Arrest. *Journal of Medicinal Chemistry,* 46: 5790-5802

Wexler LH, and Helman LJ. (1997) Rhabdomyosarcoma and the undifferentiated sarcomas. In *Principles and Practice of Pediatric Oncology* (eds. Pizzo. P and Poplack DG) pp. 799-829, *Lippincott-Raven Publishers,* Philadelphia.

Wolf S, Wakelin LPG, He Z, Stewart BW, Catchpoole DR. (2009) In vitro assessment of novel transcription inhibitors and topoisomerase poisons in rhabdomyosarcoma cell lines., *Cancer Chemotherapy and Pharmacology*, 64(6), 1059-1069.

Wolf SJ, Huynh T, Bryce NS, Hambley T, Wakelin LPG, Stewart BW, Catchpoole DR (2011) Intracellular trafficking as a determinant of AS-DACA cytotoxicity in rhabdomyosarcoma cells. *BMC Cell Biology*, In Press.

Yang WCT, Strasser FF, and Pomerat CM. (1965) Mechanism of drug-induced vacuolization in tissue culture. *Experimental Cell Research,* 38, 495-506

Yang XL, and Wang AHJ. (1999) Structural studies of atom-specific anticancer drugs acting on DNA. *Pharmacology and Therapeutics.* 83, 181-215

Zihlif M, Catchpoole DR, Wakelin LPG, and Stewart BW. (2006) Altered patterns of global gene expression as a basis for inferences concerning different topoisomerase poisons., *Gordon Conference on Molecular Therapeutic in Cancer*, Oxford, United Kingdom.

2

Telomere Maintenance Mechanisms in Soft Tissue Sarcomas

Matthew J. Plantinga and Dominique Broccoli
Memorial University Medical Center
USA

1. Introduction

1.1 Telomeres and tumorigenesis

1.1.1 Telomere structure

Human chromosomes, which are composed of linear double-stranded DNA, are capped at their ends by nucleoprotein complexes called telomeres (reviewed in (Martinez & Blasco, 2011)). This telomeric cap prevents end-to-end fusion events between chromosomes, and protects chromosome ends from being recognized as double-stranded breaks by the DNA damage machinery in the cell. Telomeric DNA is composed of tandem 5'TTAGGG repeats at each end of the chromosome, extending up to tens of kilobases. Poorly understood end-processing reactions after replication result in a 3' overhang on the G-rich strand, which invades the upstream double-stranded telomeric DNA to form a displacement (D)-loop such that the end of the chromosome is buried thereby preventing detection by the cellular DNA damage response (Greider, 1999). Telomeric DNA is in complex with a number of proteins that act to stabilize the structure and mediate telomeric functions of capping and length regulation (Figure 1). Double-stranded (ds) telomeric repeats are bound directly by TRF1 (Zhong et al., 1992) and TRF2 (Bilaud et al., 1997; Broccoli et al., 1997), while the POT1-TPP1 heterodimer binds to the single-stranded (ss) telomeric DNA (de Lange, 2005; Lei et al., 2002). The ds- and ss-telomeric DNA complexes are linked through their interaction with TIN2 (Abreu et al., 2010; Kim et al., 1999; O'Connor et al., 2006), together forming the telomeric shelterin complex (de Lange, 2005). Additional proteins necessary for telomeric function are recruited by interactions with components of the shelterin complex (reviewed in (Martinez & Blasco, 2011)).

Mammalian telomeres have been shown to contain characteristics of heterochromatin, including the presence of homologues of the heterochromatin binding protein HP1 (Koering et al., 2002; Sharma et al., 2003), enriched tri-methylation of histone H3 lysine 9 (H3K9) and histone H4 lysine 20 (H4K20) (Garcia-Cao et al., 2004), and methylation of CpG dinucleotides in subtelomeric DNA repeats (Gonzalo et al., 2006). Studies in telomerase knockout mice demonstrated that as telomeres become shorter the heterochromatic marks are lost and replaced by marks characteristic of open chromatin, such as increased acetylation of histone tails (Benetti et al., 2007), suggesting that a minimum telomere length is necessary to maintain the appropriate chromatin structure at chromosome ends. Alterations in the level of epigenetic modifications, such as tri-methylation of H3K9 and H4K20 via knockout of the relevant modifying enzymes, led to increased telomere length without effect on telomere end-capping function (Garcia-Cao et al., 2004). Intriguingly, evidence of increased telomeric recombination is also a result of altering telomeric chromatin structure (Gonzalo et al., 2006).

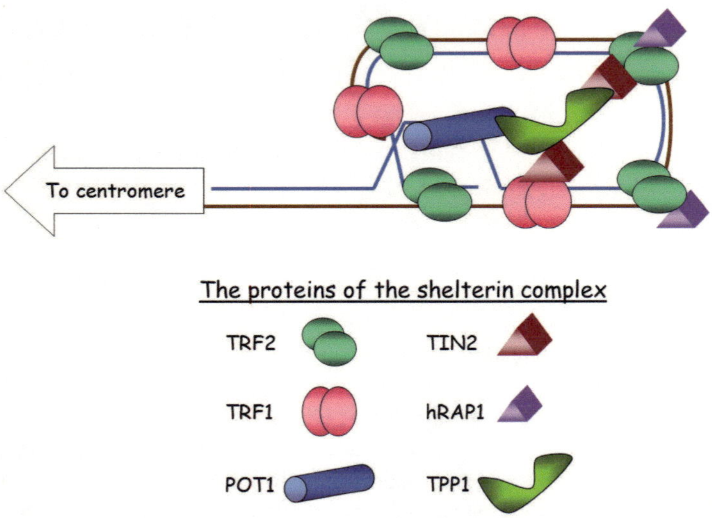

Fig. 1. Proteins of the shelterin complex. TRF1 and TRF2 bind directly to double-stranded telomeric sequence, with TRF2 recruiting RAP1. The POT1-TPP1 binds to single-stranded regions. Interactions with TIN2 link the single-stranded and double-stranded binding complexes.

Despite having chromatin features characteristic of heterochromatin, telomeres are now known to be transcriptionally active, giving rise to a species of long non-coding RNA (lncRNA) termed TERRA (Luke & Lingner, 2009). Long non-coding RNAs are involved in establishing and maintaining chromatin structure (Whitehead et al., 2009). TERRA has been suggested to play a role in telomere heterochromatin formation (Deng et al., 2009). TERRA associates with telomeres and may be involved in maintaining or remodeling telomere structure during development and differentiation (Luke & Lingner, 2009).

1.1.2 Telomere dynamics

Linear DNA molecules use RNA to prime replication by DNA polymerase. At the completion of synthesis, these primers are degraded and gaps are filled, but the regions at the 5′ ends of the newly synthesized strands cannot be filled in. Thus, with each replication cycle, telomeric sequences shorten at their 5′ ends (Figure 2). End processing events subsequent to replication (Sfeir et al., 2005) may also contribute to sequence loss. Excessive shortening of telomeres disrupts the shelterin complex through loss of binding sites for shelterin complex proteins, which exposes chromosome ends to DNA damage machinery. In the presence of an active DNA damage response (DDR), telomere uncapping activates DNA damage checkpoints, leading to cell cycle arrest or apoptosis (Martinez & Blasco, 2011). Thus, telomere length acts as a molecular clock, limiting the total number of divisions any given cell may undergo. In the absence of a robust DDR, such as often occurs on the road to transformation, exposed telomere ends result in increased genomic instability through breakage-fusion-bridge cycles induced by joining of chromosome ends. This 'telomere crisis' can only be resolved by restoring telomeres to a length sufficient for functional shelterin complex assembly. Therefore, to circumvent the effects of telomere attrition and attain unlimited replicative potential, cancer cells must solve the so-called 'end replication problem.'

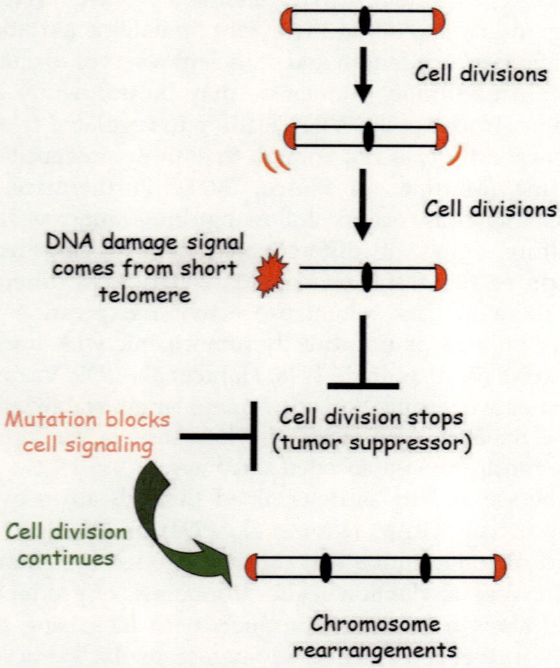

Fig. 2. Telomere attrition from subsequent cell divisions continues until critically short telomeres result in a DNA damage response and the cessation of cell division. In cancer cells, mutations in key regulatory proteins block DNA damage signaling, allowing cell division to continue, potentially leading to chromosome rearrangements from chromosome end-to-end fusions.

Telomere extension occurs by activation of a telomere maintenance mechanism (TMM), via either telomerase or a recombination-based mechanism called alternative lengthening of telomeres (ALT). Activation of either mechanism is sufficient to recover from telomere crisis, thus enabling continued growth of the cancer cells. Resolution of telomere crisis is not a prerequisite to tumor formation, however, as some adult cells contain adequate telomeric reserves to form tumors requiring clinical intervention before loss of telomeric DNA becomes sufficient to induce crisis (Reddel, 2000). Nevertheless, telomere attrition will ultimately limit tumor growth. TMM activation, because it increases replicative potential, is often associated with higher grade tumors and poorer patient prognosis (Costa et al., 2006; Matsuo et al., 2009; Ulaner et al., 2003). Indeed, progress through telomere crisis with its associated genome instability has been suggested to contribute to tumorigenicity by generating a hypermutability environment (Chin et al., 2004), analogous to the tumorigenic potential of cells with microsatellite instability.

2. Telomere maintenance mechanisms

2.1 Telomerase

Telomerase is a ribonucleoprotein complex that adds telomeric DNA *de novo* onto chromosome ends (Greider & Blackburn, 1987). The catalytic component of the holoenzyme, TERT, is a reverse transcriptase (RNA-dependent DNA polymerase) that uses the RNA component, TR (aka TERC), as a template for telomere extension (Figure 3). Telomerase is commonly active in germline and some stem cell populations (Artandi & DePinho, 2010), ensuring species-specific telomere length and sufficient reserves to complete developmental programs, respectively. In addition, telomerase may be transiently active during certain differentiation programs (Hodes et al., 2002), leading to regulated telomere extension prior to expansion. Telomerase activity is not enough to entirely prevent telomere attrition over an individual's lifetime (Martinez & Blasco, 2011). Furthermore, stressing stem cell compartments, for example as occurs following bone marrow transplantation, may contribute to premature aging of differentiated cells arising from those stem cell compartments (Allsopp et al., 2001; Lewis et al., 2004). Most differentiated cells do not express hTERT and therefore lack telomerase activity. Expression of telomerase, while conferring immortality on cells, is not directly tumorigenic with transformation requiring additional genetic changes (Bodnar et al., 1998; Hahn et al., 1999; Vaziri & Benchimol, 1998). However, as discussed above, acquisition of telomere length stabilization removes a critical tumor suppressor mechanism. Activation of telomerase is the primary TMM in most carcinomas as well as translocation-associated sarcomas.

Experimentally, telomerase activity is determined through an assay called the telomere repeat amplification protocol (TRAP) (Kim et al., 1994). In this assay, protein extracts are incubated with a short oligonucleotide that can be extended by telomerase, if it is present. After PCR amplification and acrylamide gel electrophoresis of products, extracts containing active telomerase will show a ladder of products with increasing numbers of telomeric TTAGGG repeats. The presence of active telomerase in the extract does not necessitate cellular activity, as *in vitro* activity can be achieved without the additional factors required *in vivo* to support extension of chromosome ends. Indeed, mutants that are catalytically active in vitro but unable to maintain telomeres in vivo, have been described (Counter et al., 1998) and highlight the multiple levels of regulation associated with telomere maintenance by telomerase (Osterhage & Friedman, 2009). The absence of activity by TRAP is also not definitive, as telomerase activity can be easily destroyed by technical challenges during extract isolation and soluble inhibitors of either the initial extension reaction or the PCR amplification step may be present. A definitive lack of activity can be attained by demonstrating the absence of the TERT mRNA by quantitative PCR, as activity cannot occur in the absence of the catalytic component of telomerase.

2.2 ALT

Alternative lengthening of telomeres is an umbrella term for all non-telomerase mechanisms for telomere maintenance (Cesare & Reddel, 2010; Henson & Reddel, 2010). Telomeres in ALT cells are often heterogeneous in length, ranging from very short (<6 kb) to very long (>20 kb), which are easily visualized either by southern blot or quantitative FISH. Despite the broad range of sizes, the average telomere length, as measured by quantitating southern blots, is longer than that observed in normal adult or telomerase-positive cancers (Bryan et al., 1995). ALT cells also frequently show mini-satellite instability (Jeyapalan et al., 2008;

Jeyapalan et al., 2005) and increased telomere sister chromatid exchange (T-SCE) (Londono-Vallejo et al., 2004), which presumably arises from increased recombination at telomeres. Both assays are of limited use in tumor tissue as the mini-satellite instability assay requires the ability to PCR long (~4KB) DNA fragments that may have significant degradation in archival tumor samples and the T-SCE assay relies on the ability to label cells in culture. Also found in ALT cells are double-stranded circular DNA molecules called t-circles that are generated from telomeric DNA and may function in telomere elongation via recombination-independent rolling circle replication (Tomaska et al., 2004). Single-stranded circles, called either c-circles or g-circles based on sequence, are also present in these cells, with c-circles being much more abundant (Henson et al., 2009). The ability to detect these circles with high specificity in archival tumor tissue has not been demonstrated. Perhaps the most frequently assayed characteristic of ALT cells is the appearance of ALT associated PML bodies (APBs), in which telomeric DNA co-localizes with the PML nuclear body (Yeager et al., 1999).

The role of APBs in ALT remains controversial. Conflicting reports have suggested that APBs are a marker of ALT cells that are irreversibly arrested or, conversely, are required for telomere maintenance by ALT. Early studies of ALT-positive cell lines immortalized *in vitro* suggested that perturbation of the p53 pathway might be a common element (Opitz et al., 2001; Rogan et al., 1995). We have previously demonstrated that forced expression of a transactivation-dead p53 suppresses growth of ALT-positive, but not telomerase positive, cells (Razak et al., 2004). We reported that this caused an increase in APB frequency in the absence of downstream effectors of p53, such as p21. We concluded that abrogation of p53 suppression of recombination function was required for ALT activation. In contrast, the Reddel group has reported that over-expression of transactivation competent p53 leads to an increase in APBs, and that this increase in APBs requires p21 (Jiang et al., 2009). These authors conclude that APBs arise in arrested cells rather than cells undergoing telomere elongation by recombination. Furthermore, although ATM is constitutively active in p53-positive ALT-positive cell lines, activation of p53 and downstream effectors only occurs when telomeres are uncapped via perturbation of the shelterin complex (Stagno D'Alcontres et al., 2007). PML is essential for p21 induced cellular senescence in this context, although it is not required for p53 to associate with telomeres.

In contrast to experiments suggesting that APBs only occur in arrested cells, we and others have shown that DNA replication occurs in APB-positive cells, suggesting that these structures are present in actively cycling cells (Grobelny et al., 2000). Others have found that disruption of APBs prevents telomere maintenance by ALT and leads to loss of culture viability, arguing for an active role of APBs in telomere maintenance by ALT (Jiang et al., 2005). The spatio-temporal dynamics of telomeric DNA association with PML bodies have been recently described, and the authors of this study conclude that telomere recombination takes place in these structures (Draskovic et al., 2009). Furthermore, new PML bodies form at telomeric DNA regardless of which TMM is active (Brouwer et al., 2009) and APBs form transiently in human diploid fibroblasts following high LET radiation (Berardinelli et al., 2010), suggesting that the association of telomeric DNA with PML bodies may be a component of a DNA damage response. Indeed, telomeres are transiently recognized as DNA damage during normal DNA replication (Verdun & Karlseder, 2006). The consistent theme within these data is that uncapped/short telomeres are localized to the PML body.

TERRA expression is increased in ALT cell lines and is accompanied by a less dense, albeit variable, pattern of sub-telomeric CpG methylation relative to telomerase positive and normal cells (Ng et al., 2009). It is not clear if the increase in TERRA occurs subsequent to altered sub-telomeric chromatin (i.e., as a consequence) or contributes to generating changes in sub-telomeric chromatin (i.e., as a cause). Recent work implicates TERRA as being critical for telomere structure in the ALT-positive U2OS cell line and telomerase positive HCT116 cells (Deng et al., 2009). TERRA was shown to interact with the end-capping protein TRF2, and decreasing TERRA expression levels led to loss of heterochromatin marks and telomere instability. On the surface, then, one might expect the increased TERRA in ALT cells to increase heterochromatin-associated chromatin condensation making telomeres less accessible to recombination. Conversely, we have shown that TERRA levels increase as telomeres shorten (associated with gaining histone marks consistent with an open chromatin structure) and in response to telomere uncapping (Caslini et al., 2009). The increase in TERRA, in this context, requires activity of the histone H3K4 methyltransferase MLL and the p53 DNA damage response. How might these observations be reconciled? It is likely based on published results that a minimum level of TERRA expression is necessary to support functional end-capping. However, TERRA may play additional roles in ALT-positive cells. Increased TERRA may be necessary to propagate and maintain a more open chromatin structure, which in turn promotes telomeric recombination, by titrating essential factors and modulating the formation of telomeric heterochromatin. Alternatively, increased TERRA in ALT cells may simply reflect the presence of ultra-long telomeres present in these cells. Future studies will elucidate the role of TERRA in telomere stability and telomere maintenance mechanisms.

Many questions remain about the nature of the ALT mechanism. A single ALT cell may show only some of the features associated with ALT, and may show a different subset of features than other ALT cells (Fasching et al., 2005; Slatter et al., 2010). This may result from the existence of multiple mechanisms currently described as ALT. It is unclear to what extent these different mechanisms rely on similar or overlapping pathways for telomere maintenance, and thus whether and to what extent they share genetic requirements for activation and regulation. For example, if the appearance of APBs is related to DNA damage and repair, does the lack of APBs in some ALT cells indicate lower levels of DNA damage and thus lower levels of genome instability? Or are APBs associated with a specific recombination-based pathway for telomere maintenance? An essential step on the pathway to understanding ALT regulation, and the pathways leading to telomere stabilization through recombination, would be the development of an ALT cell line lacking APBs. It remains essential as further work is done to characterize ALT to be cognizant of the potential impact the features used to define cells as ALT-positive have on any conclusions about the characteristics of ALT in general.

ALT seems to be more common in tumors of mesenchymal origin and with complex karyotypes when compared to those of epithelial origin and translocation-driven, respectively (Johnson & Broccoli, 2007; Montgomery et al., 2004; Ulaner et al., 2004), which may provide some insight into the genetic origins of ALT. Both ALT and telomerase can be active in a single tumor (Costa et al., 2006; Hakin-Smith et al., 2003; Johnson et al., 2005; Ulaner et al., 2003), suggesting that lack of functional telomerase is not a prerequisite for ALT activation, although it is not known whether both mechanisms can be active in a single cell. Studies investigating TMM in tumors rely upon a variety of assays to identify telomerase-positive and ALT-positive tumors, respectively (Costa et al., 2006; Montgomery et al., 2004; Ulaner et al., 2003). At least some of the tumors without characteristics of either mechanism are also ALT-positive based upon increased mini-satellite instability (Jeyapalan et al., 2008; Jeyapalan et al., 2005). However, a substantial fraction of mesenchymal tumors defy TMM characterization using the currently available techniques. In part this is due to many assays not being consistent with the quality of DNA isolated from tumor tissue, particularly archival tissues that are only available as formalin-fixed, paraffin-embedded samples. An alternative possibility is that only a rare subset of tumor cells, e.g. tumor stem cells, actively maintain telomeres while the bulk of the cells comprising the tumor do not have active telomere maintenance.

3. Telomere maintenance mechanisms in tumorigenesis

Although it is used in a considerable proportion of cell lines (~35%), until recently ALT had only rarely been documented in human tumors (Bryan et al., 1997). Accordingly, comparative studies have relied largely upon cell culture systems or investigation of tumors arising in late generation telomerase-deficient mouse models, which are thus forced to use ALT. Although each system has inherent limitations with respect to extrapolation to human cancer, several key insights have come from these studies. Most importantly, the two mechanisms of telomere maintenance are not equivalent with respect to their contribution to the tumorigenic phenotype. Exogenous expression of hTERT, the catalytic subunit of telomerase, in combination with activated Ras and the SV40 early region is sufficient to transform human cells and render them tumorigenic in nude mice (Hahn et al., 1999). In contrast, human cells which rely on ALT instead of telomerase for telomere maintenance, while immortal, are unable to form tumors in nude mice when injected subcutaneously, although they are competent to form tumors when injected under the renal capsule (Sun et al., 2005). If hTERT is introduced into these cells, tumorigenicity is restored in the subcutaneous setting even though telomerase is not required for telomere maintenance *per se*. Likewise, immortalized mouse embryo fibroblasts (MEFs) that use telomerase are readily able to colonize lungs and proliferate when injected into tail veins, while MEFs that use ALT are not (Chang et al., 2003). Thus, while telomere maintenance by either TMM is sufficient to ensure replicative immortality, these studies suggest that telomerase may provide additional growth advantages during *in vivo* tumorigenesis.

Both ALT and telomerase can be active in a single tumor, suggesting that lack of functional telomerase is not a prerequisite for ALT activation, although it is not known whether both mechanisms can be active in a single cell. Given tumor heterogeneity it is possible that distinct regions of a tumor utilize telomerase and ALT respectively. In cell based studies in which telomerase expression was forced in an ALT background, telomerase specifically elongated the shortest telomeres in the population (Grobelny et al., 2001). Despite extensive culturing, characteristics of ALT such as APBs were not altered in the presence of telomerase. This suggests that reconstitution of telomerase, and associated telomere stabilization, is not sufficient to suppress the ALT mechanism once it has been activated.

4. Telomere maintenance mechanisms in liposarcomas

Soft tissue sarcomas (STS) are rare malignancies of mesenchymal origin, with approximately 10 500 cases in 2010 (Jemal et al., 2010). Given the rarity of mesenchymal tumors, studies assessing TMM activation have either used multiple histological types or focused on the more common STS types. The most common adult STS, accounting for ~20% of cases, is liposarcoma, named for its morphological resemblance to adipose tissue. Liposarcomas are divided into several subtypes based on histological features: well-differentiated (WDLS), de-differentiated (DDLS), pleomorphic (PLS), myxoid (MYXLS), and round cell (RCLS). Based upon expression profiling, it has been suggested that these tumors can be further classified along a developmental pathway from the mesenchymal stem cell to mature adipocytes based on their state of differentiation (Matushansky et al 2008), with de-differentiated liposarcomas most closely resembling mesenchymal stem cells, and well-differentiated liposarcomas most closely resembling mature adipocytes. The remaining histotypes fall between these, with pleomorphic liposarcomas appearing less differentiated than myxoid/round cell tumors. Due to their relatively high frequency among adult STS, several studies of TMM have focused on liposarcomas. Intriguingly, the frequency of specific TMM utilization appears to vary with histological subtype within this category of STS (Figure 3).

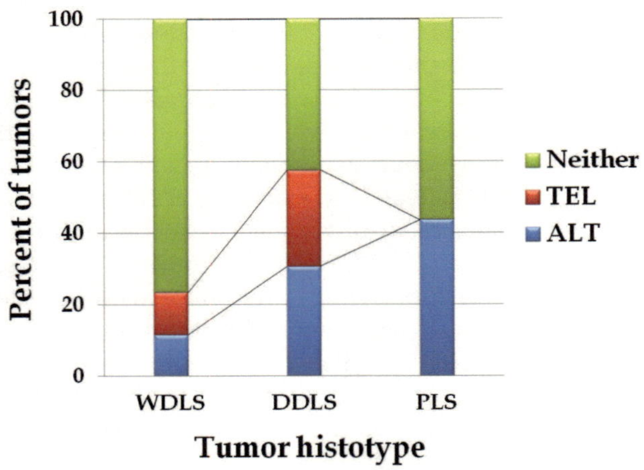

Fig. 3. TMM utilization varies among histological subtypes of liposarcoma.

WD/DDLS together account for 55% of all LS (40% and 15% respectively) (Conyers et al., 2011). Both WDLS and DDLS may contain a diagnostic Chr12q13-15 amplification (Rieker et al., 2010; Tap et al., 2011), although this genetic change is found more frequently in DDLS. WDLS are not typically included among the complex karyotype malignancies; however, upon dedifferentiation this tumor is included in the complex karyotype subdesignation. Combined, these tumors are called atypical lipotomous tumors, which, like alternative lengthening of telomeres, is commonly abbreviated ALT. WDLS are low grade tumors that are histologically similar to adipose tissue, showing primarily local recurrence with limited metastasis, in contrast to DDLS, which are higher grade tumors with greater propensity for metastasis. The WD/DDLS that have an active TMM use ALT and telomerase with similar frequency, but WDLS have a higher fraction of malignancies with no evidence of telomere maintenance (75% for WDLS, 50% for DDLS) (Costa et al., 2006).

MYX/RC LS, which together account for ~40% of all LS, are characterized by the TLS/CHOP (aka FUS/CHOP) translocation (Conyers et al., 2011). This translocation is transformative when over-expressed in mice (Perez-Losada et al., 2000) and other cell lines (Riggi et al., 2006; Schwarzbach et al., 2004), indicating that FUS/CHOP drives tumorigenesis in these malignancies. Of the two, MYX LS is the lower grade, and RC LS is the higher grade. To our knowledge, no malignancies containing the characteristic translocation have been shown to use ALT. Thus, if one uses this molecular alteration to classify MYX/RC LS, then these tumors use only telomerase for telomere maintenance. This is consistent with early reports suggesting that, as a whole, translocation-associated sarcomas utilize telomerase, rather than ALT, for telomere maintenance.

The rarest form of liposarcoma, PLS, accounts for only 5% of all LS cases (Conyers et al., 2011). Like WD/DDLS, PLS is a complex karyotype malignancy. Unlike the lower grade tumors, PLS are highly metastatic and do not contain the chromosome 12q13-15 amplification characteristic of DDLS. Thus far, no PLS tested in our hands have shown telomerase activity, using the stringent criteria of not only absence of enzymatic activity using TRAP but also absence of hTERT expression. Using the presence of APBs as a marker for ALT activation, we have found that PLS exclusively use ALT for telomere maintenance or fall in the category of tumors without evidence of either pathway. Given the advanced nature of PLS, their high likelihood to metastasize relative to other types of liposarcoma, and poor prognosis for patients (Guillou & Aurias, 2010), it is likely that these tumors have active telomere maintenance even in the absence of APBs. However, the rarity of PLS has limited the ability to test this hypothesis as most tumors are only available as archival formalin-fixed, paraffin-embedded samples, which will not provide DNA of sufficient size to allow testing for microsatellite instability. Archival samples are also not amenable to analysis for T-SCE, which requires hemi-substitution of the DNA molecule with BrdU and therefore dividing cells. Additional markers of ALT activation/utilization await a better understanding of the various recombination-based pathways utilized for telomere maintenance.

4.1 Genome instability and TMM

Telomeres serve the essential function of providing stability to the ends of linear chromosomes. The cyclical behavior of a single marked telomere in ALT cells (gradual shortening over time in culture, punctuated by rapid increases in length and resumption of telomere attrition) suggests that ALT may act after telomeres reach a critically short length. Thus, it is possible that a steady state level of compromised telomere function might be a feature of cells that utilize ALT for telomere maintenance. Consistent with this possibility, a number of chromosome ends in any given metaphase cell of ALT-positive cell lines do not contain detectable telomeric DNA when analyzed by FISH (Cerone et al., 2001; Perrem et al., 2001). Furthermore, comparison of osteosarcoma-derived cell lines that used either ALT or telomerase for telomere maintenance, using both telomere and multiplex fluorescence in-situ hybridization (FISH), revealed telomere length heterogeneity and increased chromosomal rearrangements in ALT-positive cell lines compared to telomerase-positive cell lines (Scheel et al., 2001). One phenotype exhibited by cells that have lost telomere end-protection function is the end-to-end fusion of chromosomes (Counter et al., 1992; van Steensel et al., 1998). During anaphase, these fusions are manifested as bridges of unresolved DNA between the separating daughter nuclei. Although such bridges can also arise through telomere independent mechanisms, an increase in anaphase bridges is characteristic of the loss of telomere capping function (Blasco et al., 1997; van Steensel et al., 1998). It is noteworthy that ALT-positive sarcomas that were identified in archival sections by virtue of having APBs are reported to have higher levels of genome instability as measured by anaphase bridge index (Montgomery et al., 2004). These tumors also tended to have a complex karyotype. In contrast, tumors with translocations were predominantly non-ALT (i.e., APB negative) and had lower instability.

As discussed above, shortening of telomeres leads to DNA damage and fusion-bridge-break cycles that result in increased genome instability in cancer cells with compromised DNA damage response. We previously reported that tumors using ALT for telomere maintenance have, on average, higher levels of genome instability than those using telomerase, and that tumors with any TMM active have, on average, higher genome instability than those falling in the category without evidence of either telomerase or ALT (Johnson et al., 2007). Genome instability in this study was defined as the percentage of SNPs deviating from diploid copy number. Intriguingly, genome instability was also increased in peritelomeric regions in ALT tumors, i.e., within 200 kb of the most telomeric SNP. These results are consistent with many tumors passing through telomere crisis prior to activation of a TMM.

We have re-evaluated our conclusions regarding genome instability as a function of TMM in the light of our recent realization of histological bias in TMM. Of the 32 tumors included in the study, 9 used ALT, 6 used telomerase, 1 used both ALT and telomerase, and 16 did not show characteristics of either mechanism. Within each category, tumors are distributed among multiple histological types, minimizing the effect of histology. Thus, it is likely that the differences observed in genome instability between ALT and TEL occur despite differences in histological bias rather than because of it. The more uniform telomere length and DNA damage protection conferred by telomerase may help control genome instability in telomerase-positive tumors.

4.2 TMM and survival

Previous work has shown a link between ALT activation and decreased survival in liposarcomas (Costa et al., 2006). The authors of this study did consider the potential contribution of histological type to this result, and concluded that the survival decrease associated with ALT was significant even when tumor grade, location, and histotype were taken into account. It is unclear from the methods in the paper how these factors were accounted for in the statistics. What is clear is that approximately two thirds (20/33) of the ALT-positive tumors are DDLS/other (potentially PLS), and greater than two thirds (27/34) of the telomerase-positive tumors are MYX/RC. Thus, this tumor set contains a histological bias. The authors do note that histology still needs to be considered when interpreting their multivariable analysis given the obvious bias. Further, they comment that the reduced prognostic value of telomerase-positivity is due to round cell tumors already having poor prognosis. This study, therefore, highlights the need for single histotype (and possibly even single-grade) data for survival.

In light of the discussion above regarding differences in characteristics of ALT-positive cell lines, it is important to note that Costa *et al.* defined tumors with 0.5% of nuclei containing APBs as ALT-positive. This is a fairly relaxed definition as co-localization of telomeric components with PML nuclear bodies is assayed by immunofluorescence and there is a possibility that signals will overlap by chance. We define ALT-positive as tumors in which at least 35% of the nuclei exhibit co-localization of telomeric components and PML nuclear bodies. This criterion is likely overly stringent and will exclude some ALT-positive tumors. Some of the differences may be resolved if clear criteria could be established to ensure a rigorous and consistent definition for APB-positive (and therefore ALT-positive) cells.

We recently performed a new analysis of the relationship between histotype, TMM, and survival, using 52 tumors from complex karyotype liposarcomas (WDLS, DDLS, PLS). Our analysis did not include any myxoid/round cell tumors, which comprised about a third of the samples in the earlier work. Consistent with the previous study, tumors that had activated a telomere maintenance mechanism were associated with poorer survival, but the survival difference between ALT and telomerase tumors was not significant (p=0.06). However, as the majority of tumors with a detectable TMM are higher grade, i.e., DDLS and PLS, it is possible that the difference in survival observed between TMM-positive and TMM-negative tumors reflects differences in tumor grade rather than an independent marker of patient prognosis. Within DD-LS, which use both TMMs with similar, high frequency, there was no survival difference associated with TMM (p = 0.64). Thus, it is possible that the apparent poorer prognosis for ALT seen in the larger population is biased by higher grade pleomorphic tumors that contribute only to the ALT survival data.

4.3 Genetic characterization of ALT versus telomerase-positive tumors

It has been reported that the hTERT promoter is repressed in mesenchymal stem cells (Zimmermann et al., 2003). In cell based studies, epigenetic silencing of hTERT expression has also been documented (Serakinci et al., 2006). Thus, it is possible that the increased use of ALT in mesenchymal tumors is a result of tight repression of hTERT expression in this lineage.

The observation of TMM-based differences in survival suggested that fundamental genetic differences might be present between telomerase-positive and ALT-positive tumors. In a genome-wide screen of liposarcomas, we identified deletion of Chr 1q32.4-44 as an ALT associated genetic alteration (Johnson et al., 2007). This deletion differentiates between telomerase positive and ALT-positive DDLS. It is also present in ALT-positive (i.e. APB-positive) PLS. This is a large deletion containing many genes that might be implicated in tumorigenesis. When prioritized on the basis of known biological activity, SMYD3 stands out. SMYD3 is a methyltransferase that modifies histone H3 on lysine 4 (H3K4) (Hamamoto et al., 2004). Methylation of H3K4 is found at actively transcribed regions in the genome (Eissenberg & Shilatifard, 2010). In fact, this chromatin mark is associated with the 5′ end of transcribed genes. Increased SMYD3 expression is associated with advanced cancers while reducing SMYD3 levels inhibits cancer cell growth and promotes apoptosis *in vitro* (Chen et al., 2007; Hamamoto et al., 2004; Hamamoto et al., 2006). Comparion of the expression profiles of cells with forced SMYD3 expression to cells with unaltered SMYD3 levels found alterations consistent with tumor progression, including activation of NF-kB pathway genes (Yamamoto et al., 2011). SMYD3 has recently been reported to be important for epigenetic modification of the hTERT promoter resulting in transcription of this locus (Liu et al., 2007). Importantly, over-expression of SMYD3 in both primary human fibroblasts and ALT-positive Saos-2 cells resulted in telomerase expression while siRNA-mediated knockdown led to inhibition of hTERT gene expression. However, hTERT expression does not necessarily lead to enzymatic activity capable of stabilizing telomeric repeats because, as discussed above, both telomerase activity and access to telomeres are regulated at multiple levels. In addition, ectopic SMYD3 expression likely affected multiple sites within the genome. Finally, SMYD3 expression in tumors utilizing different TMMs was not assessed. Thus, the relevance of SMYD3 deletion to ALT utilization in human tumors is not yet established.

Levels of H3K4 methylation at mammalian telomeres have not been determined. However, studies in yeast suggest that loss of H3K4 methylation is an intermediate step in assembly of silent chromatin. Telomeres are now known to be sites of active transcription and SMYD3 is located in a region often deleted in ALT-positive, but not telomerase-positive, liposarcomas. Decreased H3K4 methylation at ALT telomeres would be predicted to increase heterochromatin marks resulting in decreased TERRA expression. However, ALT-positive cells show increased TERRA levels, and increased heterochromatin would be expected to decrease telomeric recombination, the hallmark of telomere maintenance in ALT. Further experimentation will be required to resolve the apparent paradoxes concerning the role of H3K4 methylation in telomere maintenance.

Previous studies of telomere maintenance in liposarcomas have primarily grouped them as a single malignancy rather than separating them into histological subtypes. The histological bias in telomere maintenance mechanism, as described above, had not been fully realized, but inevitably created a strong histotype bias when separating tumors on the basis of TMM alone. The importance of this bias was highlighted by a recent publication reporting a gene expression signature distinguishing between tumors and cell lines using ALT and telomerase (Lafferty-Whyte et al., 2009). In that study, the authors combined expression data from cell lines and tumors to identify 297 genes that were differentially expressed between ALT and telomerase. When we applied this signature to an independent set of tumors, we found that our samples clustered not on the basis of TMM but rather by histological subtype (Doyle et al., 2011). A closer analysis of the samples used to generate the published gene signature revealed that the cell lines used for the telomerase cohort were primarily of epithelial origin and tumors were primarily MYX LS. In contrast, cell lines used for the ALT cohort were primarily of mesenchymal origin and tumors were primarily DDLS. Thus, the reported cell line signature contained a strong epithelial versus mesenchymal component, while the tumor signature was heavily influenced by histological type. Even when we applied this published signature within a single histological subtype, DDLS, it failed to discriminate tumors on the basis of TMM. This suggests that expression differences between ALT-positive and telomerase-positive tumors are subtle, if present at all.

4.4 TMM and drug sensitivity

A number of studies have established that inhibition of telomerase and/or compromising telomere integrity increase the chemosensitivity of cells. Telomerase-deficient mice exhibit an increased sensitivity to DNA damaging agents that is correlated with the level of telomere dysfunction (Lee et al., 2001). Because telomere dysfunction leads to widespread genome instability, it was proposed that the increased chemosensitivity is a consequence of the underlying increase in genome instability. Indeed, reconstitution of telomerase in this system resulted in genome stabilization and an increased resistance to DNA damaging agents. Experiments carried out using human cell lines have also established an increased sensitivity to DNA damaging agents following inhibition of telomerase (Cerone et al., 2006a, b; Saretzki, 2003). Furthermore, when telomere integrity is compromised by expressing a mutant template RNA that results in repeats unable to recruit the shelterin complex, this also results in increased sensitivity to DNA damage (Cerone et al., 2006a). Increased drug sensitivity may occur before detectable telomere shortening (Masutomi et al., 2005), raising the possibility that telomerase may provide a protective function independent of its role in maintaining telomeric DNA arrays (Martinez & Blasco, 2011). For example, telomerase may contribute to telomere capping function thereby enhancing telomere stability. Recent work has implicated telomerase in modulating the cellular response to DNA damage (Masutomi et al., 2005). In this study, reducing telomerase in primary human cells blocked the DNA damage response, thereby rendering cells more sensitive to damage. Exogenous expression of mutant hTERT alleles with reduced affinity for telomeric DNA rescued the DNA damage response as long as the introduced allele retained catalytic activity. These data suggest that telomerase may contribute to the cellular DNA damage response.

Drugs that target telomerase are increasingly used in cancer therapy with great success (Gilley et al., 2005). By reducing telomerase activity, treatment produces shorter telomeres and results in apoptosis and tumor shrinkage. In addition, telomerase inhibition increases the sensitivity of the cells to other chemotherapeutic agents, either directly through telomerase inhibition, as seen with imatinib (Deville et al., 2011), or indirectly via telomere shortening, as seen with cisplatin (Uziel et al., 2010). Both mechanisms may depend on the intersection of telomere maintenance and DNA repair. Thus ALT-positive tumors may be more sensitive than telomerase-positive tumors to DNA-damaging chemotherapies, as they possess higher levels of genome instability and lack the anti-apoptotic activity and DNA-damage protection of telomerase. Alternatively, ALT cells may be more resistant to DNA damage as they are able to form clinically significant tumors in a background of high genome instability. ALT cells, due to the lack of active telomerase, are expected to be entirely refractory to treatment by telomerase inhibitors. The association between telomere integrity and sensitivity to DNA damaging chemotherapeutic agents, together with the evidence implicating telomerase in the cellular response to DNA damage, is consistent with the possibility that TMM may be predictive of tumor response to chemotherapy.

Current treatments for liposarcomas act through specific over-expressed proteins; for example, doxorubicin response correlates with levels of topo2a (Mitchell et al., 2010), and nutlin acts as an antagonist to MDM2, a protein highly overexpressed in de-differentiated liposarcomas (Muller et al., 2007; Singer et al., 2007). Trabectidin has enhanced activity in myxoid/round cell liposarcomas due to the fusion protein (FUS/CHOP) characteristic to these malignancies (Conyers et al., 2011). These current treatments are thus expected to be independent of TMM. Although studies to date have failed to identify an ALT-specific expression profile, we expect that future studies will identify molecular targets specific to ALT that will enable more directed treatments. We expect that future treatments will be able to leverage knowledge about TMM for improved patient outcome.

5. Conclusions

Cancer treatment is steadily moving forward into the exciting realm of personalized medicine, targeting unique characteristics of each patient's disease for improved efficacy. Identification of the TMM active in a particular tumor provides a path to this personalization, indicating the potential benefit, or lack thereof, for telomerase inhibitors and DNA damage-inducing agents. Continuing research into the molecular mechanisms of ALT, accounting for inherent histological biases within liposarcoma, will identify molecular pathways for ALT-specific anti-cancer treatment that will increase value of TMM information in designing patient treatment.

6. References

Abreu, E., Aritonovska, E., Reichenbach, P., Cristofari, G., Culp, B., Terns, R.M., Lingner, J., & Terns, M.P. (2010). TIN2-tethered TPP1 recruits human telomerase to telomeres in vivo. Mol Cell Biol *30*, 2971-2982.

Allsopp, R.C., Cheshier, S., & Weissman, I.L. (2001). Telomere shortening accompanies increased cell cycle activity during serial transplantation of hematopoietic stem cells. J Exp Med *193*, 917-924.

Artandi, S.E., & DePinho, R.A. (2010). Telomeres and telomerase in cancer. Carcinogenesis *31*, 9-18.

Benetti, R., Garcia-Cao, M., & Blasco, M.A. (2007). Telomere length regulates the epigenetic status of mammalian telomeres and subtelomeres. Nat Genet *39*, 243-250.

Berardinelli, F., Antoccia, A., Cherubini, R., De Nadal, V., Gerardi, S., Cirrone, G.A., Tanzarella, C., & Sgura, A. (2010). Transient activation of the ALT pathway in human primary fibroblasts exposed to high-LET radiation. Radiat Res *174*, 539-549.

Bilaud, T., Brun, C., Ancelin, K., Koering, C.E., Laroche, T., & Gilson, E. (1997). Telomeric localization of TRF2, a novel human telobox protein. Nat Genet *17*, 236-239.

Blasco, M.A., Lee, H.W., Hande, M.P., Samper, E., Lansdorp, P.M., DePinho, R.A., & Greider, C.W. (1997). Telomere shortening and tumor formation by mouse cells lacking telomerase RNA. Cell *91*, 25-34.

Bodnar, A.G., Ouellette, M., Frolkis, M., Holt, S.E., Chiu, C.P., Morin, G.B., Harley, C.B., Shay, J.W., Lichtsteiner, S., & Wright, W.E. (1998). Extension of life-span by introduction of telomerase into normal human cells. Science *279*, 349-352.

Broccoli, D., Smogorzewska, A., Chong, L., & de Lange, T. (1997). Human telomeres contain two distinct Myb-related proteins, TRF1 and TRF2. Nat Genet *17*, 231-235.

Brouwer, A.K., Schimmel, J., Wiegant, J.C., Vertegaal, A.C., Tanke, H.J., & Dirks, R.W. (2009). Telomeric DNA mediates de novo PML body formation. Mol Biol Cell *20*, 4804-4815.

Bryan, T.M., Englezou, A., Dalla-Pozza, L., Dunham, M.A., & Reddel, R.R. (1997). Evidence for an alternative mechanism for maintaining telomere length in human tumors and tumor-derived cell lines. Nat Med *3*, 1271-1274.

Bryan, T.M., Englezou, A., Gupta, J., Bacchetti, S., & Reddel, R.R. (1995). Telomere elongation in immortal human cells without detectable telomerase activity. EMBO J *14*, 4240-4248.

Caslini, C., Connelly, J.A., Serna, A., Broccoli, D., & Hess, J.L. (2009). MLL associates with telomeres and regulates telomeric repeat-containing RNA transcription. Mol Cell Biol *29*, 4519-4526.

Cerone, M.A., Londono-Vallejo, J.A., & Autexier, C. (2006a). Mutated telomeres sensitize tumor cells to anticancer drugs independently of telomere shortening and mechanisms of telomere maintenance. Oncogene *25*, 7411-7420.

Cerone, M.A., Londono-Vallejo, J.A., & Autexier, C. (2006b). Telomerase inhibition enhances the response to anticancer drug treatment in human breast cancer cells. Mol Cancer Ther *5*, 1669-1675.

Cerone, M.A., Londono-Vallejo, J.A., & Bacchetti, S. (2001). Telomere maintenance by telomerase and by recombination can coexist in human cells. Hum Mol Genet *10*, 1945-1952.

Cesare, A.J., & Reddel, R.R. (2010). Alternative lengthening of telomeres: models, mechanisms and implications. Nat Rev Genet *11*, 319-330.

Chang, S., Khoo, C.M., Naylor, M.L., Maser, R.S., & DePinho, R.A. (2003). Telomere-based crisis: functional differences between telomerase activation and ALT in tumor progression. Genes Dev *17*, 88-100.

Chen, L.B., Xu, J.Y., Yang, Z., & Wang, G.B. (2007). Silencing SMYD3 in hepatoma demethylates RIZI promoter induces apoptosis and inhibits cell proliferation and migration. World J Gastroenterol *13*, 5718-5724.

Chin, K., de Solorzano, C.O., Knowles, D., Jones, A., Chou, W., Rodriguez, E.G., Kuo, W.L., Ljung, B.M., Chew, K., Myambo, K., *et al.* (2004). In situ analyses of genome instability in breast cancer. Nat Genet *36*, 984-988.

Conyers, R., Young, S., & Thomas, D.M. (2011). Liposarcoma: molecular genetics and therapeutics. Sarcoma *2011*, 483154.

Costa, A., Daidone, M.G., Daprai, L., Villa, R., Cantu, S., Pilotti, S., Mariani, L., Gronchi, A., Henson, J.D., Reddel, R.R., *et al.* (2006). Telomere maintenance mechanisms in liposarcomas: association with histologic subtypes and disease progression. Cancer Res *66*, 8918-8924.

Counter, C.M., Avilion, A.A., LeFeuvre, C.E., Stewart, N.G., Greider, C.W., Harley, C.B., & Bacchetti, S. (1992). Telomere shortening associated with chromosome instability is arrested in immortal cells which express telomerase activity. EMBO J *11*, 1921-1929.

Counter, C.M., Hahn, W.C., Wei, W., Caddle, S.D., Beijersbergen, R.L., Lansdorp, P.M., Sedivy, J.M., & Weinberg, R.A. (1998). Dissociation among in vitro telomerase activity, telomere maintenance, and cellular immortalization. Proc Natl Acad Sci U S A *95*, 14723-14728.

de Lange, T. (2005). Shelterin: the protein complex that shapes and safeguards human telomeres. Genes Dev *19*, 2100-2110.

Deng, Z., Norseen, J., Wiedmer, A., Riethman, H., & Lieberman, P.M. (2009). TERRA RNA binding to TRF2 facilitates heterochromatin formation and ORC recruitment at telomeres. Mol Cell *35*, 403-413.

Deville, L., Hillion, J., Pendino, F., Samy, M., Nguyen, E., & Segal-Bendirdjian, E. (2011). hTERT Promotes Imatinib Resistance in Chronic Myeloid Leukemia Cells: Therapeutic Implications. Mol Cancer Ther *10*, 711-719.

Draskovic, I., Arnoult, N., Steiner, V., Bacchetti, S., Lomonte, P., & Londono-Vallejo, A. (2009). Probing PML body function in ALT cells reveals spatiotemporal requirements for telomere recombination. Proc Natl Acad Sci U S A *106*, 15726-15731.

Eissenberg, J.C., & Shilatifard, A. (2010). Histone H3 lysine 4 (H3K4) methylation in development and differentiation. Dev Biol *339*, 240-249.

Fasching, C.L., Bower, K., & Reddel, R.R. (2005). Telomerase-independent telomere length maintenance in the absence of alternative lengthening of telomeres-associated promyelocytic leukemia bodies. Cancer Res *65*, 2722-2729.

Garcia-Cao, M., O'Sullivan, R., Peters, A.H., Jenuwein, T., & Blasco, M.A. (2004). Epigenetic regulation of telomere length in mammalian cells by the Suv39h1 and Suv39h2 histone methyltransferases. Nat Genet *36*, 94-99.

Gilley, D., Tanaka, H., & Herbert, B.S. (2005). Telomere dysfunction in aging and cancer. Int J Biochem Cell Biol *37*, 1000-1013.

Gonzalo, S., Jaco, I., Fraga, M.F., Chen, T., Li, E., Esteller, M., & Blasco, M.A. (2006). DNA methyltransferases control telomere length and telomere recombination in mammalian cells. Nat Cell Biol *8*, 416-424.

Greider, C.W. (1999). Telomeres do D-loop-T-loop. Cell *97*, 419-422.

Greider, C.W., & Blackburn, E.H. (1987). The telomere terminal transferase of Tetrahymena is a ribonucleoprotein enzyme with two kinds of primer specificity. Cell *51*, 887-898.

Grobelny, J.V., Godwin, A.K., & Broccoli, D. (2000). ALT-associated PML bodies are present in viable cells and are enriched in cells in the G2/M phase of the cell cycle. Journal of Cell Science *113*, 4577-4585.

Grobelny, J.V., Kulp-McEliece, M., & Broccoli, D. (2001). Effects of reconstitution of telomerase activity on telomere maintenance by the alternative lengthening of telomeres (ALT) pathway. Hum Mol Genet *10*, 1953-1961.

Guillou, L., & Aurias, A. (2010). Soft tissue sarcomas with complex genomic profiles. Virchows Arch *456*, 201-217.

Hahn, W.C., Counter, C.M., Lundberg, A.S., Beijersbergen, R.L., Brooks, M.W., & Weinberg, R.A. (1999). Creation of human tumour cells with defined genetic elements. Nature *400*, 464-468.

Hakin-Smith, V., Jellinek, D.A., Levy, D., Carroll, T., Teo, M., Timperley, W.R., McKay, M.J., Reddel, R.R., & Royds, J.A. (2003). Alternative lengthening of telomeres and survival in patients with glioblastoma multiforme. Lancet *361*, 836-838.

Hamamoto, R., Furukawa, Y., Morita, M., Iimura, Y., Silva, F.P., Li, M., Yagyu, R., & Nakamura, Y. (2004). SMYD3 encodes a histone methyltransferase involved in the proliferation of cancer cells. Nat Cell Biol *6*, 731-740.

Hamamoto, R., Silva, F.P., Tsuge, M., Nishidate, T., Katagiri, T., Nakamura, Y., & Furukawa, Y. (2006). Enhanced SMYD3 expression is essential for the growth of breast cancer cells. Cancer Sci *97*, 113-118.

Henson, J.D., Cao, Y., Huschtscha, L.I., Chang, A.C., Au, A.Y., Pickett, H.A., & Reddel, R.R. (2009). DNA C-circles are specific and quantifiable markers of alternative-lengthening-of-telomeres activity. Nat Biotechnol *27*, 1181-1185.

Henson, J.D., & Reddel, R.R. (2010). Assaying and investigating Alternative Lengthening of Telomeres activity in human cells and cancers. FEBS Lett *584*, 3800-3811.

Hodes, R.J., Hathcock, K.S., & Weng, N.P. (2002). Telomeres in T and B cells. Nat Rev Immunol *2*, 699-706.

Jemal, A., Siegel, R., Xu, J., & Ward, E. (2010). Cancer statistics, 2010. CA Cancer J Clin *60*, 277-300.

Jeyapalan, J.N., Mendez-Bermudez, A., Zaffaroni, N., Dubrova, Y.E., & Royle, N.J. (2008). Evidence for alternative lengthening of telomeres in liposarcomas in the absence of ALT-associated PML bodies. Int J Cancer *122*, 2414-2421.

Jeyapalan, J.N., Varley, H., Foxon, J.L., Pollock, R.E., Jeffreys, A.J., Henson, J.D., Reddel, R.R., & Royle, N.J. (2005). Activation of the ALT pathway for telomere maintenance can affect other sequences in the human genome. Hum Mol Genet *14*, 1785-1794.

Jiang, W.Q., Zhong, Z.H., Henson, J.D., Neumann, A.A., Chang, A.C., & Reddel, R.R. (2005). Suppression of alternative lengthening of telomeres by Sp100-mediated sequestration of the MRE11/RAD50/NBS1 complex. Mol Cell Biol *25*, 2708-2721.

Jiang, W.Q., Zhong, Z.H., Nguyen, A., Henson, J.D., Toouli, C.D., Braithwaite, A.W., & Reddel, R.R. (2009). Induction of alternative lengthening of telomeres-associated PML bodies by p53/p21 requires HP1 proteins. J Cell Biol *185*, 797-810.

Johnson, J.E., & Broccoli, D. (2007). Telomere maintenance in sarcomas. Curr Opin Oncol *19*, 377-382.

Johnson, J.E., Gettings, E.J., Schwalm, J., Pei, J., Testa, J.R., Litwin, S., von Mehren, M., & Broccoli, D. (2007). Whole-genome profiling in liposarcomas reveals genetic alterations common to specific telomere maintenance mechanisms. Cancer Res *67*, 9221-9228.

Johnson, J.E., Varkonyi, R.J., Schwalm, J., Cragle, R., Klein-Szanto, A., Patchefsky, A., Cukierman, E., von Mehren, M., & Broccoli, D. (2005). Multiple mechanisms of telomere maintenance exist in liposarcomas. Clin Cancer Res *11*, 5347-5355.

Kim, N.W., Piatyszek, M.A., Prowse, K.R., Harley, C.B., West, M.D., Ho, P.L., Coviello, G.M., Wright, W.E., Weinrich, S.L., & Shay, J.W. (1994). Specific association of human telomerase activity with immortal cells and cancer. Science *266*, 2011-2015.

Kim, S.H., Kaminker, P., & Campisi, J. (1999). TIN2, a new regulator of telomere length in human cells. Nat Genet *23*, 405-412.

Koering, C.E., Pollice, A., Zibella, M.P., Bauwens, S., Puisieux, A., Brunori, M., Brun, C., Martins, L., Sabatier, L., Pulitzer, J.F., *et al.* (2002). Human telomeric position effect is determined by chromosomal context and telomeric chromatin integrity. EMBO Rep *3*, 1055-1061.

Lafferty-Whyte, K., Cairney, C.J., Will, M.B., Serakinci, N., Daidone, M.G., Zaffaroni, N., Bilsland, A., & Keith, W.N. (2009). A gene expression signature classifying telomerase and ALT immortalization reveals an hTERT regulatory network and suggests a mesenchymal stem cell origin for ALT. Oncogene *28*, 3765-3774.

Lee, K.H., Rudolph, K.L., Ju, Y.J., Greenberg, R.A., Cannizzaro, L., Chin, L., Weiler, S.R., & DePinho, R.A. (2001). Telomere dysfunction alters the chemotherapeutic profile of transformed cells. Proc Natl Acad Sci U S A *98*, 3381-3386.

Lei, M., Baumann, P., & Cech, T.R. (2002). Cooperative binding of single-stranded telomeric DNA by the Pot1 protein of Schizosaccharomyces pombe. Biochemistry *41*, 14560-14568.

Lewis, N.L., Mullaney, M., Mangan, K.F., Klumpp, T., Rogatko, A., & Broccoli, D. (2004). Measurable immune dysfunction and telomere attrition in long-term allogeneic transplant recipients. Bone Marrow Transplant *33*, 71-78.

Liu, C., Fang, X., Ge, Z., Jalink, M., Kyo, S., Bjorkholm, M., Gruber, A., Sjoberg, J., & Xu, D. (2007). The telomerase reverse transcriptase (hTERT) gene is a direct target of the histone methyltransferase SMYD3. Cancer Res *67*, 2626-2631.

Londono-Vallejo, J.A., Der-Sarkissian, H., Cazes, L., Bacchetti, S., & Reddel, R.R. (2004). Alternative lengthening of telomeres is characterized by high rates of telomeric exchange. Cancer Res *64*, 2324-2327.

Luke, B., & Lingner, J. (2009). TERRA: telomeric repeat-containing RNA. EMBO J *28*, 2503-2510.

Martinez, P., & Blasco, M.A. (2011). Telomeric and extra-telomeric roles for telomerase and the telomere-binding proteins. Nat Rev Cancer *11*, 161-176.

Masutomi, K., Possemato, R., Wong, J.M., Currier, J.L., Tothova, Z., Manola, J.B., Ganesan, S., Lansdorp, P.M., Collins, K., & Hahn, W.C. (2005). The telomerase reverse transcriptase regulates chromatin state and DNA damage responses. Proc Natl Acad Sci U S A *102*, 8222-8227.

Matsuo, T., Shay, J.W., Wright, W.E., Hiyama, E., Shimose, S., Kubo, T., Sugita, T., Yasunaga, Y., & Ochi, M. (2009). Telomere-maintenance mechanisms in soft-tissue malignant fibrous histiocytomas. J Bone Joint Surg Am *91*, 928-937.

Mitchell, M.A., Johnson, J.E., Pascarelli, K., Beeharry, N., Chiourea, M., Gagos, S., Lev, D., von Mehren, M., Kipling, D., & Broccoli, D. (2010). Doxorubicin resistance in a novel in vitro model of human pleomorphic liposarcoma associated with alternative lengthening of telomeres. Mol Cancer Ther *9*, 682-692.

Montgomery, E., Argani, P., Hicks, J.L., DeMarzo, A.M., & Meeker, A.K. (2004). Telomere lengths of translocation-associated and nontranslocation-associated sarcomas differ dramatically. Am J Pathol *164*, 1523-1529.

Muller, C.R., Paulsen, E.B., Noordhuis, P., Pedeutour, F., Saeter, G., & Myklebost, O. (2007). Potential for treatment of liposarcomas with the MDM2 antagonist Nutlin-3A. Int J Cancer *121*, 199-205.

Ng, L.J., Cropley, J.E., Pickett, H.A., Reddel, R.R., & Suter, C.M. (2009). Telomerase activity is associated with an increase in DNA methylation at the proximal subtelomere and a reduction in telomeric transcription. Nucleic Acids Res *37*, 1152-1159.

O'Connor, M.S., Safari, A., Xin, H., Liu, D., & Songyang, Z. (2006). A critical role for TPP1 and TIN2 interaction in high-order telomeric complex assembly. Proc Natl Acad Sci U S A *103*, 11874-11879.

Opitz, O.G., Suliman, Y., Hahn, W.C., Harada, H., Blum, H.E., & Rustgi, A.K. (2001). Cyclin D1 overexpression and p53 inactivation immortalize primary oral keratinocytes by a telomerase-independent mechanism. J Clin Invest *108*, 725-732.

Osterhage, J.L., & Friedman, K.L. (2009). Chromosome end maintenance by telomerase. J Biol Chem *284*, 16061-16065.

Perez-Losada, J., Pintado, B., Gutierrez-Adan, A., Flores, T., Banares-Gonzalez, B., del Campo, J.C., Martin-Martin, J.F., Battaner, E., & Sanchez-Garcia, I. (2000). The chimeric FUS/TLS-CHOP fusion protein specifically induces liposarcomas in transgenic mice. Oncogene *19*, 2413-2422.

Perrem, K., Colgin, L.M., Neumann, A.A., Yeager, T.R., & Reddel, R.R. (2001). Coexistence of Alternative Lengthening of Telomeres and telomerase in hTERT-transfected GM847 cells. Molecular and Cellular Biology *21*, 3862-3875.

Razak, Z.R., Varkonyi, R.J., Kulp-McEliece, M., Caslini, C., Testa, J.R., Murphy, M.E., & Broccoli, D. (2004). p53 differentially inhibits cell growth depending on the mechanism of telomere maintenance. Mol Cell Biol *24*, 5967-5977.

Reddel, R.R. (2000). The role of senescence and immortalization in carcinogenesis. Carcinogenesis *21*, 477-484.

Rieker, R.J., Weitz, J., Lehner, B., Egerer, G., Mueller, A., Kasper, B., Schirmacher, P., Joos, S., & Mechtersheimer, G. (2010). Genomic profiling reveals subsets of dedifferentiated liposarcoma to follow separate molecular pathways. Virchows Arch *456*, 277-285.

Riggi, N., Cironi, L., Provero, P., Suva, M.L., Stehle, J.C., Baumer, K., Guillou, L., & Stamenkovic, I. (2006). Expression of the FUS-CHOP fusion protein in primary mesenchymal progenitor cells gives rise to a model of myxoid liposarcoma. Cancer Res *66*, 7016-7023.

Rogan, E.M., Bryan, T.M., Hukku, B., Maclean, K., Chang, A.C., Moy, E.L., Englezou, A., Warneford, S.G., Dalla-Pozza, L., & Reddel, R.R. (1995). Alterations in p53 and p16INK4 expression and telomere length during spontaneous immortalization of Li-Fraumeni syndrome fibroblasts. Mol Cell Biol *15*, 4745-4753.

Saretzki, G. (2003). Telomerase inhibition as cancer therapy. Cancer Lett *194*, 209-219.

Scheel, C., Schaefer, K.L., Jauch, A., Keller, M., Wai, D., Brinkschmidt, C., van Valen, F., Boecker, W., Dockhorn-Dworniczak, B., & Poremba, C. (2001). Alternative lengthening of telomeres is associated with chromosomal instability in osteosarcomas. Oncogene *20*, 3835-3844.

Schwarzbach, M.H., Koesters, R., Germann, A., Mechtersheimer, G., Geisbill, J., Winkler, S., Niedergethmann, M., Ridder, R., Buechler, M.W., von Knebel Doeberitz, M., *et al.* (2004). Comparable transforming capacities and differential gene expression patterns of variant FUS/CHOP fusion transcripts derived from soft tissue liposarcomas. Oncogene *23*, 6798-6805.

Serakinci, N., Hoare, S.F., Kassem, M., Atkinson, S.P., & Keith, W.N. (2006). Telomerase promoter reprogramming and interaction with general transcription factors in the human mesenchymal stem cell. Regen Med *1*, 125-131.

Sfeir, A.J., Shay, J.W., & Wright, W.E. (2005). Fine-tuning the chromosome ends: the last base of human telomeres. Cell Cycle *4*, 1467-1470.

Sharma, G.G., Hwang, K.K., Pandita, R.K., Gupta, A., Dhar, S., Parenteau, J., Agarwal, M., Worman, H.J., Wellinger, R.J., & Pandita, T.K. (2003). Human heterochromatin protein 1 isoforms HP1(Hsalpha) and HP1(Hsbeta) interfere with hTERT-telomere interactions and correlate with changes in cell growth and response to ionizing radiation. Mol Cell Biol *23*, 8363-8376.

Singer, S., Socci, N.D., Ambrosini, G., Sambol, E., Decarolis, P., Wu, Y., O'Connor, R., Maki, R., Viale, A., Sander, C., *et al.* (2007). Gene expression profiling of liposarcoma identifies distinct biological types/subtypes and potential therapeutic targets in well-differentiated and dedifferentiated liposarcoma. Cancer Res *67*, 6626-6636.

Slatter, T., Gifford-Garner, J., Wiles, A., Tan, X., Chen, Y.J., MacFarlane, M., Sullivan, M., Royds, J., & Hung, N. (2010). Pilocytic astrocytomas have telomere-associated promyelocytic leukemia bodies without alternatively lengthened telomeres. Am J Pathol *177*, 2694-2700.

Stagno D'Alcontres, M., Mendez-Bermudez, A., Foxon, J.L., Royle, N.J., & Salomoni, P. (2007). Lack of TRF2 in ALT cells causes PML-dependent p53 activation and loss of telomeric DNA. J Cell Biol *179*, 855-867.

Sun, B., Chen, M., Hawks, C.L., & Hornsby, P.J. (2005). Immortal ALT+ human cells do not require telomerase reverse transcriptase for malignant transformation. Cancer Res *65*, 6512-6515.

Tap, W.D., Eilber, F.C., Ginther, C., Dry, S.M., Reese, N., Barzan-Smith, K., Chen, H.W., Wu, H., Eilber, F.R., Slamon, D.J., *et al.* (2011). Evaluation of well-differentiated/de-differentiated liposarcomas by high-resolution oligonucleotide array-based comparative genomic hybridization. Genes Chromosomes Cancer *50*, 95-112.

Tomaska, L., McEachern, M.J., & Nosek, J. (2004). Alternatives to telomerase: keeping linear chromosomes via telomeric circles. FEBS Lett *567*, 142-146.

Ulaner, G.A., Hoffman, A.R., Otero, J., Huang, H.Y., Zhao, Z., Mazumdar, M., Gorlick, R., Meyers, P., Healey, J.H., & Ladanyi, M. (2004). Divergent patterns of telomere maintenance mechanisms among human sarcomas: sharply contrasting prevalence of the alternative lengthening of telomeres mechanism in Ewing's sarcomas and osteosarcomas. Genes Chromosomes Cancer *41*, 155-162.

Ulaner, G.A., Huang, H.Y., Otero, J., Zhao, Z., Ben-Porat, L., Satagopan, J.M., Gorlick, R., Meyers, P., Healey, J.H., Huvos, A.G., *et al.* (2003). Absence of a telomere maintenance mechanism as a favorable prognostic factor in patients with osteosarcoma. Cancer Res *63*, 1759-1763.

Uziel, O., Beery, E., Dronichev, V., Samocha, K., Gryaznov, S., Weiss, L., Slavin, S., Kushnir, M., Nordenberg, Y., Rabinowitz, C., *et al.* (2010). Telomere shortening sensitizes cancer cells to selected cytotoxic agents: in vitro and in vivo studies and putative mechanisms. PLoS One *5*, e9132.

van Steensel, B., Smogorzewska, A., & de Lange, T. (1998). TRF2 protects human telomeres from end-to-end fusions. Cell *92*, 401-413.

Vaziri, H., & Benchimol, S. (1998). Reconstitution of telomerase activity in normal human cells leads to elongation of telomeres and extended replicative life span. Curr Biol *8*, 279-282.

Verdun, R.E., & Karlseder, J. (2006). The DNA damage machinery and homologous recombination pathway act consecutively to protect human telomeres. Cell *127*, 709-720.

Whitehead, J., Pandey, G.K., & Kanduri, C. (2009). Regulation of the mammalian epigenome by long noncoding RNAs. Biochim Biophys Acta *1790*, 936-947.

Yamamoto, K., Ishida, T., Nakano, K., Yamagishi, M., Yamochi, T., Tanaka, Y., Furukawa, Y., Nakamura, Y., & Watanabe, T. (2011). SMYD3 interacts with HTLV-1 Tax and regulates subcellular localization of Tax. Cancer Sci *102*, 260-266.

Yeager, T.R., Neumann, A.A., Englezou, A., Huschtscha, L.I., Noble, J.R., & Reddel, R.R. (1999). Telomerase-negative immortalized human cells contain a novel type of promyelocytic leukemia (PML) body. Cancer Res *59*, 4175-4179.

Zhong, Z., Shiue, L., Kaplan, S., & de Lange, T. (1992). A mammalian factor that binds telomeric TTAGGG repeats in vitro. Mol Cell Biol *12*, 4834-4843.

Zimmermann, S., Voss, M., Kaiser, S., Kapp, U., Waller, C.F., & Martens, U.M. (2003). Lack of telomerase activity in human mesenchymal stem cells. Leukemia *17*, 1146-1149.

Part 2

Diagnosis and Investigations in Soft Tissue Tumors

3

Classification of Soft Tissue Tumors by Machine Learning Algorithms

Jaber Juntu[1], Arthur M. De Schepper[2], Pieter Van Dyck[2], Dirk Van Dyck[1], Jan Gielen[2], Paul M. Parizel[2] and Jan Sijbers[1]

[1]*Universiy of Antwerp, Physics Department, Vision Lab.*
[2] *Dept. of Radiology, Antwerp University Hospital, University of Antwerp*
Belgium

1. Introduction

MR imaging is currently regarded as the standard diagnostic tool for detection and grading of soft tissue tumors (STT) (De Schepper et al. (2005)). Soft tissue is a term describing all the supporting, connecting or tissues surrounding other structures and organs of the body such as fat, muscle, blood vessels, deep skin tissues, nerves and the tissues around joints (synovial tissues). Soft tissue tumors can grow almost anywhere in the human body. Soft tissue sarcomas, which are the malignant type of STT, are grouped together because they share certain microscopic characteristics, have similar symptoms, and are generally treated in similar ways. Radiologists often look for certain features in the MR image to differentiate benign from malignant STT tumors (Juan et al. (2004); Mutlu et al. (2006)). Although the signal characteristics of both benign and malignant tumors frequently overlap, some MR image features are more highly correlated to the benign or the malignant types of STT, see De Schepper et al. (2000) and De Schepper & Bloem (2007). For example, the most commonly used individual parameters for predicting malignancy are the inhomogeneity (texture) and the intensity (gray level) of the MRI signal with different pulse sequences (De Schepper et al. (2005); Hermann et al. (1992)). Inhomogeneity of the tumor region on T1-weighted MR images is a very good indicator of the malignancy of the tumor because 90% of malignant tumors are inhomogeneous and show a disorganized textured pattern of the MRI signal intensity (Weatherall (1995)). This pattern is formed as a result of the losses of tissue structure and the changes of the extracellular matrix (ECM) by cancer. The study by (Hermann et al. (1992)) reported a sensitivity of 72% and specificity of 87% in predicting malignancy based on visual comparison of texture in the tumor regions in T1-MR images. The reason for the large difference between the sensitivity and the specificity in this study is the difficulty of perceiving texture in some of the malignant tumors. The limited ability for human to perceive and discriminate between textures is well known for quite some time (Julesz (1975); Julesz et al. (1973)). Computer aided diagnostic systems can improve the radiologists performance in identifying the pathological type (i.e. benign or malignant) of a soft tissue tumor from MR images (Meinel et al. (2007)). Eventhough visually comparing the textures of benign tumor and malignant tumor sometimes show no difference, the extracted numerical values by texture analysis are quite different. Figure 1 shows subimages of a benign and a malignant tumors and the values of some of the extracted texture features. Such an example shows that texture analysis can be used for obtaining information that is not visible to the human eye. The reader can refer to (Materka & Strzelectky (1998); Tuceryan & Jain (1998); Wagner (1999)) as excellent references to texture analysis.

In the last few years there has been growing interest in the use of machine learning classifiers for analyzing MRI data. The main aim of this chapter is to train and test several machine learning classifiers with texture analysis features extracted from MR images of soft tissue tumors. The present chapter will also serve as an introductory tutorial by providing a systematic procedure to build and evaluate a machine learning classifier that can be used for practical applications. The typical steps to build machine learning classifier consist of feature extraction, feature selection, classifier training and evaluation of the results. Several studies have tackled the problem of texture analysis for discriminating between benign and malignant tumors for specific type of malignancy, for example, the brain (Mahmoud-Ghoneim et al. (2003)) the liver (Jirák et al. (2002)) and the breast (Huang et al. (2006)). However, most papers did not follow the recommended approach for building machine learning systems (for an example see Salzberg (1997)) and left some unanswered questions. This research aims at answering some questions related to the problem of texture analysis of STT, such as the classifiers complexity, the effect of the training data set on the classifier behaviour and the appropriate size of the training data that can be used to train a machine learning classifier and obtain good generalization performance. In the following sections, we will go through the process of building and testing several machine learning classifiers as shown in Fig. 2.

We warn the reader that the training dataset is not meant to train the classifier *per se*, as the name implies, but should be considered as a representative statistical sample from the population of STT. We assume that the training and testing data samples are randomly, identically and independently sampled from the population of STT (i.e, it is an *idd* sample). The process of training and testing the classifier is a sort of statistical parameter estimation problem where in that case the parameter of interest is the error rate of the classifier performance in unseen data. As such, all the experiments in the following sections are in fact to study how the classifier perform in other unseen data from the same STT population. To put a classifier in real practice, the classifier should be trained and tested with several datasets sampled from the same population with the same procedure as outlined in the following sections. Once the classifier evaluation is finished, all the available data can be used to train the final classifier. The classifier should be comprehensively tested based on a prospective study before using the classifier. A shorter preliminary version of this chapter was published in Juntu et al. (2010).

2. Patients data set and the MR images

A large database of multicenter, multimachine MR images was collected by the *University Hospital Antwerp (UZA)* from different radiology centers for the purpose of conducting scientific research. At the start of this study, there was a real concern that texture features could be more sensitive to image variation due to imaging with different MRI systems or changes in MRI acquisition parameters than variation due to changes in texture as a result of pathological changes. However, a recent study by Mayerhoefer et al. (2005), clearly showed that the difference in texture features extracted from MR images obtained with different machine units seems to have only small impact on the results of tissue discrimination. In the present study, a database of T1-MR images of 86 patients having benign soft tissue tumors and 49 patients having malignant tumors were used in this retrospective study. All malignant and benign masses were histologically confirmed. We discarded all MR images that showed severe

(a) ROI from a benign tumor (b) ROI from a malignant tumor

Features	Skewness	Perc 1%	Perc 10%	Perc 50%	s(0,2) SumVariance	s(0,4) Contrast	Horzl_fraction	dgr_LngRemph45	GrSkewness	Teta2	Sigma	WavEnHH_s1
Benign ROI	0.26	106	112	119	9.62	2.94	0.49	4.38	0.90	0.71	0.18	0.10
Malignant ROI	0.21	93	45	51	5.78	2.11	0.58	3.41	0.73	0.54	0.25	0.16

Fig. 1. An example of benign and malignant tumors texture

imaging artifacts or that were corrupted by a high level of bias field inhomogeneity signal. From the tumor regions in the MR images, we cut square subimages of size 50×50 pixels for texture features computation. The physical size of that area is not fixed but it depends on the image acquisition parameters. However, the actual size of that area will not effect the values of the extracted features. To increase the size of the training dataset, we selected several tumor regions from the MR images for every patient. Hence, the total size of the dataset available for training consisted of 253 benign and 428 malignant subimages of size 50×50 pixels each. In order to preserve texture information, we avoid preprocessing the subimages. However, histogram equalization was applied to all the tumor subimages since some texture features such as the first order texture features are sensitive to graylevel variation.

3. Texture computation

Texture can be characterized and described in different ways using various sets and combinations of parameters. Most texture features computation was done using the software package MaZda 3.20 which allows the computation of texture features based on statistical, wavelet filtering, and model-based methods of analyzing texture (Castellano et al. (2004)). We also wrote other Matlab programs to calculate some texture features such as the Haralick's texture features to have a better and fine control of adjusting the parameters that effect the extracted features. To ensure the consistency of the calculated texture feature across all the tumor subimages, we wrote a MaZda macro script that reads the tumor subimages and calculates tumor texture with the same texture analysis parameters setting. The extracted texture features were saved in a text file for feature selection and classification. The following is a short description of the texture features that were computed from the tumor subimages, which are also summarized in Table 1 for easy reference:

- *First order statistics:* extract texture statistics based on a function of a single pixel. The simplest approach is to construct a histogram for the image of interest. The histogram is converted into probability function by dividing the values in the histogram by the total

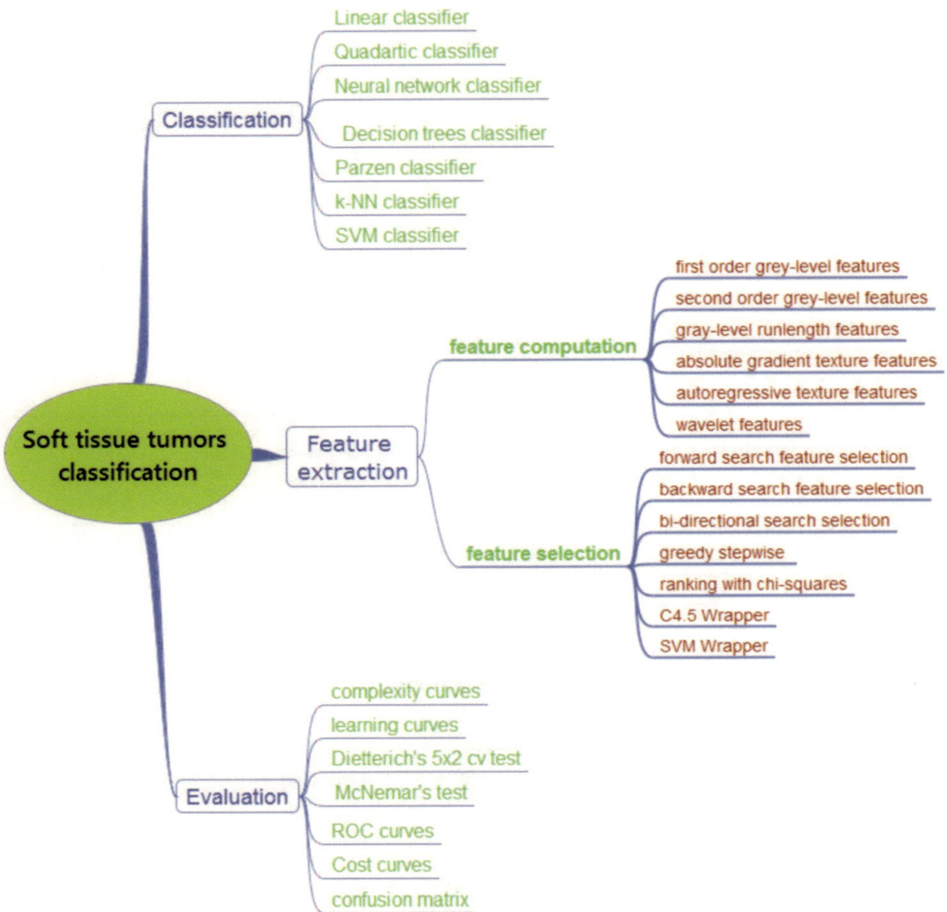

Fig. 2. Block diagram of the chapter

number of pixels in the image. A set of statistical parameters from the probability density function are calculated such as the mean, the variance, the skewness, and the kurtosis.

- *Second order statistics:* the Haralick's texture features and the absolute gradient distribution are used in this study. In this method of texture analysis the correlation between two or more neighborhood pixels is taken into account. Since complex texture patterns are formed by the interaction between more than one pixel, second order statistics might provide extra texture information that can not be extracted based on first order statistics of the texture. The Haralick's texture analysis (Haralick et al. (1973)) is probably the most famous technique of second order texture analysis methods. It is based on the calculation of statistics from a function of two variables that measures the probability of occurrence of a pair of pixels that are separated by d pixels with an angle θ. We calculated 11 different Haralick's features from the co-occurrence matrix. The co-occurence matrix is calculated for every two pixels inclined by an angle θ and separated by a distance d. To take the scaling and rotation of texture into account, we calculated the Haralick's features from the co-occurrence matrices calculated with angles $\{0°, 45°, 90°, 135°\}$ and distances of $\{1, 2, 3, 4, 5\}$ pixels. The absolute gradient texture features are also included to incorporate texture features that are invariant to gray-level scaling caused by bias field inhomogeneity. Every pixel in the image was replaced by the absolute gradient which was calculated from a window of size 3×3 around the pixel by calculating the absolute of the squared summation of the difference between the two pixels above and down the center pixel and the two pixels on the right and left. Doing that for all pixels resulted in a gradient image from which several statistical parameters could be obtained: the mean, the variance, the skewness, and the kurtosis.

- *Higher order statistics:* used to capture texture information which are dependent on the interaction between several neighborhood pixels. We selected two different approaches,
  - the run-length gray-level matrix approach were a consecutive set of pixels with the same gray level value are counted and the result is stored in a 2D matrix indexed by the gray-level value and length of the gray-level run. Several statistics are calculated from the 2D matrix.
  - write a mathematical function or model that describes the texture, for example the autoregressive texture model. The basic idea of autoregressive models for texture is to express a gray level of a pixel as a function of the gray levels of its neighborhood pixels Mao & Jain (1992). The related model parameters for one image are calculated using a least squares technique and are used as texture features. This approach is similar to the Markov random fields.
- *Filtering method:* The image is split into subbands with bandpass filters such as the wavelet transform. The energy of the sub-bands are used as a texture features.

After the texture analysis step, each tumor subimage is encoded by a feature vector as shown in Fig. 3. The texture features are labeled as $\{f_1, f_2, ..., f_{290}\}$ (see Table 1).

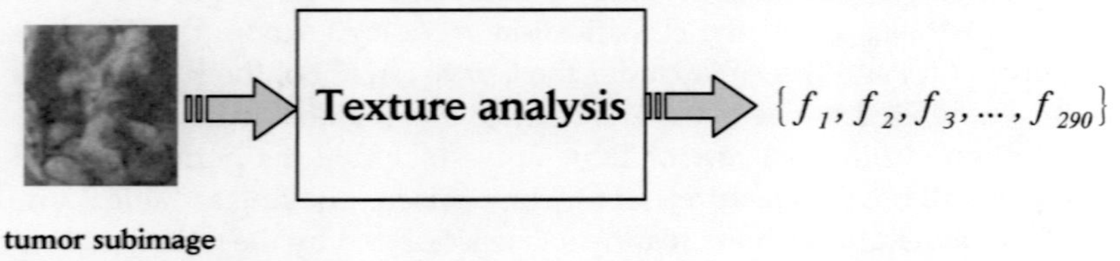

Fig. 3. Texture analysis features

4. Feature selection

Feature selection was used to remove redundant features. This step is very important because it improves the performance of the learning models and reduces the effect of the curse of dimensionality. Feature selection also speeds the learning process and improves the model interpretability. Deciding which feature to keep, because it is relevant, and which one to discard, is largely dependent on the context. To perform an unbiased feature selection, we tested several feature selection techniques. We experimented with the following feature selection methods:

Methods	Calculated parameters
First order: $\{f_1,\ldots,f_{10}\}$	
histogram	mean, minimum, variance, skewness, kurtosis 1%, 10%, 50%, 90% and 99% percentiles.
Second Order: $\{f_{11},\ldots,f_{250}\}$ & $\{f_{271},\ldots,f_{277}\}$	
coocurrence matrix { angles=$\theta = 0°, 45°, 90°, 135°$ and distances=1,2,3,4,5 }	angular second moment, contrast, sum of squares, inverse difference moment, sum average, correlation, entropy, difference variance, difference entropy.
absolute gradient distribution	mean of absolute gradient, variance of absolute gradient skewness of absolute gradient, kurtosis of absolute gradient.
Higher order: $\{f_{251},\ldots,f_{270}\}$ & $\{f_{278},\ldots,f_{282}\}$	
runlength graylevel matrix	short run emphasis moment, long run emphasis moment, run length nonuniformity, fraction of image in run.
autoregressive texture model	$\theta_1, \theta_2, \theta_3, \theta_4, \sigma$.
Filtering technique: $\{f_{283},\ldots,f_{290}\}$	
wavelet	energies of wavelet coefficients of subbands at successive scales.

Table 1. Texture analysis methods used in this study and the corresponding texture features

- *Unsupervised feature selection techniques:* these methods do not use the class labels and the selected features are strongly dependent on the sample distribution of the pixels graylevel values. We selected texture features subsets by forward, backward, bidirectional, and greedy stepwise search methods and two feature ranking methods, namely, the chi-squares statistics and the information gain criteria ranking methods.
- *Supervised selection techniques:* these techniques use class labels for guiding the feature selection process, thus, the selected features are the ones that improve the discrimination between benign and malignant tumors. We used the C4.5 decision tree algorithm and the support vector machines as a wrappers.

Table 2 lists all the feature selection techniques that were tested in this study and their selected subset features. It is not surprising that the 8 feature selection methods selected different features subsets because each one has a different measure for feature relevance. However, feature selection methods that belong to the same group generally selected almost similar features. The selected features subsets were used as an input to a simple Bayes classifier to evaluate the efficacy of the texture features subsets. The results of the classification are listed in Table 2. We also listed the classification accuracy ($Acc\%$), the True Positive (TP), the True Negative (TN) and the Area Under the Curve (AUC) of the ROC. The measure that is generally recommended to use is the AUC, since it is a global measure and insensitive to the data distribution. In the last row of Table 2, we included the performance of the Bayes classifier using the full textures features set for comparison. Looking at Table 2, one can notice that the classification results with the feature subsets selected by the feature ranking methods are worse than classification using the full texture feature since their AUC values are 0.72 and 0.75, respectively, while the full texture features classification has an AUC value of 0.78. The best texture features subset was the one that had the highest AUC value. The texture features subset with the highest AUC is the forward selection method which was used for training and testing the classifiers.

5. The trained classifiers

The main purpose of the training data is to infer a mathematical decision function or an algorithm for making prediction. Thereby, a given training data set is used to optimize the parameters of a machine learning classifier, which then results in a simple mathematical function or expression that can be used for making prediction. If the same classifier is trained

Method	The best selected features	ACC%	TP	TN	AUC
Forward selection	$f_4, f_6, f_7, f_8, f_{66}, f_{169}, f_{255}, f_{263}, f_{274}, f_{279}, f_{282}, f_{286}$	76.80	0.80	0.74	**0.87**
Backward selection	$f_4, f_6, f_7, f_8, f_{114}, f_{253}, f_{263}, f_{274}, f_{279}, f_{281}, f_{282}, f_{286}$	77.70	0.80	0.74	0.85
Bidirectional search	$f_4, f_6, f_7, f_8, f_{66}, f_{169}, f_{255}, f_{263}, f_{274}, f_{279}, f_{282}, f_{286}$	77.10	0.79	0.73	0.86
Greedy stepwise search	$f_4, f_6, f_7, f_8, f_{66}, f_{253}, f_{f263}, f_{274}, f_{279}, f_{282}, f_{286}$	78.00	0.83	0.69	0.83
Ranking with chi-squares statistics	$f_7, f_{16}, f_{37}, f_{45}, f_{46}, f_{52}, f_{251}, f_{253}, f_{255}, f_{263}, f_{265}, f_{268}$	67.99	0.65	0.73	0.72
Ranking with information gain	$f_7, f_{16}, f_{37}, f_{45}, f_{46}, f_{52}, f_{251}, f_{253}, f_{254}, f_{255}, f_{268}, f_{282}, f_{286}$	65.34	0.56	0.81	0.75
C4.5 decision tree wrapper	$f_6, f_{21}, f_{38}, f_{49}, f_{56}, f_{64}, f_{118}, f_{164}, f_{253}$	70.77	0.70	0.73	0.78
Best features with SVM wrapper	$f_5, f_6, f_{13}, f_{98}, f_{172}, f_{178}, f_{216}, f_{217}, f_{256}$	78.00	0.86	0.64	0.84
Full texture features set	$f_1, f_2, ..., f_{290}$	73.71	0.74	0.73	0.78

Table 2. Bayes classifier results for the best selected texture features subsets

on a different training data drawn independently and identically from the same problem domain, we expect to obtain a decision function with a similar performance. If the classifier performance stays the same independent of training with a specific training dataset, the classifier then learned how to differentiate benign from malignant tumors from the training data. However, if the classifier performance changes considerably by changing the training dataset, then that classifier can not be used for prediction. However, in principle the decision function (i.e. the classifier) can not be made completely independent from the structure of the training data and the complexity of the learning algorithm. To isolate all contributing factors that might interfere with training the classifier and to minimize the bias in the stated results, we systematically applied several machine learning evaluation strategies. First, we trained several classifiers that belong to different machine learning algorithms on the same texture features data. The selected classifiers are trained with crossvalidation procedure to make better use of the training data. The crossvalidation procedure also tries to minimize the effect of the probability distribution of a specific training dataset on the classifier performance. Second, we study the effect of changing the size of the training data set on the classifiers performance by plotting the learning curves that show the error rate of the trained classifiers as a function of the size of the training data set. Third, we used some statistical tests for comparison between the classifiers performance. We also plotted the ROC (Receiver Operating Curve) and the Cost curves to analyze the classifiers' performance. Finally, we applied the McNemar's statistical test to compare the performance of the best classifier against the radiologists' performance.
From several machine algorithm groups, we selected the following classifiers:

Linear classifier: This classifier assumes that the benign and the malignant classes have the same covariance matrix but different means. It estimates the covariance matrix from the full training data and assigns a new case to the class with the highest probability. Such classifier is able to separate benign and malignant tumors by a simple linear decision surface. The probability distribution of the full training dataset is assumed to be normally distributed.

Quadratic classifier: This classifier is more complex than the linear classifier since it estimates different matrices for the means and covariance of the benign and the malignant classes. Such classifier is able to separate the benign and the malignant tumors by a quadratic nonlinear decision surface. The probability distributions of the benign and the malignant classes are assumed to be normally distributed but not necessary with the same covariance matrices.

Nonparametric density estimation classifiers: Parzen classifier and k-NN nearest neighborhood classifier. Both classifiers estimate the empirical probability density function of the benign and the malignant classes from the training data instead of assuming certain probability distribution function such as the linear and quadratic classifiers.

Decision trees classifier: Such classifier uses logical rules to separate the benign form the malignant tumors regardless of the probability distribution of the training data.

Back-propagation neural network: The *NN*-classifier separates the tumors by high nonlinear decision surface. The neural network uses an iterative optimization algorithm to find the weights of the neural network from the training data.

Support vector machine classifier: The SVM classifier simplifies the classification problem by transforming the input space into high dimensional space such that the classification problem become a linear one and easier to solve. The SVM classifier does not depend on the probabilistic distribution of the training dataset and has the ability to generalize quite well for classification problems of varied degrees of complexities. During the training process, a quadratic optimization algorithm is used to iteratively adjust the complexity of the decision function to adopt to the problem domain.

In the following sections, we describe several tests that were performed to study the effect of the size of the training data set on the classifier performance. Additionally, we tested the complexity of the decision function, analyzed the classifier performance and statistically compared the performance of two classifiers. Finally, we tested the classifier performance against the radiologists' performance.

6. The size of the training data and the classifiers performance

The classifier learns the classification function from the training data. The training data represents a small sample from the population of soft tissue tumors and hence the size of the training data has an impact on the trained classifier. We run the learning curve test to study the effect of the size of the training data set on the classifier performance. Using a small subset of the training data, we tuned the parameters for each classifier as follows. The back-propagation neural network has two hidden layers, an input layer of 12 nodes (i.e, number of selected texture features by the forward selection method) and an output layer with two nodes corresponding to the benign and the malignant classes. The SVM classifier is trained with an RBF kernel which is tuned with a grid search algorithm that resulted in a ($\sigma = 10000$) and a cost coefficient ($C = 1.0$). We used the PRTOOLS 4.0 matlab toolbox to run this experiment. We left the parameters of the decision trees and the Parzen classifier to their default values, which forces the PRTOOLS toolbox to tune them automatically to their best values. We trained the 7 classifiers with different sizes of the training data set. At each specific size of the training data set, we measured the error rate of all the classifiers. For each specific size of the training data, we repeated the experiment 10 times and the average error rate was calculated. Figure 4 shows the learning curves of the 7 trained classifiers. The learning curves show some interesting facts about the problem domain. First, the learning curves are smooth which is a good indicator of the classifiers stability against changes in the training data distribution . The smoothness of the learning curves is also a necessary condition for carrying some statistical tests that we used to compare the classifiers performance(Dietterich (1998)). Second, the 7 classifiers learned very well with few training samples. Most classifiers achieved an error rates between 0.251 and 0.198 after training with as few as 50 training samples. As we increase the size of the training data set, the error rate decreases very slowly after training by 50 samples. This observation indicates that a small training data set is sufficient to get good generalization performance. Increasing the size of the training set after certain limit seems to have little impact on improving the classifiers performance any further. The third observation is related to the complexity of the classifiers. Simple classifiers such as the k-NN nearest neighborhood classifier and the SVM with an RBF kernel with large bandwidth achieved lower error rates compared to the neural network classifier. This observation is an indication that the decision surface that separates the benign from the malignant tumors based on texture features is a very simple mathematical function which we investigate further in the following section. Classification problems that procedure linear or simple decision function are less likely to overfit the training data and often generalize and predict very well in unseen data.

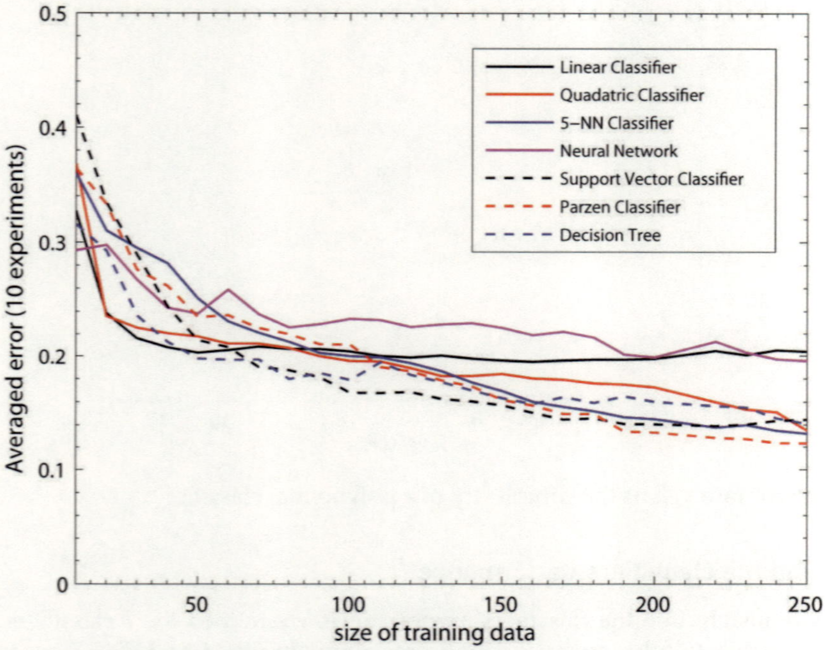

Fig. 4. The learning curves of the 7 trained classifiers

7. The complexity of the decision function

The learning curves from the last section showed that classifiers which produce simple decision functions generalize better since they have the smallest error rate on the testing samples. To check that conclusion we ran a test using an SVM classifier with a polynomial kernel that produces a polynomial decision function with a varied degree of complexity. We varied the degree of the polynomial kernel gradually from 1 to 20 and at each degree of the polynomial, we run the experiment 10 times using a crossvalidation procedure. Each point in the learning curves is the average of the error rates of ten different experiments. Figure 5 shows the error rate of the polynomial classifier versus the degree of the polynomial kernel function. The plot clearly shows that the error rate is minimum at a polynomial decision function of the 4th degree. The error rates for the linear classifier (a 1st degree polynomial) and the quadratic classifier (a 2nd degree polynomial) are large since they under-fit the training data. A polynomial classifier higher than the 4th degree also have high error rate since it overfit the training data. This explains why in Fig. 4 that the simple linear classifier and the neural network classifier both have high error rates compared to other classifiers, because the linear classifier is too simple and the neural network classifier is too complex for the problem domain. That also explains why the SVM classifier has a good classification performance because it is very flexible and can adept to classification problems of varied complexity.

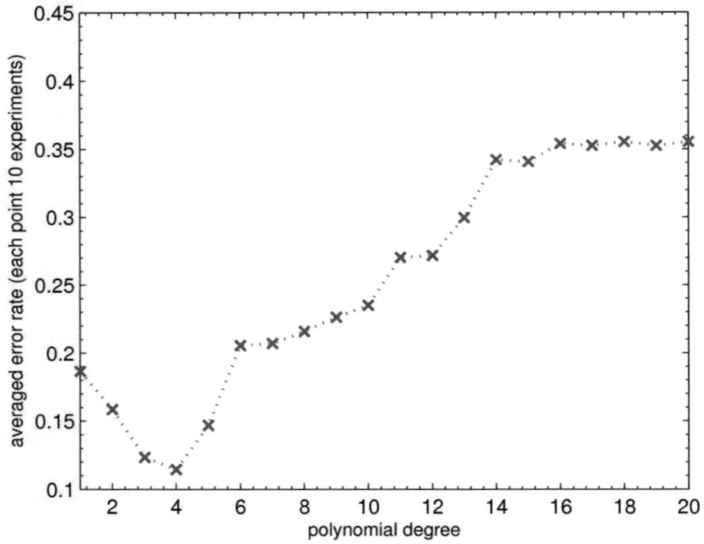

Fig. 5. The error rate versus the complexity of a polynomial classifier

8. Analyzing the classifiers performance

To gain more insight into the classifiers' performance, we trained the 7 classifiers using the full data set with a 10-folds crossvalidation procedure. In Fig. 6 and Fig. 7, we plotted the ROC curves and the Cost curves of the 7 classifiers. In the ROC curves plot, the best curves are at the top of the plot. In the ROC curves, we see that the classifiers are ranked, according to an increase in performance, as follow: the decision trees, the neural networks, the linear classifier, the quadratic classifier and the k-NN classifier. However, there is an ambiguity about the ranking of the Parzen and SVM classifiers because their ROC curves intersect. In the Cost-curve plot, the classifiers are ranked in the same order as the ROC curves. However, this time the curves of the best classifiers are at the bottom of the plot. The Cost-curves of the Parzen classifier and the SVM classifier have the same normalized expected cost value for a probability cost function (PCF) between 0.45-0.75 where both curves intersect. For a value of PCF < 0.45, the SVM classifier performance is better than the Parzen classifier while for the value of PCF > 0.75 the Parzen classifier performance is better. In other words, both classifiers perform equally well if the cost of classifying benign and malignant tumors is kept the same. However, if we would like to change the cost of classifying benign and malignant tumors, for example, we decided to give more cost for missing malignant tumors than missing benign tumors then both classifiers perform differently (see Holte & Drummond (2011)). The later observation explains why the SVM and Parzen classifier have an overlapping performance which is easy to explain from the ROC curves.

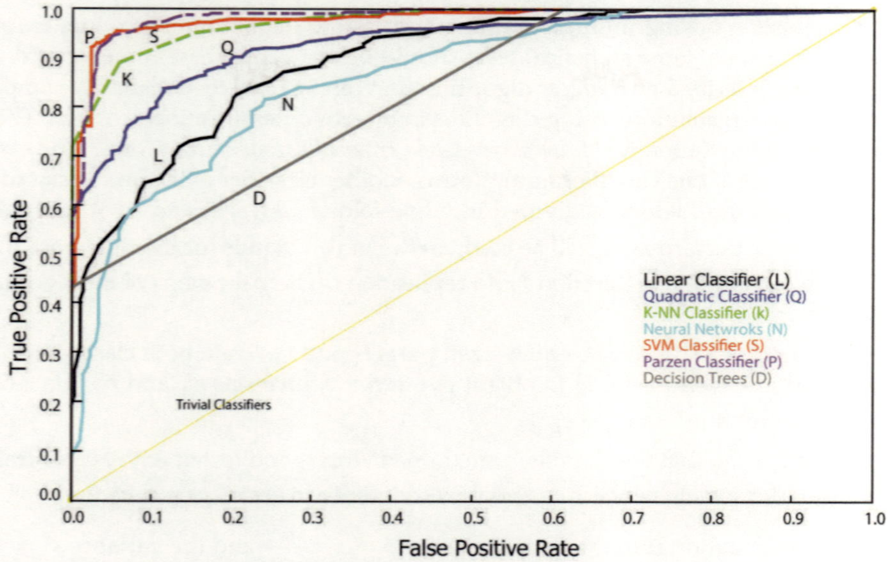

Fig. 6. ROC curves of the trained classifiers

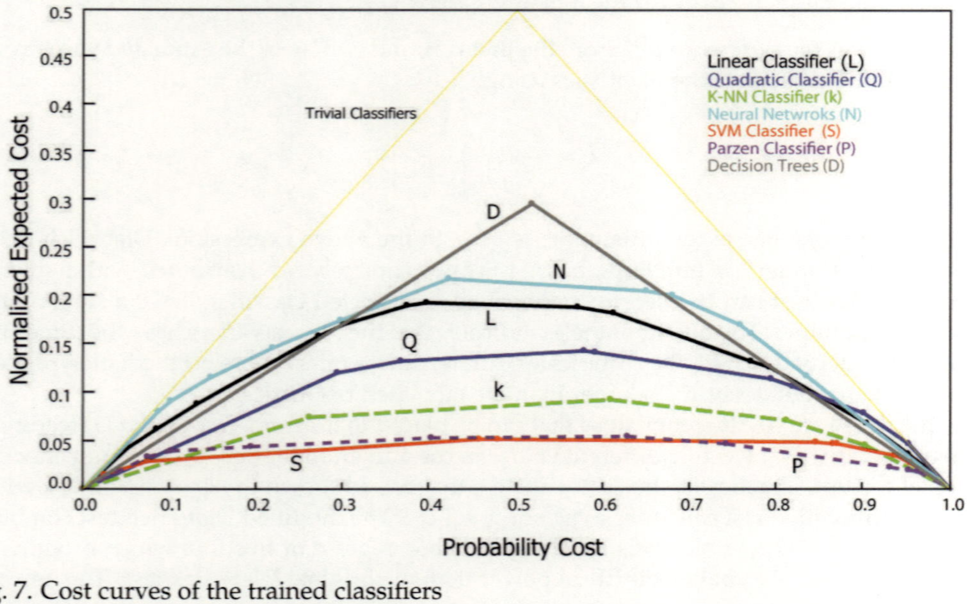

Fig. 7. Cost curves of the trained classifiers

9. Statistical comparison between two classifiers

Classifier performance is a function of several factors including the statistical distribution of the training and testing data, the internal structure of the classifier and the inherent randomness in the training process. Even if we train two different classifiers with the same dataset their classification error rates will not be necessary the same. That is because classifiers are trained with different algorithms and with different optimizations criteria and different parameter settings. The most effective way to compare classifiers is to empirically train and test the classifiers using multiple training and testing data. This procedure is repeated several times and then some statistical tests should be applied to assess their performance. Dietterich (1998) described an 5×2 *cv* algorithm that can be used to statistically compare the performance of two machine learning classifiers in the same classification problem. The name of the test is an abbreviation for "*5 iterations 2-fold crossvalidation paired t-Test*". The same test can be used to check if one classifier outperforms another classifier on a specific classification task. Let D be a dataset which is divided into five folds $F_1, F_2, .., F_5$ and let A and B be two classifiers that their performance will be compared. Let $p_j^{\{i\}}$ stands for the difference in errors between the two classifiers in iteration j fold replication i. Then, the steps of the algorithm are as follows:

- divide the first fold F_1 into two equal-sized parts t_1 and t_2. Train both classifiers A and B using t_1 and test them using t_2 to obtain two error estimations e_A^1 and e_B^1. Calculate the difference in errors $p^{(1)} = e_A^1 - e_B^1$
- swap t_1 and t_2 such that the classifiers are trained with t_2 and tested with t_1 . Re-train both classifiers and calculate new errors and new difference in errors $p^{(2)} = e_A^2 - e_B^2$
- for this crossvalidation run, calculate the mean $\bar{p} = \frac{p^{(1)}+p^{(2)}}{2}$ and the variance $s^2 = (p^{(1)} - \bar{p})^2 + (p^{(2)} - \bar{p})^2$
- repeat the same procedure for the remaining folds $\{F_2, ..., F_5\}$

Let $p_1^{(1)}$ denotes the difference $p^{(1)}$ from the first run, and s_i^2 denote the estimated variance for run $i, i = 1, ..., 5$. Calculate the $\tilde{t}$-statistics using:

$$\tilde{t} = \frac{p_1^{(1)}}{\sqrt{(1/5)\sum_{i=1}^{5} s_i^2}} \tag{1}$$

Note that only one of the ten differences is used in the above expression. Dietterich (1998) has shown that under the null hypothesis, $\tilde{t}$ is approximately a t-distributed with 5 degrees of freedom. The test can be used to check if two constructed classifiers have a similar error rate on new example. The null hypothesis indicates that the two classifiers have the same error rate and the alternative hypothesis indicates different error rates. We reject the null hypothesis with 95 percent confidence if $\tilde{t}$ is larger than the tabulated t-statistics.
Note that, there are 10 different values that can be placed in the numerator of Eq.(1) leading to 10 possible statistics. Selecting different values in the numerator of Eq.(1) should not effect the results of the test. Practically, this is not always the case as shown in Alpaydin (1999), which proposed a modified test called *the combined* 5×2 *cv* . The modified Dietterich test combines the results of the 10 possible statistics and uses more degrees of freedom which promises to be more robust and has better statistical power than the original Dietterich test. The new test calculates:

$$\tilde{f} = \frac{\sum_{i=1}^{5} \sum_{j=1}^{2} \left(p_i^{(j)}\right)^2}{2\sum_{i=1}^{5} s_i^2} \sim F_{n,m} \tag{2}$$

and tests the estimated $\tilde{f}$ against an F-statistics with 10 and 5 degrees of freedom. Reject the null hypothesis if $\tilde{f}$ is larger than the tabulated F-statistics value (i.e., $F = 4.74$), otherwise, accept the null hypothesis.

Exp#	$e_A^{(1)}$	$e_B^{(1)}$	$p^{(1)}$	$e_A^{(2)}$	$e_B^{(2)}$	$p^{(2)}$	s^2
1	0.3853	0.1618	0.2235	0.3588	0.2029	0.1559	0.0023
2	0.3382	0.1735	0.1647	0.1353	0.1706	-0.0353	0.0200
3	0.4265	0.1794	0.2471	0.3176	0.2000	0.1176	0.0084
4	0.3824	0.1735	0.2088	0.3618	0.1529	0.2088	0.0
5	0.3912	0.1794	0.2118	0.3529	0.1647	0.1882	0.0003

Table 3. Error rates, differences and variances s^2 of the SVM classifer (A) and the Parzen (B) using 5×2-fold crossvalidation on tumors' texture.

We selected two classifiers from Fig. 7, namely, the SVM and the neural networks classifiers. We run the test to check whether both classifiers have similar performance or have different performance. The results of running the 5-iterations 2-fold crossvalidation algorithm are summarized in Table 3. Using Eq.(2), we calculated $\tilde{f} = 5.58$ which is larger than the the theoretical F-statistics value. Hence, the null hypothesis that both classifiers have similar error rates was rejected. Therefore, according to *the combined* 5×2 *cv* test, the SVM classifier had better performance than the neural network classifier with 95% statistical confidence. In conclusion, the test shows that some classifiers can have better performance than other classifier when trained with the same training dataset.

10. Machine learning versus radiologists performance

An important question is how machine learning classifiers perform compared to radiologists. In the previous section, we used the modified 5×2 *cv* Dietterich test to compare two classifiers. However, we can not use the same test to compare a classifier performance against the radiologists diagnosis since the radiologist results can not be repeated. Instead, we applied the McNemar's test (Alpaydin (2001)). To apply McNemar's test, we first have to express the results of the radiologists and the SVM classifier as depicted in Table 4: Second, we

N_{00}: Number of examples misclassified by both	N_{01} : Number of examples misclassified by the classifier but not the radiologists
N_{10}: Number of examples misclassified by radiologists but not the classifier	N_{11}: Number of examples correctly classified by both

Table 4. A table used to perform McNemar's test.

construct two hypothesis: the null hypothesis H_0 is that there is no difference between the error rates or accuracies of the radiologists and the classifier and the alternative hypothesis H_1 is that the radiologists and the classifier have different performance. If the null hypothesis is correct, then the expected counts for both off-diagonal entries in Table(4) are $\frac{1}{2}(N_{01} + N_{10})$. The discrepancy between the expected and the observed counts is measured by the following statistics:

$$\frac{(|N_{01} - N_{10}| - 1)^2}{N_{01} + N_{10}} = \tilde{\chi}^2, \qquad (3)$$

which is, approximately, distributed as χ^2 with 1 degree of freedom. First, we run several experiments to find an optimal classifier. The best classifier so far was the SVM classifier. The results of the SVM classifier against the radiologists are summarized in Table 5. Using Eq.3, we obtained $\tilde{\chi}^2 = 12.85$ which is larger than the tabulated $\chi^2 = 3.48$. Hence, we rejected

	laboratory results		
SVM results		*malignant*	*benign*
	malignant	405	23
	benigin	25	228

	laboratory results		
physician results		*malignant*	*benign*
	malignant	134	45
	benigin	32	552

Fig. 8. The SVM and the radiologists confusion matrices

$N_{00} = 39$	$N_{01} = 16$	$N_{00} + N_{01} = 55$
$N_{10} = 45$	$N_{11} = 581$	$N_{10} + N_{11} = 625$
$N_{00} + N_{10} = 84$	$N_{01} + N_{11} = 597$	$N = 681$

Table 5. A table constructed for the McNemar's test

the null hypothesis that both the radiologists and the SVM classifier have similar error rates. Therefore, the SVM seems to perform slightly better than the radiologist. This last conclusion should, however, be taken with a grain of salt because it is based on statistical analysis of the SVM classifier with a limited training data set that does not represent the full distribution of the soft tissue tumors.

The McNemar's test does not tell us about the strength between the agreement or the disagreement between the radiologists and the SVM classifier to validate the previous test so we evaluated the kappa statistics ($\kappa = 0.5$) which is larger than 0 which shows that the results of the McNemar's test is correct. Finally, the confusion matrix of the SVM classifier is shown in Fig. 8. The radiologist performance is also shown in Fig. 8.

11. Conclusions

We demonstrated that texture analysis of soft tissue tumors and machine learning algorithms can be used as a tool for objective evaluation of MR images and the results correlate well with the laboratory results. We ran several tests and come up with some interesting observation related to the problem of texture analysis of soft issue tumors. First, texture features combined with machine learning algorithms seems to perform as well as radiologists since computer can extract more information related to signal homogeneity in T1-MRI than what human can do based only on visual perception. Second, we do not need a large training data set to train a machine learning classifier and obtain a good classification performance since texture features correlate very well with the pathology of the tumor. Moreover, simple classifiers such as a Parzen classifier or an SVM classifier can effectively separate benign from malignant tumors.

12. Acknowledgments

Thanks to the *University Hospital Antwerp (UZA), Dept. of Radiology* for providing the MR images. The authors would like to thank Prof. Robert Holte for providing the Cost Curve software.

13. References

Alpaydin, E. (1999). Combined 5 x 2 cv F test for comparing supervised classification learning algorithms, *Neural Computation* 11(8): 1885–1892.

Alpaydin, E. (2001). Assessing and comparing classification algorithms.

Castellano, G., Bonilha, L., Li, L. & Cendes, F. (2004). Texture analysis of medical images, *Clinical Radiology* 59: 1061–1069.

De Schepper, A. M. & Bloem, J. L. (2007). Soft tissue tumors : grading, staging, and tissue-specific diagnosis, *Topics in Magnetic Resonance Imaging* 18(6): 431–444.

De Schepper, A. M., De Beuckeleer, L., Vandevenne, J. & Somville, J. (2000). Magnetic resonance imaging of soft tissue tumors, *European Radiology* 10(2): 213–223.

De Schepper, A., Vanhoenacker, F., Parizel, P. & Gielen, J. (eds) (2005). *Imaging of Soft Tissue Tumors*, 3rd edn, Springer.

Dietterich (1998). Approximate statistical tests for comparing supervised classification learning algorithms., *Neural Computation* 10(7): 1895–1923.

Haralick, R.M., Shanmugan, K. & Dinstein, I. (1973). Textural features for image classification, *IEEE Transactions on Systems, Man and Cybernetics* 3(6): 610–621.

Hermann, G., Abdelwahab, I., Miller, T., Kelin, M. & Lewis, M. (1992). Tumor and tumor-like conditions of the soft tissue: Magnetic resonance imaging features differentiating benign from malignant masses, *Br J Radiol* 65: 14–20.

Holte, R. C. & Drummond, C. (2011). Cost-sensitive classifier evaluation using cost curves, *Proceedings of The 24th Florida Artificial Intelligence Research Society Conference (FLAIRS-24)*.

Huang, Y., Wang, K. & Chen, D. (2006). Diagnosis of breast tumors with ultrasonic texture analysis using support vector machines, *Neural Computing & Applications* 15(2): 164–169.

Jirák, D., Dezortová, M., Taimr, P. & Hájek, M. (2002). Texture analysis of human liver, *Journal of Magnetic Resonance Imaging* 15(1): 68–74.

Juan, M., García-Gómez, Vidal, C., Luis Martí-Bonmatï£¡, Joaquín, G. & et al. (2004). Benign/malignant classifier of soft tissue tumors using MR imaging, *Magnetic Resonance Materials in Physics, Biology and Medicine* 16: 194–201.

Julesz, B. (1975). Experiments in visual perception of texture, *Sci Am* 232: 34–43.

Julesz, B., Gilbert, E., Shepp, L. & Frisch, H. (1973). Inability of humans to discriminate between visual textures that agree in second-order statistics, *Perception* 2: 391–405.

Juntu, J., Sijbers, J., De Backer, S., Rajan, J. & Van Dyck, D. (2010). Machine learning study of several classifiers trained with texture analysis features to differentiate benign from malignant soft-tissue tumors in T1-MRI images, *J. Magn. Reson. Imaging* 31(3): 680–689.

Mahmoud-Ghoneim, D., Toussaint, G. & Jean-Marc, C. (2003). Three dimensional texture analysis in MRI: a preliminary evaluation in gliomas, *Magnetic Resonance Imaging* 21(9): 983–987.

Mao, J. & Jain, A. K. (1992). Texture classification and segmentation using multiresolution simultaneous autoregressive models, *Pattern Recognition* 25(2): 173 – 188.

Materka, A. & Strzelectky, M. (1998). Texture analysis methods- a review, *Technical University of Lodz 1998, COST B11-techincal report* 11: 873–887.

Mayerhoefer, M. E., Breitenseher, M. J., Kramer, J., Aigner, N., Hofmann, S. & Materka, A. (2005). Texture analysis for tissue discrimination on T1-weighted MR images of knee joint in a multicenter study: Transferability of texture features and comaprison of feature selection methods and classifiers, *J Mag Reson Imaging* 22: 674–680.

Meinel, L. A., Stolpen, A. H., Berbaum, K. S., Fajardo, L. L. & Reinhardt, J. M. (2007). Breast MRI lesion classification: Improved performance of human readers with a backpropagation neural network computer-aided diagnosis (CAD) system, *Journal of Magnetic Resonance Imaging* 25(1): 89 –95.

Mutlu, H., Silit, E., Pekkafali, Z., Basekim, C., Ozturk, E., Sildiroglu, O., Kizilkaya, E. & Karsli, A. (2006). Soft-tissue masses: Use of a scoring system in differentiation of benign and malignant lesions, *Clinical Imaging* 30(1): 37–42.

Salzberg, S. L. (1997). On comparing classifiers: Pitfalls to avoid and a recommended approach, *Data Mining and Knowledge Discovery* 1: 317–327.

Tuceryan, M. & Jain, A. K. (1998). Texture analysis, *in* C. H. Chen and L. F. Pau and P. S. P. Wang (ed.), *The Handbook of Pattern Recognition and Computer Vision (2nd Edition)*, World Scientific Publishing Co., pp. 207–248.

Wagner, T. (1999). Texture analysis, *in* B. Jane, H. Haubecker & P. Geibler (eds), *Handbook of Computer Vision and Applications, Vol.2, Signal Processing and Pattern Recognition*, Academic Press, chapter 12, pp. 275–308.

Weatherall, P. (1995). Benign and malignant masses, MR imaging differentiation, *Mag Reson Clin N Am* 3: 669–694.

4

Medical Theory on Orthopedics Combining Molecular Imaging with Clinical Practice

Jing jing Peng
Dept. Beijing Institute of Traumatology and Orthopaedics
Beijing Ji Shui-Tan Hospital
The 4th Clinical Hospital of Peking University
China

1. Introduction

Soft tissue is defined as the supportive tissue of various organs,the term soft tissue tumors defines neoplasms derived from soft tissue. At the clinical level, a mass is the most common sign of a soft tissue tumor. However, the clinical manifestations and signs of parathyroid adenoma are not in the neck at first since, very often, there are patients who's neck is normal at primary physical examination. Bone pain or dysfunction fractures are the main reason for the parathyroid tumor patients to visit the hospital. Parathyroid tumor (Figure 1) is an endocrine tumor, mainly associated with bone metabolism therefore the patients go to the orthopedic department first. Although the parathyroid tumor is benign if patients do not get timely and accurate diagnosis and effective treatment(surgical removal of parathyroid adenoma), they will not only receive the delayed treatment but also, a significant decline of life quality will occur. The loss of ability to work increases the burden on families and society.

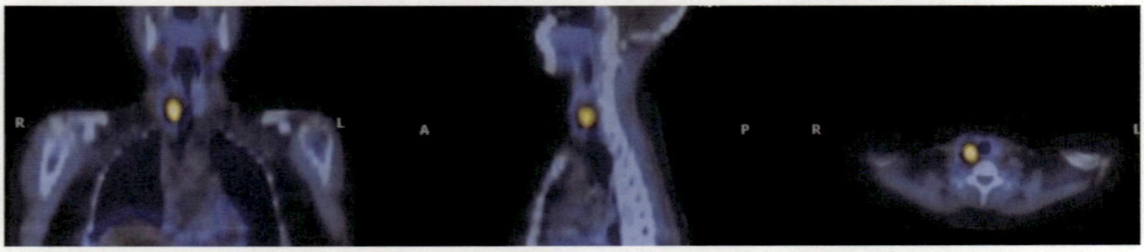

Fig. 1. Parathyroid adenoma
The neck SPECT/CT scan function-anatomy fused Imaging reveals A focus of increased ^{99m}Tc-MIBI activity at the posterior inferior of the right lobe of the thyroid which consistent with parathyroid adenoma

Effective treatment for parathyroid tumors depends on timely, accurate diagnosis.Doctor Peng Jing Jing, <Advancement in the Application of Nuclear Medicine> published in

Apr.2001 V7N4:59-61 Journal of "China Contemporary Medicine", reported the use of nuclear medicine, that is molecular imaging, which enables early diagnosis and successful treatment of patients with parathyroid adenoma. The cases in clinical with SPECT for ^{99m}Tc-MDP whole body bone scan and ^{99m}Tc-MIBI parathyroid tumor imaging, in which patients receive timely diagnosis and successful treatment, recover and live a happy life[3]. In recent years, as the clinic study of new technology and equipment in bone-joint disorders, orthopedic clinical applications of molecular imaging and promotion of the Chinese doctors for parathyroid tumor diagnosis and treatment, medical science has made a positive contribution [4].

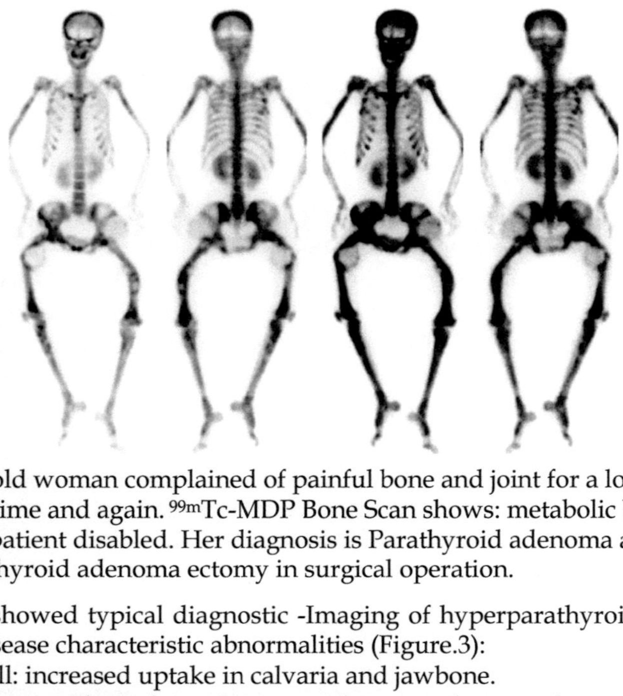

Fig. 2. A 39 years-old woman complained of painful bone and joint for a long time with occurred fracture time and again. ^{99m}Tc-MDP Bone Scan shows: metabolic bone disease which causes the patient disabled. Her diagnosis is Parathyroid adenoma and she was performed a parathyroid adenoma ectomy in surgical operation.

The contribution showed typical diagnostic -Imaging of hyperparathyroidism- resulted in metabolic bone disease characteristic abnormalities (Figure.3):

1. The Black skull: increased uptake in calvaria and jawbone.
2. Generalized increased uptake with increased contrast between bone and soft tissue due to bone turnover speed and subtracted kidney image.
3. Tie sternum and Cage beads.
4. Foci of increased uptake due to fracture or brown tumor in rib cage.
5. Decreased uptake brown tumor in the right ilium as doughnut .
6. Whole body Bone scan patterns in advanced metabolic bone disease and insufficiency fracture in right neck of femur.

There are two main features of metabolic bone disease due to hyperparathyroidism in ^{99m}Tc-MDP bone imaging: (1) Increased uptake in calvaria and jawbone showed "the Black skull". (2) Bone scan is clear showed total body as "Super Scan": Generalized increased uptake with increased contrast between bone and soft tissue: increased uptake in long bones and increased uptake in axial skeleton, increased uptake in periarticular areas, increased uptake in costochondral junctions (beads) and increased uptake in sternum (tie sternum).The patient right leg was shorten with foci of increased uptake due to dysfunction fracture, brown tumor due to fibrocystic changes.

JST Beijing JST hospital 31st Xin Jie-kou East Street, Beijing, P.R. China
Dear Dr. Sun: 1999.01.11
RE: Mis. Liang beauty DOB1958.07.09 Age: 40
ID: 305447 SPECT: 981193 Address: Hebei China

I saw this pleasant lady in my inpatients clinic on 1998.12 .09
She was C/O painful hip radiating to her legs.
Mrs. Liang was admitted into hospital on 1998.12.07 her X-Ray showed the Femoral neck pathological fracture of the right femur. ? metastatic bone disease.
On questioning her, I found that Mrs. liang had been C/O leg pain for 3 years, Also she felt severe right hip pain before my seeing her 2 /52.
On examination, I found her right leg was external rotated and shorten, there was tenderness in the hip joint and mildly swollen. Her Vital signs were normal (Temp\ pulse \Resp \B/P).
Tests carried out were:
Hip X-ray BMD (bone mineral density)
ECT: bone scan and parathyroid tumor image
Ultra scan
Blood tests:
Serum Ca (calcium), P (phosphorus), AKP, PTH, ESR
The results showed she had a hypercalcemia and hypophosphatemia:
Serum Ca was high 3.11(2.25-2.75) mmol/L,
Serum P was lower 0.85(0.97-1.6) mmol/L.
AKP was high 502(25-90) IU/L.
PTH (parathyroid hormone) was high.
Hip X-ray showed: The intertrochanter's fracture of the right femur.
BMD was low: T scores of < 2.5SD
Bone scan(^{99m}Tc-MDP)patterns in advanced metabolic bone disease (please see attached picture):

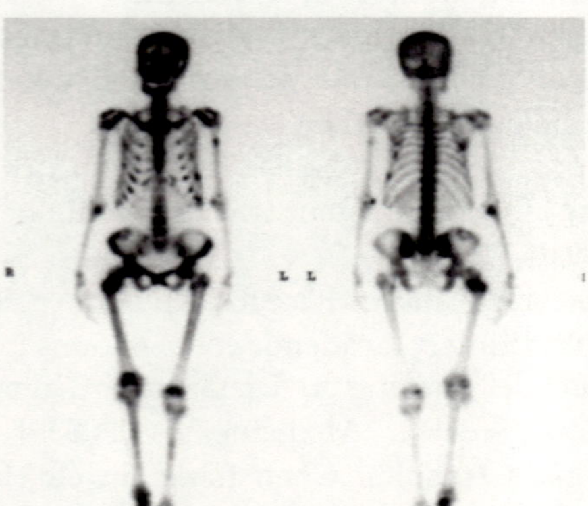

^{99m}Tc-MDP Bone scan showed metabolic disease

Fig. 3. Diagnostic Imaging of hyperparathyroidism resulted in metabolic bone disease characteristic abnormalities.

The right leg was dysfunction fracture of the right femur. In conclusion, I think that diagnosis is hyperparathyroidism.
So, I have had ^{99m}Tc-MIBI parathyroid tumor double-phase imaging. ^{99m}Tc-MIBI parathyroid tumor imaging not only can observe the shape and location, but can also display functional status for parathyroid tumor.

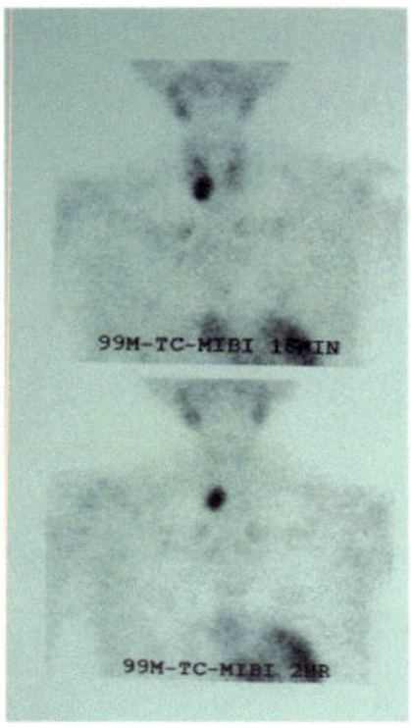

Fig. 4. ^{99m}Tc-MIBI parathyroid tumor (double-phase) imaging.

Immediate (upper) and Delayed (lower) ^{99m}Tc-MIBI imaging reveals a focus of increased activity at the inferior tip of the right lobe of the thyroid, Consistent with parathyroid adenoma.
^{99m}Tc-MIBI scan showed: right lower parathyroid adenoma (Please see attached).

Ultra scan also showed: Parathyroid tumor
Diagnosis:Primary hyperparathyroidism caused by a parathyroid adenoma
Metabolic bone disease Osteoporosis
Dysfunction fracture (the right femur).
Mrs. Liang was given operating treatments on 1998.12.21:
First, was performed parathyroid adenoma' ectomy in surgical operating theatre.
Then, Reduction of fracture and internal fixation was performed by orthopedic doctor.
Finally, the diagnosis in pathology (98-X1095) was:
Parathyroid adenoma
Focus which lead to fracture of the right femur was brown tumor
She was discharged on 1999.01.11.
She was given diet and some medication advice to help her to gain full recovery.
JST' doctor Peng Jing Jing etc. Primary Academic contributions to this project
< Application of Radionuclide Imaging in Diagnosis of hyperfunctioning Parathyroid tumors>journal of Chinese Nuclear Medicine Dec.2003[2] .Cited by Zhuhai City, Guangdong Province People's Hospital Chen Jiang lin etc. in Anthology of Medicine Apr.2006[5], the paper reported a case Qualitative and locational diagnosis with nuclear medicine of primary hyperparathyroidism and successful surgery of parathyroid adenoma: Peng Jingjing et al thought, there are two main features of metabolic bone disease due to hyperparathyroidism in ^{99m}Tc-MDP bone imaging: (1) Bone scan is clear showed total body as "Super Scan"; (2) Increased uptake in calvaria and jawbone for

^{99m}Tc-MDP showed “the Black skull”. ^{99m}Tc- MIBI parathyroid tumor imaging not only can observe the shape and location, but also display hyper-functional status for parathyroid tumor.

Achiever said: Primary hyperparathyroidism is rare in clinic. Because of occult onset and symptoms varied, misdiagnosis is made sometimes. A clear diagnosis of hyperparathyroidism and parathyroid tumors localization is the key for successful treatment. ^{99m}Tc-MDP bone scintigraphy and ^{99m}Tc -MIBI parathyroid tumor imaging has certain advantages. To be used clinically, those principal achieves can reduce misdiagnosis of primary hyperparathyroidism.

2. Clinical features of parathyroid adenoma

2.1 Definition

Primary hyperparathyroidism incidence rate is about 27/100000 per year, of which 80% is parathyroid tumor, 20% is benign hyperplasia, and parathyroid carcinoma is extremely rare. Because of the parathyroid hormone (PTH) secretes more than the level required to maintain normal serum calcium concentration bring about, laboratory parameters abnormal shows hypercalcemia, hypophosphatemia, elevated alkaline phosphatase and parathyroid hormone increased.

Clinical symptoms mainly in four systems

1. Bones-- musculoskeletal symptoms: bone pain, dysfunction fractures;
2. Stones--symptoms of urinary system: history of kidney stones with pain;
3. Groans--digestive symptoms: abdominal discomfort, nausea, vomiting, dyspepsia and constipation;
4. Moans—neuropsychiatric symptoms: memory loss, depression, depressed.

Diagnostic whole body bone scan image

"Super scan" of hyperparathyroidism (HPT) metabolic bone disease

Early parathyroid adenoma causing bone metabolism changes in ^{99m}Tc-MDP whole body bone scan image is generalized increased uptake with characterized by the "black skull" and very clearly as "super scan" which give expression to increased contrast between bone and soft tissue due to bone turnover speed and active bone metabolism.

Metabolic bone disease with HPTdifferent from metastasis imaging

Differential point in whole body bone scan image between "super scan" of HPT metabolic bone disease and wide range of bone metastasis is: HPT metabolic bone disease "super scan" is general uniformity high uptake in the axial skeleton and limb bones (Figure 5); and features of bone metastasis "super scan" are: high uptake of the mainly axial skeleton (Figure 6) and proximal limb bone, with point like lesions of radioactive concentration.

2.2 Fracture and brown tumor

The Patient with proceeding of parathyroid tumors, X-ray radiograph shows bone resorption caused by osteoclast, and lacy cortical thinning leading to subperiosteal bone resorption, typical in middle phalanx radial side of index finger and middle finger.

Radiology images can also show brown tumor formed by micro-fracture bleeding, local accumulation of macrophages, and replacement of fibrous tissue. Brown tumor and fractures in the whole body bone scan images showed localized uptake. Large fibrocystic changes (brown tumor) can be expressed as a radioactive defect of the "cold zone" (Figure 2, the anteposition imaging shows: brown tumor in right ilium).

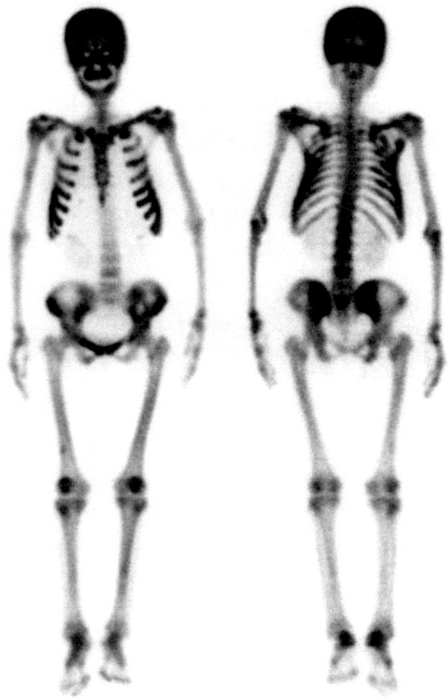

Fig. 5. "Super scan" with HPT metabolic bone disease

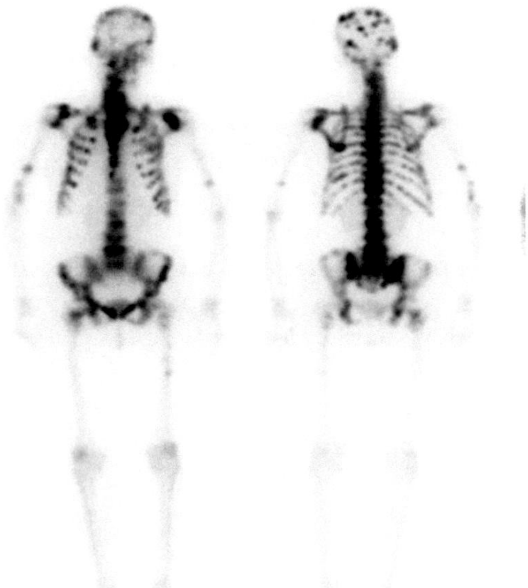

Fig. 6. "Super scan" with extensive bone metastases

2.3 Preoperative localization of parathyroid adenoma

B-ultrasonic examination: after the diagnosis of HPT metabolic bone diseases, neck ultrasound is a simple and preferred method to localize the parathyroid tumors.

^{99m}Tc-MIBI parathyroid tumor imaging: after the diagnosis of HPT metabolic bone diseases, the SPECT ^{99m}Tc-MIBI double-phase parathyroid tumor imaging is helpful to the localization diagnosis of parathyroid adenoma (especially ectopic parathyroid adenoma) which is prepared for surgical removal.

3. Diagnosis and differential diagnosis of parathyroid tumor

3.1 Clinical diagnosis of parathyroid adenoma

1. Clinical manifestations of parathyroid adenoma have diversity. There are four mainly symptoms: skeletal system, urinary tract stones, neuropsychiatric system and digestive symptoms. Bone pain and fracture is the most common complained of. Therefore, physicians and surgeons should have a basic consciousness with the diagnosis of parathyroid tumors, such as patients with long kidney stones history, have symptoms of bone pain or fractures.
2. Laboratory test is helpful to the diagnosis of hyperparathyroidism: calcium, phosphorus, alkaline phosphatase (AKP) and parathyroid hormone (PTH) was abnormal.
3. The recognition characteristic image of the "super scan " of hyperparathyroidism in ^{99m}Tc-MDP whole body bone scan is very important.
4. Neck ultrasonography and ^{99m}Tc-MIBI double-phase parathyroid imaging can diagnose and localize parathyroid tumor clearly, which contribute to parathyroid tumor surgery.

3.2 Differential diagnosis of parathyroid adenoma in clinical orthopedics

Abnormal secretion of parathyroid hormone PTH leads to changes in bone metabolism in parathyroid tumor patients .Bone pain or dysfunction fracture are always the reason for patients to the hospital. There were many patients initially diagnosed with unilateral bone cyst (Brown tumor of fibrocystic changes in local radiology images), or misdiagnosed as bone metastases (bone scan imaging features were not yet understand). In order to accurate diagnosis and effective treatment for parathyroid tumor, it is very important to familiar with the differential diagnosis of bone scan, advances of orthopedic medical imaging basic research in molecular imaging and clinical application in bone tumors and disease as a starting point, the next section focus on the bone scan imaging features and differential diagnosis between parathyroid tumor metabolic bone disease and multiple myeloma, rickets etc. eight diseases, with the aim of doctor comprehend typical characteristic distinction.

4. Advancement in fundamental researches

New concept of orthopedic molecular imaging

International medical imaging community reached a consensus on the "molecular imaging" definition In June 2007:

1. "Molecular imaging" is the imaging embodiment for the molecular level;
2. "molecular imaging" observes living body (human or animal) in vivo,which can provide dynamic observation time-varying continuously.

3. "molecular imaging" can be detected by means of instruments (such as PCT/CT and MRI, etc. equipment) and can be quantitative.

The theoretical development of orthopedic molecular imaging was based on the new understanding of bone anatomy and physiology.

Bone structure of normal adult bone can be summarized in four categories [6]:

Gross level

The skeleton consists of two major parts, the axial skeleton includes the skull, spine and rib cage (ribs and sternum), while the appendicular skeleton includes the bones of the extremities, pelvic girdle and pectoral girdle (clavicles and scapulae)

Tissue level

Bone is divided into two types of tissues forming the skeleton: compact or cortical bone and cancelous, trabecular or spongy bone. The compact bone constitutes 80% of the skeletal mass. The appendicular skeleton is composed predominantly of contical bone. The cortical bone is thicker in the diaphysis. The blood supply to the metaphysic is rich. The spine is composed predominantly of cancellous bone in the body of the vertebra and compact bone in the endplates and posterior elements. The spongy bone has a turnover rate approximately eight times greater than the cortical bones and hosts hematopoietic cells and many blood cells.

Cellular lever

Three types of cells can be seen in bone: osteoblasts, which produce the organic bone matrix; osteocytes, which produce the inorganic matrix; osteoclasts, which are active in bone resorption. Osteoclasts are derived from the hemopoietic system, in contrast to the mesenchymal origin of osteoblasts. Osteocytes are derived from osteoblasts that have secreted bone matrix around themselves.

Molecular level

At the Molecular level, bone matrix is composed primarily of organic matrix (approximately 35%), including collagen and glycoproteins, and inorganic matrix (approximately 65%), which includes hydroxyapatite, cations (calcium, magnesium, sodium, potassium and strontium) and anions (fluoride, phosphorus and chloride). The calcium in inorganic matrix of bone provid hardness to withstand pressure, and the collagen fibers in organic components provide support and tension.

^{99m}Tc-MDP bone scan can embodiment changes in the pathogenesis of the human body on the molecular level, and it is detected by SPECT, three phase imaging for patient examine dynamic change with time varying and may performed semi—quantitative analysis for lesion,so bone scan is part of within the domain of molecular imaging [7]. Orthopedic Nuclear Medicine constitutes an important component of orthopedic molecular imaging. Recent Advances in Orthopedics Combined Medical Imaging with Clinical Practice are important to the development of molecular imaging and rich of content [8, 9], [7, 10].

For example, using isotopic tracer ^{99m}Tc-MDP as a molecular probe we can tracer the oncology biological behavior of osteosarcoma[11],Bone scan can detect multiple lesions of osteosarcoma, show the lung,bone and lymph node metastasis FIGURE.7(A), and provide postoperative follow-up for painful body differential diagnosis recurrence from prosthetic loose FIGURE.7 (B) and efficacy evaluation of chemotherapy. Chemotherapy efficacy for osteosarcoma before operation may be evaluted by quantitative study of ^{18}F-FDG [12], and

^{18}F-FDG imaging (SPECT/CT) to detect what primary carcinoma lesion is from and location for biopsy pathological confirmed diagnosis metastatic carcinoma[10] FIGURE.8, to solve the medical difficult problem.

Primary Academic contributions to this project 《Application of Radionuclide Imaging in Osteosarcoma》 [11]Cited by Ruijin Hospital, Shanghai Jiao Tong University School of Medicine Feng Guo-wei etc. reported a case bone scan uptake ^{99m}Tc-MDP increased appearance in aggressive osteosarcoma with pleural,lung metastases demonstrated by operative pathological specimen[13]: Using SPECT Imaging and Molecular probe with tracer ^{99m}Tc-MDP, After following up 133 patients with osteosarcoma,Peng Jingjing et al thought, ^{99m}Tc-MDP SPECT images for detection of pulmonary and bone metastases and recurrent is useful. The usefulness of bone scintigraphy is overall in that is more sensitive than radiograph, X-ray and bone scan may be complementary in favor of the patients diagnoses, treatment and follow up.

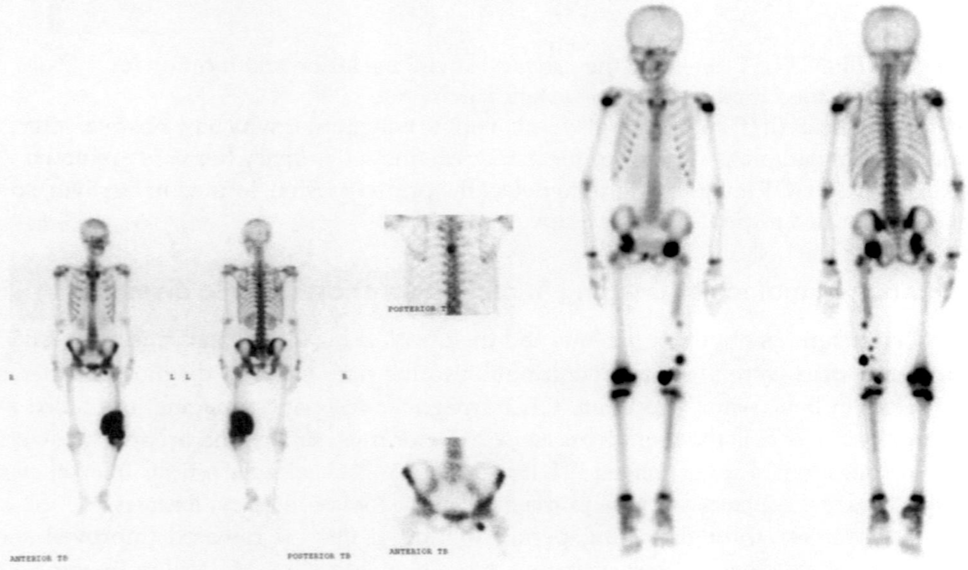

(A) (B)

Fig. 7. Bone scan showed Osteosarcoma focus for ^{99m}Tc-MDP positive imaging tracing metastases in bone and lymph node with surgical pathology confirmed (A) and recurrence indication after operation (B).

For unknown primary tumor of bone metastases performed PET/CT scan is necessary because of variety of ^{18}F-FDG, a sensitive tracer of malignant tumor, to identify the primary tumor so that patients can receive timely treatment. Unknown primary metastatic tumors occur in approximately 5% to 6.5%, according to report at least 1 / 3 of patients with PET detected the primary lesion, in which patients receive accurate and timely treatment.

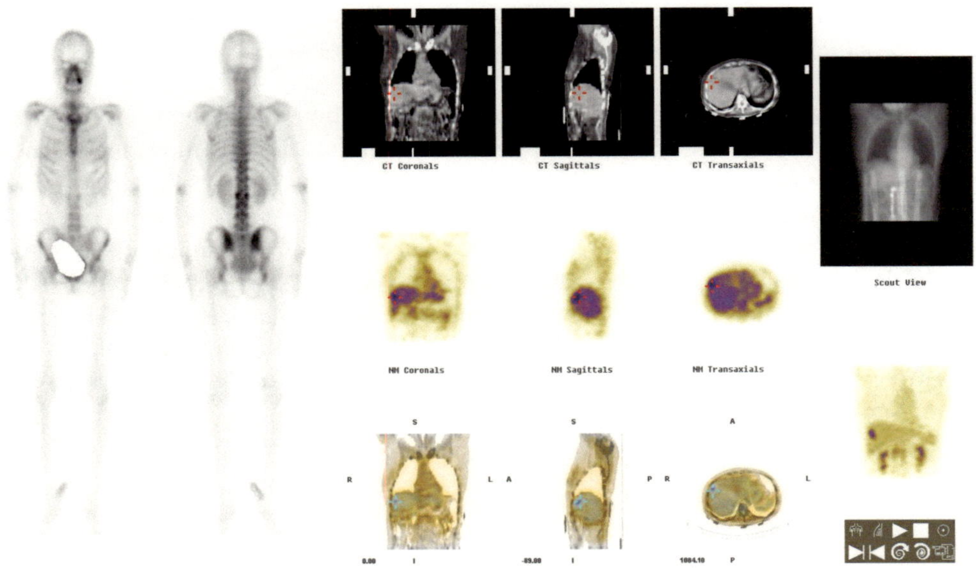

Fig. 8. ^{18}F-FDG SPECT/CT detecting the primary carcinoma lesion and location for pathological confirmed lumbar spine metastatic carcinoma.
^{99m}Tc-MDP bone scan (left) seen in single lumbar spine bone tumor which by hospital after operation surgical pathology confirmed metastatic carcinoma, primary tumor is unknown. By ^{18}F-FDG SPECT / CT imaging (right) to detect the primary lesion, located in the liver, so the patient performed a specific liver therapy.

5. Application of molecular imaging in diagnosis of orthopedic diseases

In the difficult diagnosis of puzzle patients and treatment, bring forth diagnostic ^{99m}Tc-MDP bone scan new ideas were a positive contribution to the pati. Difficult diagnosed patients were abnormal in bone scan, X-ray film, CT, or magnetic resonance imaging, but failed to identify problems .What is the real illness cause? Doctor must timely and accurate answers to diagnostic questions. Famous Beijing JST Hospital is the first choice for patients from all over the country whose first symptoms are bone pain and pathologic (or insufficiency) fractures.
JST' hospital doctors through a long period of careful clinical research improved the cognitive level of medical images, bringing the new ideas in Molecular Imaging in Diagnosis of Orthopedic Diseases. We summed up the imaging features diagnosis law of parathyroid tumor, and differentiate diagnosis regular pattern from other diseases on bone scan, used the scientific theory to guide clinical practice.
The patients complained of bone pain for unknown reasons. Fracture was diagnosed accurately by the bone scan. Patients diagnosed with metabolic bone disease primary hyperparathyroidism were treated with surgically removing of parathyroidoma, metabolic bone diseases by secondary hyperparathyroidism such as renal osteopathy or Rickets went to department of internal medicine treatment. Patients diagnosed with Multiple myeloma were treated in the hematology department. Patients diagnosed with articular disease were treated in the orthopedics [14] or rheumatology department. Patients diagnosed with benign or malignant bone primary tumor or bone disease were treated in bone oncology or

pediatrics orthopedic department. Importantly, which eliminate the burden of mind for the patients without serious diseases. Application of the research findings for imaging diagnoses can not only exclude the difficulty and anxiety for patients and get the suitable cure in a timely manner, but also provide the effective way for acquire the best economy and social performance.

The bone scans imaging differential diagnosis of parathyroid adenoma there are eight of typical image patterns which a doctor should be familiar with in clinical diagnoses. Have you had an knowledge of thereinafter imaging diagnoses Trained continued medical education[4]?

5.1 Primary hyperparathyroidism caused by a parathyroid adenoma

Metabolic bone disease

【case report】 Female patient, 29 years old complaining of pain in low back and both knees for 4 years, lower extremity weakness, vomiting and kidney stones 2 years. X-ray film showed severe osteoporosis, and fracture of the right pubic bone.

【The results of tests】 Ca ↑ 3.27 mmol / L (2.25 ~ 2.75), P ↓ 0.78 mmol / L (0.8 ~ 1.6), AKP ↑ 1002 mmol / L (25 ~ 90), parathyroid hormone (PTH) ↑ 70.1 (0.8 ~ 3.9)

【^{99m}Tc-MDP Bone scan】

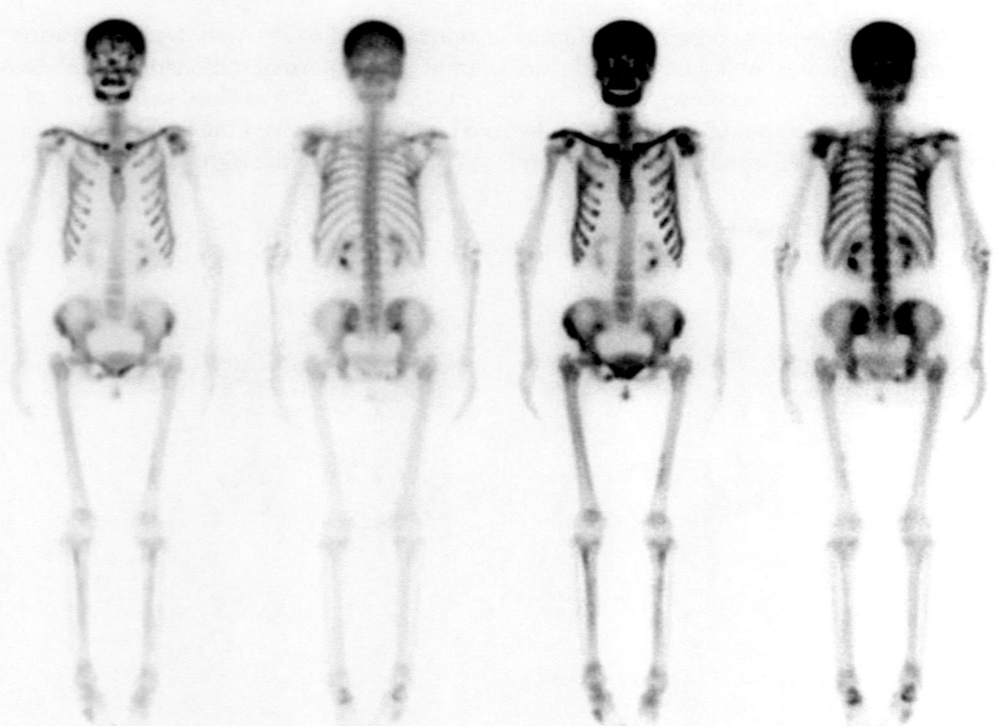

Fig. 9. ^{99m}Tc-MDP Bone scan showed metabolic disease with HPT

Whole body bone scan

After Intravenous imaging agent ^{99m}Tc-MDP 20mCi 3 hours, whole body bone scan was obtained (Fig. 9.) Bone image is very clearly. The skull showed increased radioactivity universal distribution. Axial skeleton and limb bones are visible with increased uptake - "super scan" of hyperparathyroidism Metabolism Bone disease; local increased radioactivity at the fracture site in the right pubic bone. Renal imaging was light, for radiation occlusion in double renal pelvis due to kidney stones with urinary obstruction.

【neck ultrasound】 no seen abnormal in thyroid

【diagnosis 】 Ectopic parathyroid adenoma

【Treatment】 Surgical resection of ectopic parathyroid adenoma.

Two years later, the patient recovered.

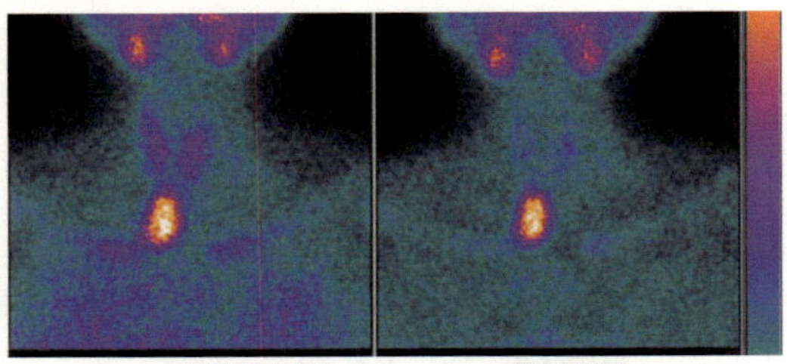

(A)15MIN (B)2HR

Fig. 10. ^{99m}Tc -MIBI parathyroid tumor imaging

^{99m}Tc-MIBI double-phase parathyroid tumor imaging: Early image (A)shows, the position and morphology of double-leaf thyroid were normal. The abnormal radioactive uptake can be seen on the right side below thyroid, the lower edge of which was close to the level of sternum .The size is about 3.8cm × 2.4cm. Delayed image (B) showed the thyroid image faded, and the oval-shaped abnormal lesion is still visible below the right side of thyroid.

5.2 Metastases “Super scan”

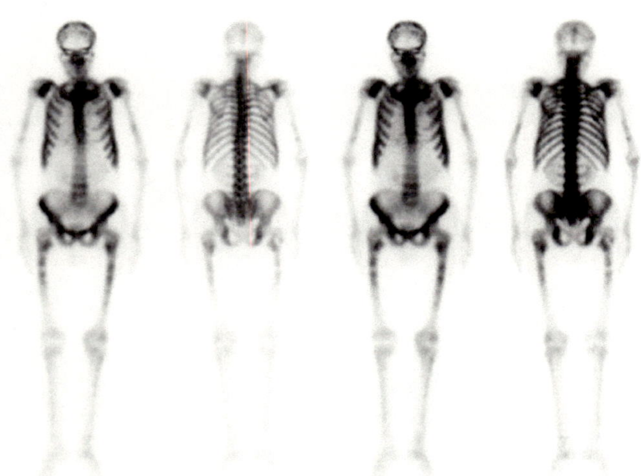

Fig. 11. Bone and bone marrows Metastases from poorly differentiated adenocarcinoma.

"Super scan" caused by extensive bone and marrow metastasis is different from the one caused by metabolic bone disease with hyperparathyroidism. The metastasis' Super scan is characterized by diffuse uptake of lesions mainly located in the axial skeleton and proximal limbs, which can be spotty radioactivity concentration.

In hyperparathyroidism resulting in metabolic bone disease, "Super scan" is involving the entire bone. "The black skull" is obviously. Radioactivity distributes diffusely and evenly.

5.3 Hypertrophic Osteoarthropathy

Hypertrophic Osteoarthropathy caused by Secondary form intrathoracic pathological condition which is a form of periostitis and may be painful. Tubular bones may show periosteal new bone formation. This pathological feature explains the typical bone scan pattern of diffusely increased uptake along the cortical margins of long bones giving the appearance of "parallel tracks".

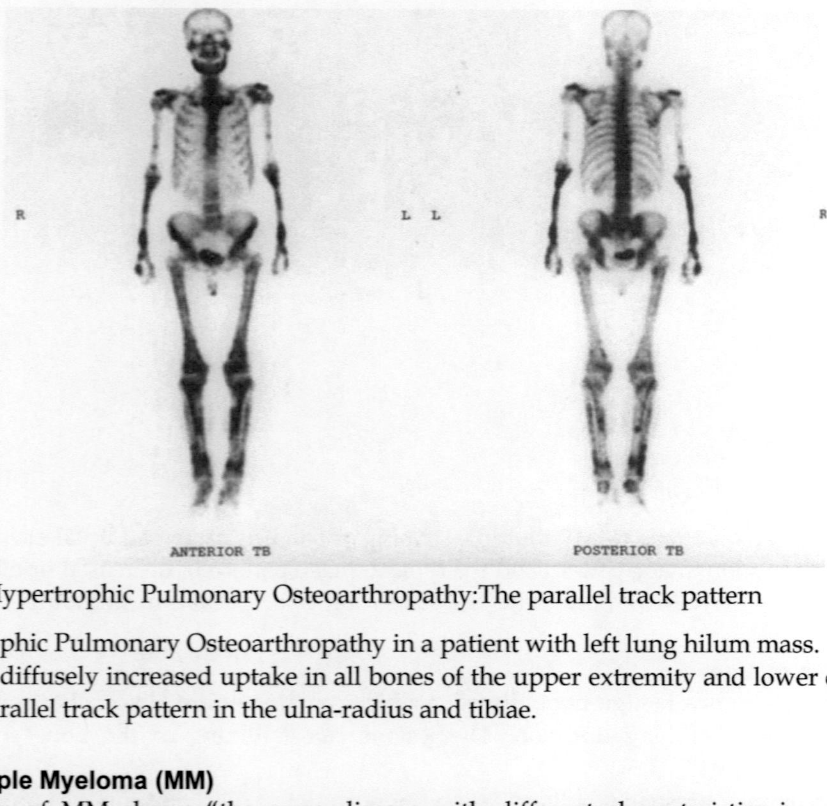

Fig. 12. Hypertrophic Pulmonary Osteoarthropathy:The parallel track pattern

Hypertrophic Pulmonary Osteoarthropathy in a patient with left lung hilum mass.

Note the diffusely increased uptake in all bones of the upper extremity and lower extremity with a parallel track pattern in the ulna-radius and tibiae.

5.4 Multiple Myeloma (MM)

Bone scan of MM shows "the same disease with different characteristics images". The patient's image can have many manifestations: multiple uptake Increase strip or banding, decreased uptake cold spot lesions [15], which mainly distribute in the spine, pelvis, ribs, skull and proximal long bone.

In clinical work, some MM bone scan image does not show the bone destruction, so bone scan revealed no abnormalities. Imaging physicians and orthopedic surgeons should pay attention to the patient's complain for bone pain, considering for multiple myeloma.

Patient's relevant laboratory tests, bone pain, anemia, infection and renal dysfunction and related organ or tissue damage (ROTI) should be recorded.

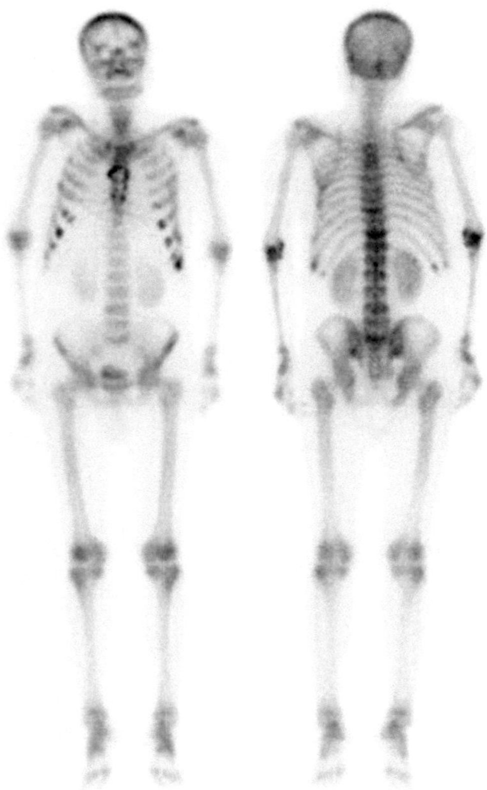

Fig. 13. Multiple Myeloma (MM) multiple striping or banding increased uptake with Spinal is the most common image pattern and the typical image pattern of decreased uptake "Cold spot" lesions on ^{99m}Tc-MDP Bone scan (Note the "Cold spot" lesions in sternum)

5.5 Fibrous dysplasia

Fibrous dysplasia is a benign bone disorder which remains essentially unchanged and can be seen in lesion of long duration. The lesions cause thining of the bone cortex and replacement marrow.

The condition may present as solitary lesion (monostotic) or with multiple foci (polyostotic). Polyostotic fibrous dysplasia may be associated with café-au-lait pigmentation and multiple endocrine hyperfunction, most commonly seen as precocious puberty in girls, Cushing's syndrome, and is called the McCune-Albrightzonght syndrome.

Standard radiographs show lucent areas with various amounts of ossification and cyst formation and may show expansion. Fibrous dysplasia, in general appears as an area of markedly increased uptake on ^{99m}Tc-MDP bone scan.

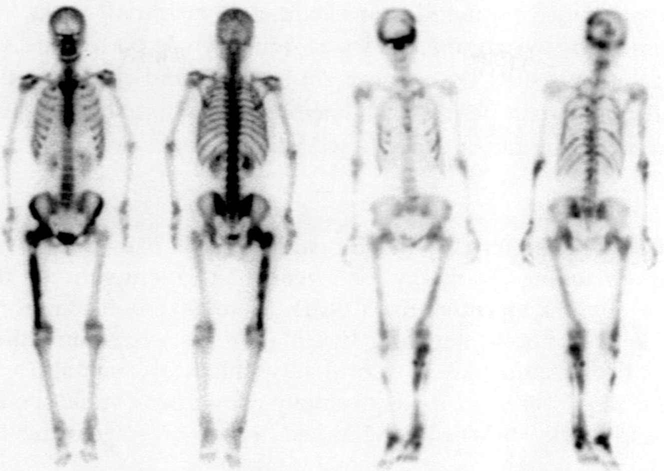

Fig. 14. Fibrous dysplasia (A) monostotic the right femur (B) polyostotic for whole body bone

Bone scan image show intensely increased uptake in lesion bones.
Whole body bone scan used for overlook the Fibrous dysplasia condition present as solitary lesion (monostotic) or with multiple foci (polyostotic).

5.6 Rheumatoid Arthritis

Rheumatoid Arthritis is the autoimmune disease causes inflammation of the connective tissue mainly in the joints. Synovitis activity is the dominant clinical variable that determines the therapeutic approachin patients with rheumatoid arthritis. ^{99m}Tc-MDP bone scan used for overlook the all joint to measure the condition present of synovitis activity and differential diagnosis from other diseases result in bone-joint pain.

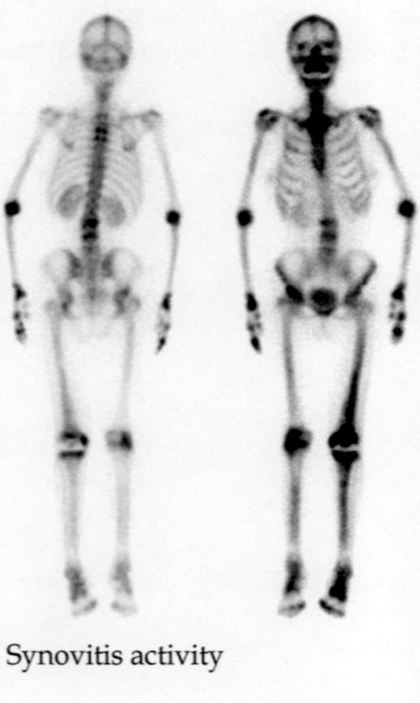

Fig. 15. Rheumatoid Arthritis Synovitis activity

A 52 years old female patient, suffered from rheumatoid arthritis 4 years. The left knee was painful and deformed for six months. TKA was done. Whole body bone scan showed that left knee joint was after treated by replacement surgery, and rheumatoid arthritis (active phase) violated elbows, wrists, hands, hips, knees, feet and thoracic and lumbar spine with Increase uptake in the areas of the joints affected Synovitis activity.

5.7 Rickets

A 41-year-old male patient suffered from joint pain and back pain more than 5 years and his lower limbs were weakening gradually for 1 year. The patient suffered from intermittent back pain with no obvious incentive for 5 years, more severe in the morning.It was also accompanied by joint stiffness, which reduced after the event, and did not affect the activities. Initially he was treated at a local hospital as rheumatoid arthritis, the pain releived. But in the past 2 years, the pain gradually got worse, double shoulder, hips, chest, leg were painful and weak. He was bound to bed, get up on stage difficultly. He was 7cm lower then when he was young.

Tests carried out and The results showed

Serum calcium (Ca) 2.4mmol / L (2.25-2.75)

Serum phosphorus (P) ↓ 0.53mmol / L (0.8-1.6)

Alkaline phosphatase (AKP) ↑ 480 IU / L (25-90)

Rheumatoid factor (RF)-negative

HLA-B27- negative

A/G were normal, renal function BUN, CRE, UA mused in the normal range.

Spine X-ray showed osteoporosis. MRI reported suspected pelvis bone destruction. Whole body bone scan (Figure16) shows skeletal clearly: Bilateral ribs show multiple hot spots, as "beaded ribs"; the spine shows multiple vertebral collapse as strip change; The agent ^{99m}Tc-MDP uptake in shoulders is increased, and the left is more; There are ribbon-like zones increased uptake in rib cage, pelvis, femora, tibia and metatarsals. Bone scintigraphy scan shows metabolic bone disease: A specific abnormality of the rickets is the presence of Looser's zones, also called Pseudofractures or Milkman's fractures.

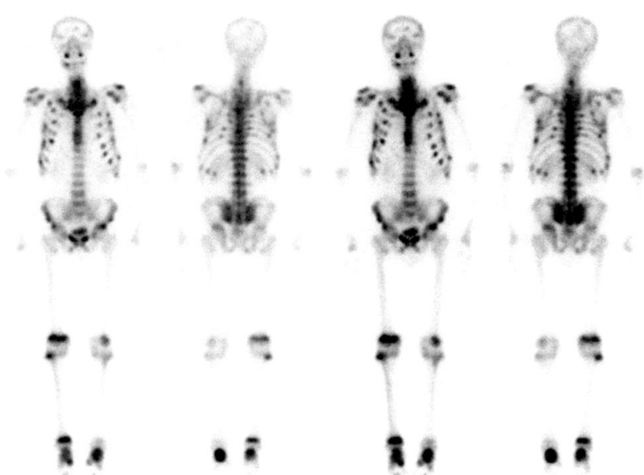

Fig. 16. Diagnostic Imaging feature of Rickets

Bone scintigraphy scan shows metabolic bone disease. Note there are ribbon-like zones multiple foci increased uptake in rib cage caused by pseudofractures on bone scans mimicking metastatic bone disease. This characterstic pseudofractures is one of specific abnormality of Rickets.

The presence of Looser's zones, also called Pseudofractures or Milkman's fractures, there are ribbon-like zones increased uptake in rib cage, pelvis, right distal femora 、tibia,Bilateral metatarsals and spinal column, Long-standing Osteomalacia result in characteristic Biconcave collapsed vertebrae.

We recommended further examination: 1.25-dihydroxyvitamin D_3 [1, 25 - (OH) $_2D_3$] 26.75pg/ml (26 -65pg/ml), Parathyroid hormone PTH ↑ 84.6 pg / ml (8.3 -68.0), 24-hour urine calcium 0.36mmol, urinary phosphorus 38.13mmol.

Diagnosis: The patient was diagnosed as hypophosphatemic rickets based on the fact of middle-aged male patients with chronic process. The bone pain and muscle weakness was the main manifestation, which progressively increased and lead to movement disorder. Laboratory tests: normal calcium, hypophosphatemia and elevated ALP. Bone scan with pseudo fractures are the characteristic of bone scan imaging finding prompted rickets. The diagnosis of hypophosphatemic rickets was established. Increased PTH caused by hyperparathyroidism was secondary to rickets.

After three years of out-patient and hospital treatment, this patient has been able to work properly.

The patient's ^{99m}Tc-MDP bone scan image shows the pseudofeatures of metabolic bone disease: rib pseudofracture site showed local radioactivity uptake; ribbon-like zones increased uptake in spine, pelvis and lower extremities which embodiment Osteomalacia reflect the pathological changes of pseudofracture in rickets.

Rickets refers that bone matrix of adults whose epiphyseal growth plate has been closed mineralized impediently. It is a metabolic bone disease that newly formed bone matrix is not mineralized in the normal manner. There are many causes responsible for decreased extracellular calcium phosphate product, and resulted in bone mineral deposition obstacles. The clinical manifestations of rickets are mainly bone pain and muscle weakness, fractures and deformities. Metabolic bone disease, pseudo fractures are the characteristic of bone scan imaging finding.

Rickets belongs to endocrine and metabolic diseases. Now there are many related diseases, including seven sets of issues: Associated with vitamin D endocrine system diseases, phosphate balance abnormalities, metabolic acidosis, abnormal calcium balance, bone matrix abnormalities, lack of primary mineralization, some factors leading to the inhibition of mineralization. Although the clinical presentation is similar, but the pathogenic mechanisms are different, relating biochemical laboratory examination and treatment are also different. Therefore, in the diagnosis of rickets, we need the systematic, in-depth inspection and analysis to clarify the etiology. Diagnosis and treatment guide of rickets refers to Cecil Medicine.

5.8 Paget's disease (Osteitis deformans)

A 54 years old male patient, complained of "left knee pain, glided into varus deformity leg 4 years, left muscle atrophy, walking inconvenience", were diagnosed as Paget's Osteitis by pathology.

Whole body bone scan showed characteristic bone expansion changes: left tibia was bending deformity; T4 vertebral body, left pelvis and tibia in the active stage of osteolysis which osteogenesis showed increased uptake. The radioactivity distribution of the left humerus was mild and uniform in sclerotic phase.

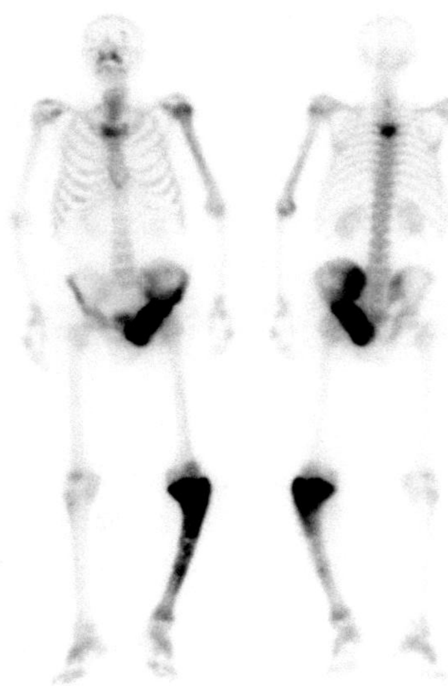

Fig. 17. Diagnostic Imaging of Paget's disease

Bone scintigraphy scan shows increased uptake in the left tibia with bending deformation, T4 and left pelvis with enlargement and bending deformans of the bones affected with lytic the active phase. The Left humerus shows no abnormal uptake of the radiopharmaceuticals with time on the sclerotic phase indicating a relatively inactive lesion.

6. Ensure patient safety preventing traumatic complication Acute Pulmonary Embolism (APE)

Beijing Ji Shui Tan Hospital is a large modern comprehensive hospital which focuses on Orthopadic and traumatology. The surgical volume reached 35000 in 2009. Clinical research in medical imaging make a positive contribution for the protection of medical quality and patient safety, during the process of exploring critical and difficult orthopadic patients and optimize the efficacy of the diagnosis.

The treatment of post-traumatic critically ill patients with acute pulmonary embolism (APE)
In Nov. 10, 2000, a 56-year-old man fell from 3 meters high and got multiple traumas (Right hip fracture, fracture of the right pubis ischium branch, open comminuted fracture of the right olecranon). On Nov. 20, when the patient received second operation of open reduction and plate fixation for the right fracture acetabular under general anesthesia, he had chest tightness, shortness of breath, PaO_2 critical situation of declining. Orthopedic surgery was stopped and the rescue was implemented in the ICU ward immediately. ECG shows sinus tachycardia and S□Q□ T□ & V_1rsr 'wave, which was believed to be acute pulmonary embolism. Lung perfusion ECT was done for the patient immediately in nuclear medicine department.
^{99m}Tc-MAA Lung perfusion Imaging showed lung with morphologic abnormalities. Right lung was lobe and segmental perfusion defects, and left lung shows segmental perfusion defects (figure 18). With normal X-ray before surgery (Nov. 18), V / Q diagnosis was done-acute pulmonary embolism. In the ICU ward the patient received anticoagulation and thrombolytic therapy. 2 weeks later (Dec. 4), pulmonary perfusion imaging (Figure 19) was reviewed, the original lobe and segmental perfusion defects had been seen the distribution of perfusion and lung morphology was normal after effectively treatment. X-ray and ECG were normal too. The patient was pulled through by accurate diagnoses and effective treatment.

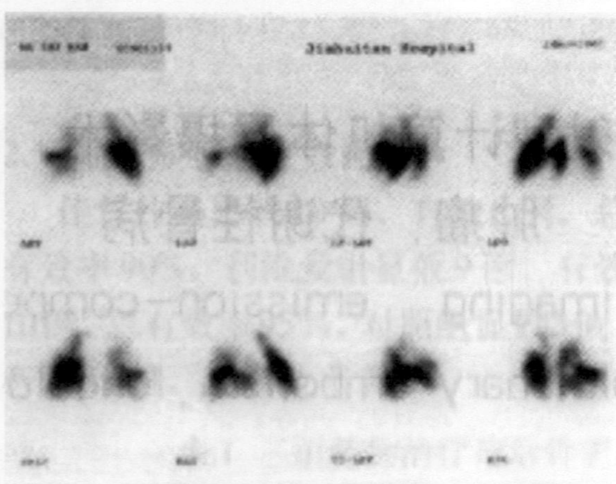

Fig. 18. Lung perfusion imaging of post-traumatic acute pulmonary embolism

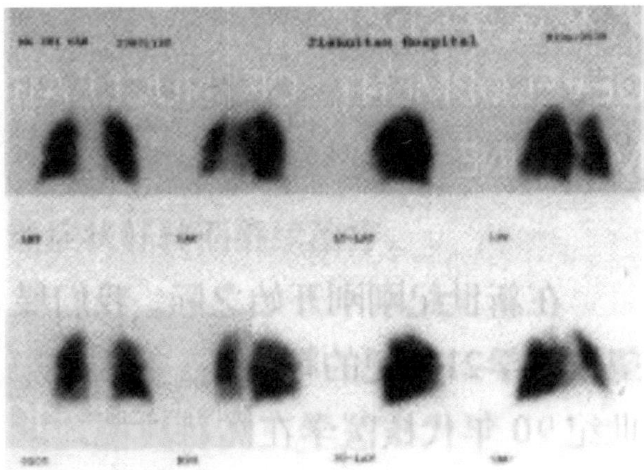

Fig. 19. 2 weeks after treatment, normal lung perfusion imaging

Timely diagnosis and successful treatment of the patient with large area of APE after injury is described in paper <Advancement in the Application of Nuclear Medicine> published in Apr.2001 V7N4:59-61 Journal of "China Contemporary Medicine". This paper inspired Beijing Ji Shui Tan Hospital on the understanding and study of acute pulmonary embolism[1. Doctors can see directly from the image: lower limb Thrombosis bring about post-traumatic pulmonary embolism is an important research topic. Early diagnosis and treatment for APE patients can prevent recurrent thromboembolism. It can improve the cure rate, reduce mortality and ensure medical safety of patients before and after surgery.

The development of molecular imaging in China should follow simple, efficient, accurate principles. Accuracy is the key]. Accurate diagnosis and effective treatment cost savings and improve quality of life. Development of medicine, science and technology reflects in significant health benefits for the people.

7. Acknowledgements

The author would like to thank the teachers at JST Hospital Orthopedic: Prof. Shu-huan Wang, Prof. Guo-wei Rong, Beijing Hospital Nuclear Medicine -Prof. Wan-ying Qu and Peking Union Medical College Hospital -Prof. Qian Zhou for their valuable contribution and inspiration.

The author would also like to express gratitude to all who have kindly helped in realization of this chapter: JST Hospital lead orthopedist Wei Tian, oncologist You bo Cai, Qing-zhang, and pathologist Hong-hong Liu,surgeon Fu rong Xia,. Thank you for your expertise and scientific efforts. Thanks to the Technologists of Dept. Nuclear Medicine JST and my students Dr. Jin Feng, Dr. Lian-na Zhang and Dr. Fang Yang for their time and scrupulous work.The author would like to express her sincerest gratitude to the patients.

8. References

[1] Jing jing Peng, Wei Tian *(corresponding author) Application of bone scintigraphy in the fracture diagnosis. Guide of China Medicine 2010; 8(5): 115-118.

[2] Jing-jing Peng, Hong-hong Liu *(corresponding author), Xia Fu-rong,Cai You-Bo ^{99m}Tc-MDP Bone Imaging Diagnoses of parathyroid tumors. Chin J Nucl Med, 2003;23(6):263-265

[3] Jing-jing Peng Advancement in application of *nuclear medicine* .China Contemporary Medicine 2001; 7(4):59-61

[4] Jing-jing Peng Advancement in clinical application of *orthopedic nuclear medicine* (lectures)Chin J of Bone Tumor and Bone Disease 2009; 8(6): 356-359

[5] Jiang-lin Chen, Zhao-chang Lin, Shu-ping Tang.Case report: Qualitative and location diagnosis with nuclear medicine of primary hyperparathyroidism. Anthology of Medicine Apr.2006; 25 2:361-362 (PEER REVIEWS AND EVALUATIONS)

[6] Book Orthopedic Nuclear Medicine, Berlin: springer, 2004 ISBN: 3-540-00614-1 Book Editor:Abdelhamid. H. Elgazzar.(translation <Orthopedic Nuclear Medicine> into Chinese Publication ISBN-978-7-117-12367-9/R·12368 Book Editor:Jing-jing Peng,Wei Tian *)

[7] Book *Diagnostic Imaging Orthopedic Nuclear Medicine* ISBN-978-7-117-13047-9/R·13048 Book Editor: Jing-jing Peng Chapter 1 Fundamental Researches: New concept of orthopedic molecular imaging

[8] Book *Clinical Orthopedics* ISBN-7-5323-7404-1 Book Editor: Shu-huan Wang: Jing-jing Peng Chapter: Radionuclide Imaging

[9] Book Chinese *Medical Imaging* ISBN-978-7-117-12740-0/R·12741 Book Editor: Qian Zhou, Wanying Qu Jing-jing Peng Chapter Bone Scintigrapy: Primary bone tumors section 4217-4221

[10] Book *Practical Orthopedics of Jishuitan* ISBN-978-7-117-09461-0 Book Editor: Wei Tian Jing-jing Peng Chapter :PET Imaging 69-76

[11] Jing-jing Peng, Guo-wei Rong * (corresponding author), Qing Zhang, You-bo Cai et,al Application of Radionuclide Imaging in Osteosarcoma. Chin J Nucl Med, 2000;20(2):65-67

[12] Jin Feng, Jing-jing Peng * (corresponding author), Hong-hong Liu Yang Fang, Xiao-hui Niu Response of osteosarcoma to chemotherapy evaluated by ^{18}F-FDG Imaging Chin J of Clinic med imaging 2010,21(9):638-640

[13] Guo-wei Feng, Zhong-yi Yang, Liang Guan, Cheng-mo Zhu Case report: Lung Metastases Diagnosis with ^{99m}Tc-MDP Bone Scan Tracing of Osteosarcoma. (PEER REVIEWS AND EVALUATIONS) Chinese Journal of Nuclear Medicine 2007;(27)6:372

[14] Jing jing Peng, Xu Fu. Radionuclide Image manifestation characteristics in osteoarthritis of knee Chin J Nucl Med, 1988;8(3):142-144 Chin J of Med Imaging Technology 2008,24(1):127-130

[15] Yan-xia Bai, Jing jing Peng *(corresponding author), Fang Yang, Min-qiu Lu. Detecting bone lesions of patient multiple myloma on scintigraphy. Chin J Med Imaging Technol. 2008;24 (7):1106-1109

[16] Zhang Yun-jian , Zhao Ning , Xia Guo-guang, Li Tian-shui, Wang Yan-xia. Prognostic factors for patients with pulmonary thromboembolism after orthopedic surgery Journal of Peking University (Health Sciences) 2010,42(6):798-710

5

Imaging Findings of Adipocytic Tumors

Jun Nishida, Shigeru Ehara and Tadashi Shimamura
Departments of Orthopaedic Surgery and Radiology,
School of Medicine Iwate Medical University, Morioka City,
Japan

1. Introduction

Adipose tissue tumors are the most common soft tissue tumors in both benign and malignant categories. A presumptive diagnosis of the adipose tissue tumors usually can be made based on the imaging findings [5]. However, there are some exceptions. Making differential diagnosis of hibernoma from lipoma-like well-differentiated liposarcoma may be difficult by imaging findings, while the making histological diagnosis is not difficult. Lipoma-like well-differentiated liposarcomas can mimic intramuscular or intermuscular lipomas in radiological as well as histological findings, and they may occasionally cause problems in establishing diagnosis and treatment planning. Although making differential diagnosis of these benign lesions from lipoma-like well-differentiated liposarcomas may be important, it may also be important to make a differential diagnosis between intramuscular lipoma, intermuscular lipoma and hibernoma for appropriate surgical treatment and follow-up, because differences in recurrence rates among these benign tumors exist.
The purpose of this section is to elucidate the differences in imaging features among these adipocytic neoplasms for appropriate treatment planning. The imaging findings of other adipocytic sarcomas are also included.

2. Intramuscular lipoma

Intramuscular lipoma is difficult to differentiate from lipoma-like liposarcoma, and imaging findings are useful for differentiating from liposarcomas. The common sites of occurrence include the thigh (particularly the quadriceps and hamstring muscles), deltoid, triceps brachii and pectoralis major muscles.; all of which are relatively large muscles. The disease is most frequently found in the lower extremities, and is also commonly found in the upper extremities. As for the symptoms, a painless mass or tumor is the most common, accounting for approximately 60% of the cases [12], and a relatively large number of patients present mainly with swelling. A possible reason is that the lesions occur in the deep muscle layers and it cannot be easily palpated as a mass or tumor. Neuropathy is rarely seen: posterior interosseous nerve palsy is sometimes caused by the intramuscular lipoma in the supinator muscle. Pain as the main complaint is rare. CT findings are particularly characteristic. Typically, imaging features are spherical to oval, sharply demarcated space-occupying lesion whose density as a whole is the same as that of fat. The lesion has a streaky structure with the same density as that of the muscle (Fig. 1A). The thickness of the streaky structures varies, and the streaks may be discontinuous. At surgery, intramuscular lipomas are often removed with a part of the surrounding muscle to ensure an adequate surgical margin, because it is difficult to separate the lesion from the surrounding muscle. The reported local recurrence rates vary from 3.0 to 62.5% when intramuscular lipomas are simply removed without attempting wide resection [2, 3, 6, 9]. Therefore, wide resection is recommended to avoid local recurrence. However, such recommendation was made partly to prevent recurrence or dedifferentiation as a result of misdiagnosis of lipoma-like liposarcoma in an era when the accurate imaging diagnosis was not made, and the differences between intramuscular lipomas and well-differentiated liposarcomas were not fully recognized. The streaky structures observed on CT macroscopically and histologically represent muscle fibers involved in the lesion, and are often difficult to separate from the lesion. Although capsule or pseudocapsule is not generally obvious macroscopically, intramuscular lipomas are multilocular elastic soft lesions, similar to normal subcutaneous lipomas. However, in approximately 15% of the cases, no streaks are observed on CT and the lesions have a capsule that allows separating easily from the surrounding muscle tissue at surgery [12]. Macroscopically, intramuscular lipomas are yellowish multilocular lesions with a smooth surface similar to normal lipomas, and have a capsule in some cases. The streaky structures are visualized as low signal intensities on T2-weighted MR images, however, it is believed that these tumors cannot be as clearly detected by MR as by CT, because of the strong high signal intensities in the lesion, representing fat (Fig. 1B).

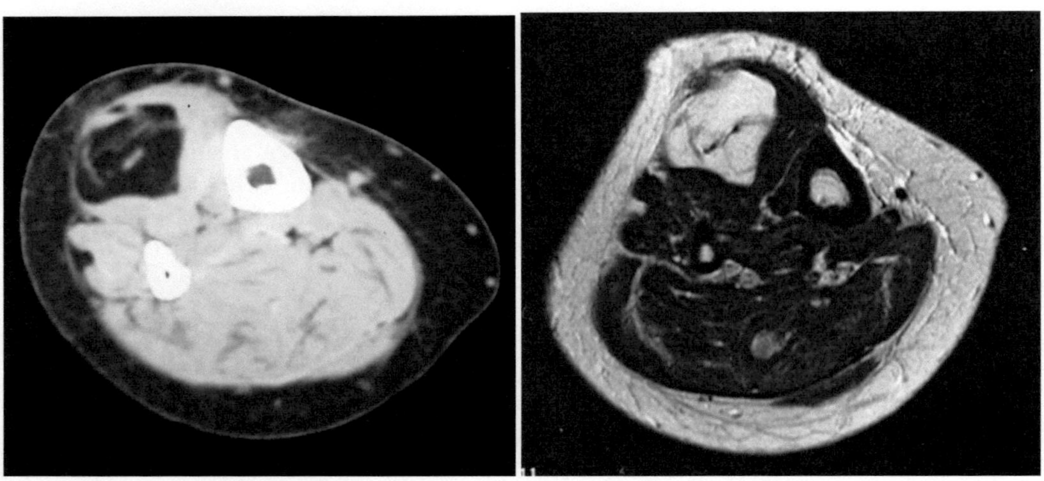

A B

Fig. 1. A. Computed tomography reveals a fat density mass containing thick streaks with occasional interruption. B. Magnetic resonance imaging (axial T2 weighted image) demonstrates a fat signal mass with streaky structures are in the tibialis anterior muscle.

3. Intermuscular lipoma

Intermuscular lipoma is a benign lesion that literally occurs between deep muscles. The thigh is the most common site of occurrence, and the chest wall, buttock, forearm, upper arm and neck are also commonly involved. A painless mass is often observed as a presenting symptom, but only a few patients present with the chief complaint of swelling, since the lesion arises between muscles and extend into regions of low tissue pressure while growing; it is often recognized as mass on the body surface. Patients rarely complain of pain. On CT, intermuscular lipomas are most often visualized as space-occupying lesions with the same density as that of fat, a dumb-bell or gourd shaped, with a narrow part, and the streakiness inside the lesions are characteristic (Fig. 2A). However, such streaky structures are thinner and more continuous and have smoother curves than those in intramuscular lipomas in many cases. Similar findings are also seen on MR imaging, but the streaky structures visualized as low signal intensities on T2-weighted images may not be so prominent due to the high signal intensity of the whole lesion, similar to intramuscular lipomas (Fig. 2B). At surgery, intermuscular lipomas can be easily manually separated from the surrounding tissues. The streaky structure on CT is fibrous tissue in the fascia and inter-tissue spaces, and can be easily detached by lifting from the margin of the lesion. Intermuscular lipomas are encapsulated and marginal resection is easily performed. Both the macroscopic and histological appearances are similar to those of normal lipomas and no muscle tissue is observed. Basically recurrence or complications are not common.

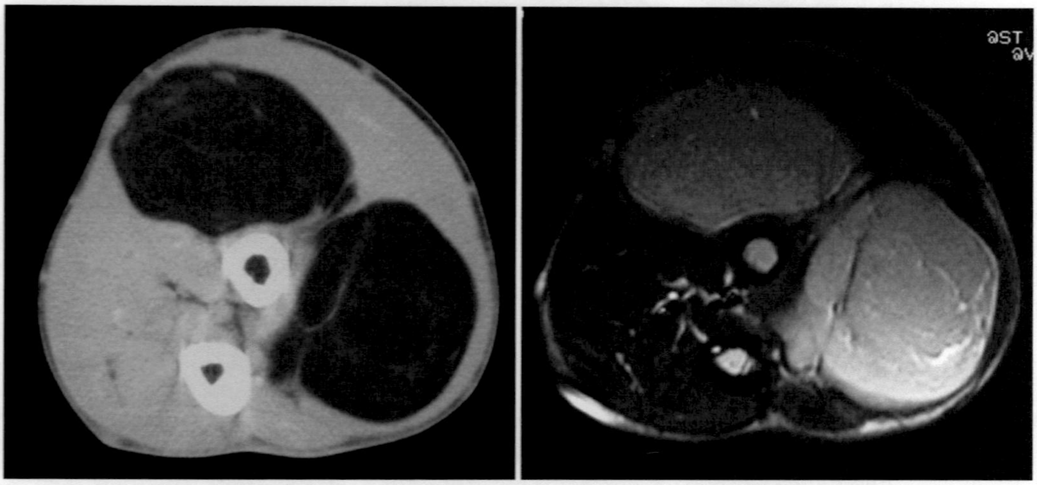

A B

Fig. 2. A. Computed tomography reveals a dumb-bell-shaped fat density tumor containing thin streaky densities in intermuscular lipoma of the forearm. B. Magnetic resonance imaging of the intermuscular lipoma (axial T2 weighted image) reveals a high signal intensity mass. The streaky structures are seen again but are less distinctive than on computed tomography.

4. Hibernoma

Hibernoma is a lesion showing proliferation of adipocytes similar to those in brown fat in hibernators. In humans, brown fat usually exists in the neck, upper back, retroperitoneum, and they are the common sites of hibernoma. On CT, hibernoma is depicted as a low-density mass with a higher density than normal subcutaneous fat, and that is the cause of easily confusion of this lesion to lipoma-like liposarcoma, because an amorphous hazy high density is also seen (Figure 3A). It has recently been reported that hibernomas show a much higher degree of accumulation than liposarcomas on PET images (Figure 3B), and PET is currently considered as a major modality for differentiation between benignity and malignancy [13]. Histologically, brown adipocytes are characteristic.

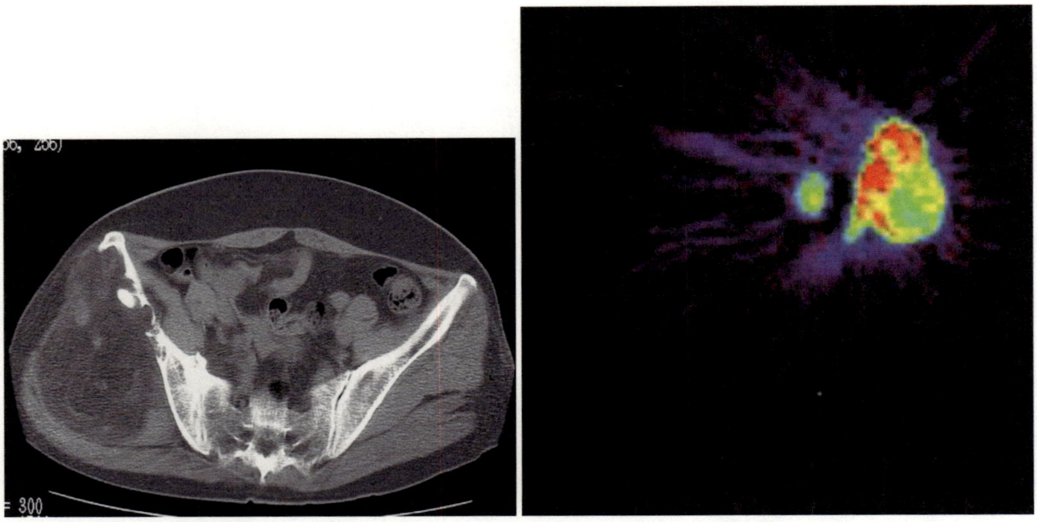

A B

Fig. 3. A. Axial slice of computed tomography of a case with hibernoma demonstrated a fat density lesion with areas of hazy amorphous density in the medial compartment of the pelvis. B. Coronal FDG PET showed the extremely intense uptake (SUV : 98.1). Used with permission from Med Sci Monit [13].

5. Well-differentiated liposarcoma

Well-differentiated liposarcoma is a locally aggressive, low-grade malignancy with some atypia in the proliferating adipocytes and stromal cells, and is classified into 3 subtypes: lipoma-like, inflammatory and sclerosing-type. The thigh is the most common site of occurrence, but the retroperitoneum, lower leg are also commonly involved. As for symptoms, a slowly growing painless mass is often seen, accompanied by neurologic symptoms in some cases. Well-differentiated liposarcoma often occurs in deep soft tissue layer, and some patients complain of swelling. Imaging findings are relatively characteristic and are often useful for differentiation, particularly from benign tumors other than hibernomas. On CT, well-differentiated liposarcomas are basically visualized as lipid-rich lesions consisting of the same density areas as fat, associated with slightly or clearly containing amorphous hazy high-density areas, and areas with other soft tissue densities (Figure 4A). The proportion of lipomatous and non-lipomatous areas, and non-lipomatous component is not clearly visualized in lipoma-like liposarcoma. Therefore, it is often difficult to differentiate between benig and malignant tumors either by imaging or histologocal findings. However, accurate evaluation of the amorphous-hazy high density is helpful for making a correct diagnosis. On T2-weighted MR image a proportion of muscle fibers, in the form of thick bundles, is often found to be incorporated into the lesion on the images. However, because of the strong fat signal, the findings are more characteristic on CT images (Figure 4B). Macroscopically, well-differentiated liposarcomas are harder than lipomas in general and contain more fibrous tissue, which occasionally involve musclular layer. However, lipoma-like liposarcoma has a cut surface similar to that of benign lipoma. In addition, well-differentiated liposarcoma is not so strongly adherent to the surrounding tissue and is often easily detached, and it makes differentiation from benign diseases difficult. Histologically, well-differentiated liposarcomas are characterized by atypical lipoblast proliferation as a part of this lesion and also spindle cell proliferation accompanied by collagen fiber proliferation among the adipocytes. Histological subtypes are determined by the degree of proliferation of the collagen fibers and spindle or fusiform cells, and the degree of inflammatory cellular infiltration, mainly lymphocytes. Well-differentiated liposarcomas are occasionally misdiagnosed as benign lesions due to a weak atypia, and when it is difficult to judge between benign or malignant nature of the lesion, imaging findings are very helpful. Well-differentiated liposarcoma is a low-grade malignancy with a low metastatic frequency. The prognosis is relatively good, however, the recurrence rate is high when wide resection is not performed. Many patients with well-differentiated liposarcoma in the retroperitoneum have a poor prognosis due to the difficulty of wide resection. In addition, patients often have huge lesions involving the femoral or sciatic nerves, and marginal resection is sometimes inevitably performed particularly in the elderly, to preserve the functions. In such cases, when the recurrence is repeated, dedifferentiated liposarcoma sometimes occurs. Therefore, particularly careful follow-up is necessary.

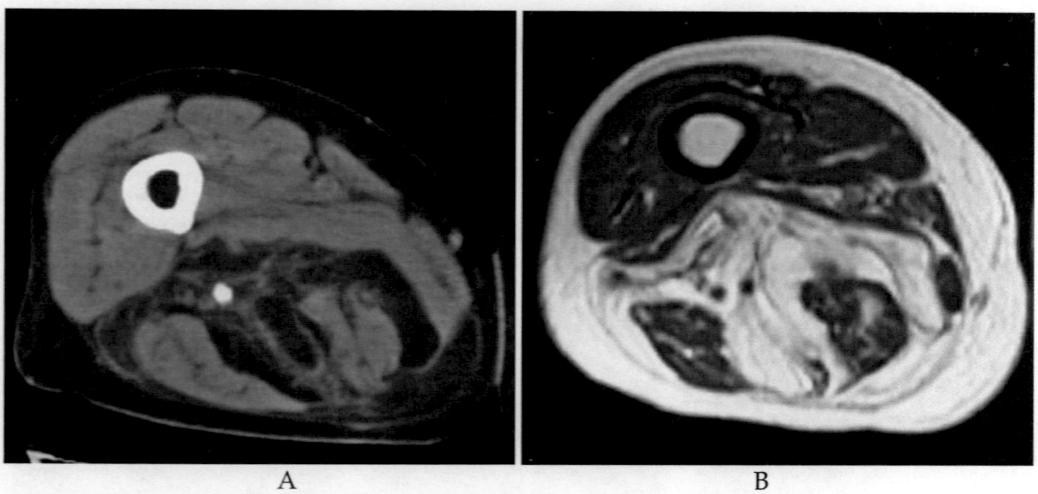

A B

Fig. 4. A. Computed tomography of a case with lipoma-like liposarcoma reveals a fat density mass spreading in the intra- and intermuscular space with amorphous hazy high density including streaky structures and septa with soft tissue density. The thickness of the streaky densities varies and is interrupted occasionally. B. Magnetic resonance imaging (axial T2 weighted image) reveals a high intensity tumor. The signal intensity is slightly lower than that of normal fat. The streaks are less distinctive than on computed tomography.

6. Dedifferentiated liposarcoma

In the WHO classification, dedifferentiated liposarcoma is a variant of well-differentiated liposarcoma transforming into high-grade sarcoma with various non-fatty tumor components. In most cases, the dedifferentiated areas show an appearance of high-grade malignant fibrous histiocytoma or fibrosarcoma. However, it has been reported that when the primary lesions were reassessed after development of the dedifferentiated liposarcoma, some patients had higher-grade malignant components than those initially seen. Thus, the precise pathology cannot be established initially in some cases with dedifferentiated liposarcoma. It is generally considered that the occurrence of dedifferentiation liposarcoma is time-dependent and that approximately 10% of well-differentiated liposarcomas dedifferentiate after at least a few years of progression. Dedifferentiated liposarcoma is often found in the retroperitoneum, and the reason is considered to be that well-differentiated liposarcomas in the retroperitoneum cannot be easily detected and cannot be radically resected, and lesions in the retroperitoneum are often found incidentally. In many cases of dedifferentiated liposarcoma in the extremities, a painless mass or tumor present for a long time suddenly grows rapidly before the patient visits the hospital. Both CT (Figure 5A) and MR imaging (Figure 5B) findings are similarly characteristic, and dedifferentiated liposarcomas are visualized as lesions in which non-fatty areas occur adjacent to lipid-rich components. The lipid-rich components show an appearance of well-differentiated liposarcoma, and areas with totally different area seen adjacent to that component. If a patient have a history of lipoma that grew rapidly after recurrence, it is relatively easy to make the diagnosis based on the history and imaging findings. However, histological diagnosis is sometimes difficult, like in the case of well-differentiated liposarcoma, unless biopsy specimens are taken precisely from the areas considered to be dedifferentiated on images. Thus, imaging findings are an important guide to the biopsy. On macroscopic examination, hard, dedifferentiated, gray to brown non-fatty areas are usually seen adjacent to fatty component areas, and it is consistent with the imaging findings. Necrosis is often

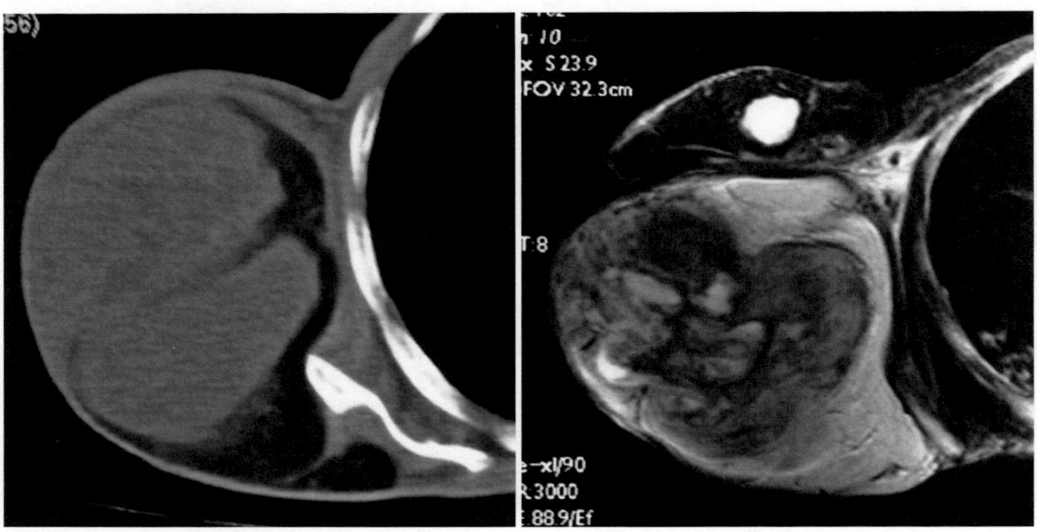

A B

Fig. 5. A. Computed tomography of dedifferentiated liposarcoma shows a muscle density mass in the fat density area. B. Magnetic resonance imaging (axial T2 weighted image) of dedifferentiated liposarcoma reveals a high and low signal intensity area adjacent to the high signal intensity area.

observed in dedifferentiated areas. Histologically, high-grade malignant component with clearly distinct histology are observed adjacent to areas of well-differentiated liposarcoma. The border between these areas is usually clear. On histological evaluation, major part of the dedifferentiated areas shows the appearances of malignant fibrous histiocytoma and fibrosarcoma, and various other features, including those of rhabdomyosarcoma and osteosarcoma, can also be observed depending on the case. Dedifferentiated liposarcoma is a high-grade malignancy and requires wide resection. Many patients with dedifferentiated liposarcoma of the retroperitoneum, a common site of occurrence, have a poor prognosis, because wide resection is not possible. However, despite the high-grade histological malignancy in the dedifferentiated areas, the probability of metastasis is not extremely high. The 5-year survival rate is approximately 70%, which is perhaps higher than the supposed rate, considering the histological malignancy and common sites of occurrence [7, 10, 16]. Nevertheless, the 10-year survival is considered to be poor.

7. Myxoid/round cell liposarcoma

According to the WHO definition, myxoid/round cell liposarcoma is a disease in which round to oval malignant mesenchymal cells proliferate in a background of proliferating signet ring-like lipoblasts and myxoid stroma. In this 2002 WHO classification, myxoid liposarcoma and round cell liposarcoma are dealt with as the same category. It has been estimated that distant metastases are seen in approximately one-third of the cases. The prognosis varies significantly depending on the histological findings: the percentage of the total area occupied by round cells of greater than 5%, the presence of a necrotic area, and overexpression of p53: all are considered to be poor-prognostic factors [1, 8, 15]. Myxoid/round cell liposarcoma often occurs in the deep layer of the extremities, and the thigh is the most commonly involved site, accounting for approximately two-thirds of all cases. Unlike other liposarcomas, myxoid/round cell liposarcoma rarely occurs in the retroperitoneum. A slowly growing, painless mass is the most common presenting complaint. In addition, as compared to other liposarcomas, myxoid/round cell liposarcoma occurs more often in younger age groups, particularly those in their 30s to 40s, and it is the most common liposarcoma seen in patients younger than 20 years. In imaging findings, myxoid/round cell liposarcoma is basically characterized by a strongly represented mucous stroma, but imaging modalities show the appearance of non-specific soft tissue tumor when the proliferation of the round cells is predominant. On CT, myxoid/round cell liposarcomas show densities between those of fat and muscle, with lipid-rich areas having a density similar to that of fat and areas with densely proliferating cells having a density similar to that of muscle (Fig. 6A). Myxoid/round cell liposarcomas are visualized as low signal intensities on T1-weighted MR images (Fig. 6B) and as high signal intensities on T2-weighted images, and it also shows areas of high T2-weighted signal intensity mixed with those of a low signal intensity, reflecting the degree of proliferation of the fatty component (Fig. 6C). These findings make differenitation difficult from other mucous tumors, including myxoma, extraskeletal myxoid chondrosarcoma and myxofibrosarcoma. Macroscopically, myxoid/round cell liposarcomas are solid multilocular tumors with a relatively clear border. Myxoid/round cell liposarcomas are characterized by a myxoid cut surface, however, the myxoid stroma is sometimes not macroscopically visible in cases with predominant round cell proliferation. Histologically, myxoid/round cell liposarcomas are characterized by the proliferation of signet ring-like lipoblasts, round to oval malignant mesenchymal cells, in a background of myxoid stroma, and blood vessels with a dendritic or chicken-wire appearance. The mucus consists of hyaluronic acid. This liposarcoma was previously classified as myxoid liposarcoma and round cell liposarcoma, according to the degree of round cell proliferation. The proliferative activity of the round cells has been shown to vary from almost none to marked, depending on the case or the site. Extensive resection is the treatment of choice. It has been reported that the higher the proportion of round cells, the higher the metastatic frequency [8]. However, in occasional cases of multiple occurrences, the prognosis is poor even if the histological grade is low.

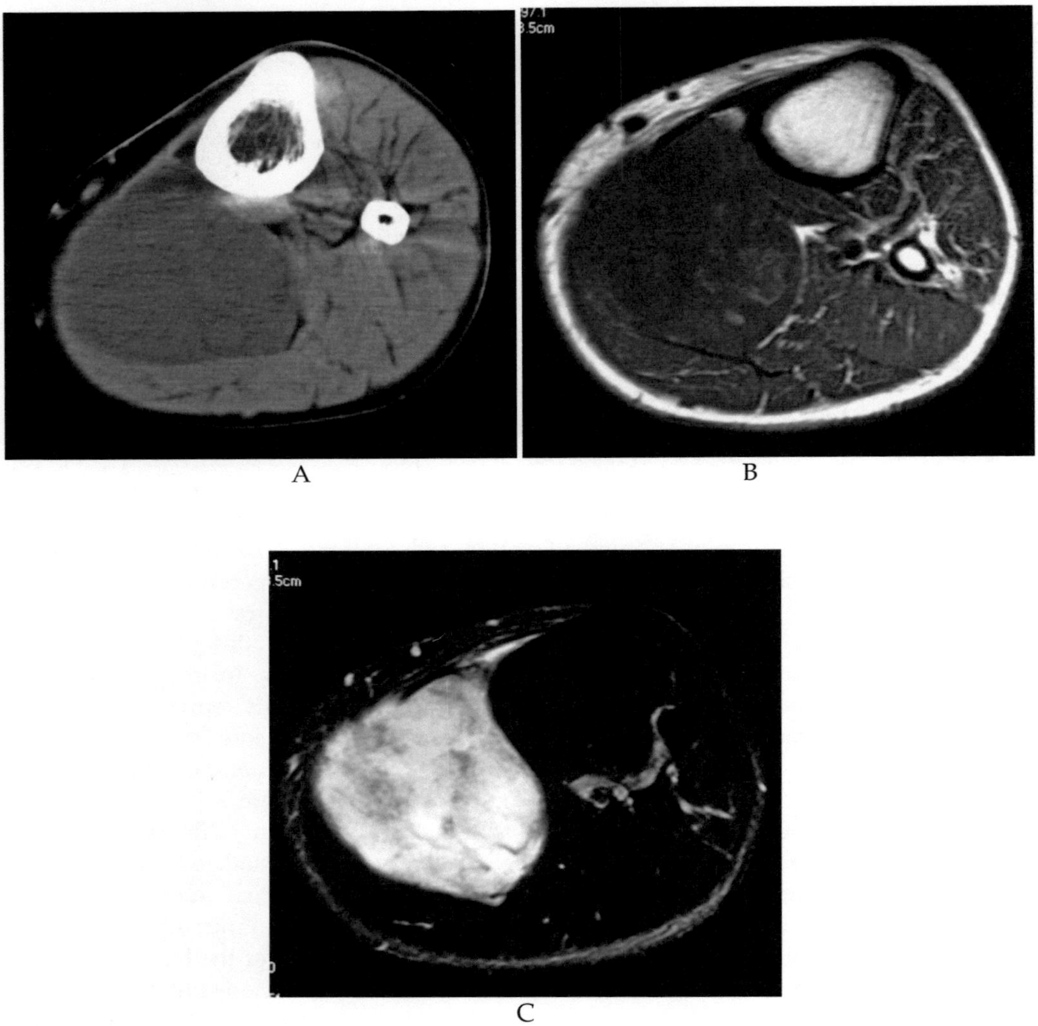

Fig. 6. A. Axial slice of computed tomography of myxoid/round cell liposarcoma demonstrated a densities between those of fat and muscle. B. MR (T1 weighted images) findings of myxoid/round cell liposarcoma showed low signal intensity areas. C. MR (fat suppressed T2 weighted images) findings of myxoid/round cell liposarcoma showed high signal intensity lesion mixed with those of a low signal intensity area.

8. Pleomorphic liposarcoma

Pleomorphic liposarcoma is a rare condition composed of proliferating lipoblasts with various morphologies. Lesions showing the appearance of well-differentiated liposarcoma or having a tendency to differentiate into other mesenchymal tumors are excluded. A rapidly growing, hard mass or tumor is the main presenting complaint in many cases. Pleomorphic liposarcoma frequently occurs in the extremities, particularly in the lower extremities, but it may also occur in the retroperitoneum; it does not often occur in the trunk. Both CT and MR imaging findings are characterized by multilocular growth, although varying depending on the extent of fatty components (Fig. 7). Imaging features depend on the presence and distribution of lipid-rich component. Non lipid component has non specific feature on CT and MR images. Pleomorphic liposarcoma contains less fatty components as compared to other types of liposarcoma, and the appearance of a non-specific soft tissue mass is seen in some cases. Detection of lipid-rich components helps in making diagnosis. Macroscopically, pleomorphic liposarcoma is a multilocular solid lesion, with the cut surface being white to yellow in color. A necrotic appearance is more often seen in pleomorphic liposarcoma than in other liposarcomas. In addition, large lesions measuring more than 10 cm in diameter are often found. The border with the surrounding tissues varies, clear, encapsulated, and ill-defined, because of invasion into the surrounding tissues. Histologically, pleomorphic liposarcomas are high-grade malignancy containing polymorphic lipoblasts in varying amounts. The prognosis is obviously poor as compared with that of other liposarcomas, but there have been no reports yet of analysis of a sufficiently large number of cases. The prognosis is particularly poor in cases with deeply located, larger size and having distinctive mitotic activities [4, 11, 14].

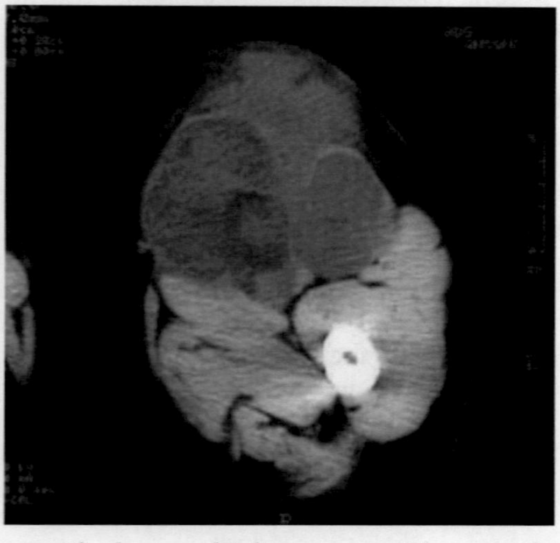

Fig. 7. CT findings of a case with pleomorphic liposarcoma. The mass showed multilocular lesion with a densities between those of fat and muscle. Used with permission from Clin Imagiol [14].

9. Conclusions

There are differences in the configuration, and the thickness and shape of the streaky structures between intramuscular and intermuscular lipomas on images, particularly on CT. When observed carefully, lipoma-like liposarcomas are characterized by an amorphous-hazy high density and show invasive, spherical expansion into the surrounding tissues in many cases. Imaging findings of well-differentiated liposarcomas are clearly different from those of benign lesions, and differentiation is usually possible on imaging features. Clinical or imaging differentiation of high-grade malignancy, including dedifferentiated liposarcoma, from benign lesions is often possible. When performing biopsy, the imaging guidance for establishing a precise diagnosis is important.

10. References

[1] Antonescu CR, et al. Prognostic impact of P53 status, TLS-CHOP fusion transcript structure, and histological grade in myxoid liposarcoma: a molecular and clinicopathologic stud of 82 cases. Clin Cancer Res 7: 3977-3987, 2001.

[2] Bjerregaard P, et al. Intramuscular lipoma of the lower limb. J Bone Joint Surg 71-B: 812-5, 1989.

[3] Dionne G P, et al. Infiltrating lipomas and angiolipomas revisited. Cancer 33: 732-8, 1974.

[4] Downes KA, et al. Pleomorphic liposarcoma. Clinicopathologic study of 19 cases. Mod Pathol 14. 179-184, 2001.

[5] Ehara S, et al. Atypical lipomas, liposarcomas, and other fat-containing sarcomas. CT analysis of fat element. Clin Imaging 19: 50-3, 1995.

[6] Fletcher C D, et al. Martin-Bates E. Intra-muscular and intermuscular lipoma: neglected diagnoses. Histopathology 12: 275-87, 1988.

[7] Henricks WH, et al. Dedifferentiated liposarcoma: a clinicopathological analysis of 155 cases with proposal for an expanded definition of differentiation. Am J Surg Pathol 21, 271-281, 1997.

[8] Kilpatrick SE, et al. The clinicopathologic spectrum of myxoid and round cell liposarcoma. A study of 95 cases. Cancer 77 1450-1458 1996.

[9] Kindblom L G, et al. Intermuscular and inter-muscular lipomas and hibernomas. A clinical, roentgenologic, histologic, and prognostic study of 46 cases. Cancer 33: 754-62, 1974.

[10] McCormic D, et al. Dedifferentiated liposarcoma. A clinico-pathologic analysis of 32 cases suggesting a better prognostic subgroup among pleomorphic sarcomas. Am J Surg Pathol 18, 1213-2123, 1997.

[11] Miettinen M, et al. Epithelioid variant of pleomorphic liposarcoma. Study of 12 cases of distinctive variant of high-grade liposaecoma. Mod Pathol 12: 722-728, 1999.

[12] Nishida J, et al. Imaging characteritics of the deep-seated lipomatous tumors: Intramuscular lipoma, intermuscular lipoma and lipoma-like liposarcoma. J.Orthop. Sci 12: 533-541, 2007.

[13] Nishida J, et al. Clinical findings of Hibernoma of the buttock and thigh: Rare involvements and extremely high uptake of FDG-PET. Med Sci Monit 15. CS117 - 122, 2009.

[14] Nishida J, et al. Transition of the concept of adipose tissue tumors and imaging diagnosis. Clinical Imagiol. 25. 54 -61, 2009.

[15] Smith TA, et al. Myxoid /round cell liposarcoma of the extremities. A clinicopathologic study of 29 cases with particular attention to extent of round cell liposarcoma. Am J Surg Pathol 20, 171-180, 1996.

[16] Weiss SW, et al. Well-differentiated liposarcoma (atypical lipoma) of deep soft tissue of the extremities, retroperitoneum, and miscellaneous sites. A follow-up study of 92 cases with analysis of incidence of "dedifferentiation". Am J Surg Pathol 16, 1051-1058, 1997.

Part 3

Types of Soft Tissue Tumors

6

Pediatric Soft Tissue Tumors

Ezequiel Trejo-Scorza[1], Belinda Beatriz Márquez Álvarez[2], Carlos José Trejo-Scorza[3] and Simón Paz- Ivannov[3]
[1]*Department of Pediatric Surgery Maternity "Concepción Palacios"*
[2]*Department of Pathology of Maternity "Concepción Palacios"*
[3]*Universidad Central de Venezuela*
Venezuela

1. Introduction

The literature on cancer, of the Children Hospital "JM de los Ríos", allowed us to distinguish two series of solid tumors in children. The first serie (1, 2, 3), from 1937 to 1976, with 581 cases of malignant solid tumors, 75 of which were sarcomas (Table N° 1) and a second serie (4, 5), from 1985 to 2001, with 1.796 cases of solid tumors, with 280 cases of soft tissue tumors (Table N° 2). In both series, soft tissue tumors ranked the third in frequency with the 12.90% and 15.96% of cases, respectively. We refer to these statistics, since they are the base of our discussion.

	1937-1962 (1)	1963-1971 (2)	1972-1976 (3)	1937-1976
Lymphoma / Hodgkin	41(13)	104(21)	39(12)	184(46) (31.66%)
Central nervous system tumors	20	56	19	95 (16.35%)
Wilms' tumor.	35	40	11	86 (14.80%)
Sarcomas	27 (soft tissue sarcomas 20, osteosarcomas 7), (fibrosarcomas of soft tissue 6, bone fibrosarcomas 2)	30	18 (soft tissue sarcomas 12, osteosarcomas 6)	75 (12.90%)
Neuroblastoma	10	21	12	43 (7.40%)
Bone tumors				
Retinoblastoma	16	19	2	37 (6.36%)

Teratomas	17	11	12	40 (6.88%)
Carcinoma	8	10	2	20 (3.44%)
Ovarian dysgerminoma			1	1 (0.17%)
Liver tumors				
Other tumors				
Total	174	291	116	581

Table 1. Solid tumors in the Children´s Hospital "JM de los Ríos" 1937-1976 (1, 2, 3)

	1985-1995 (4)	1996-2001	1985-2001 (5)
Lymphoma / Hodgkin	304/135	86/7	390/142 (21.71%)
Central nervous system tumors	199	189	388 (21.60%)
Renal Tumors / Wilms' tumor.	115/98	80/71	195/169 (10.85%)
Soft tissue tumors /Rhabdomyosarcomas	178/114	102/54	280/168 (15.59%)
Neuroblastoma	79	62	141 (7.85%)
Bone tumors	58	67	125 (6.95%)
Retinoblastoma	35	19	54 (3.00%)
Germ cell tumors Germ	111	16	127 (7.07%)
Carcinoma	31	15	46 (2.56%)
Ovarian dysgerminoma			
Liver tumors	25	18	43 (2.39%)
Other tumors	12	-5	7 (0.38%)
Total	1147	649	1796

Table 2. Solid tumors in the Children´s Hospital "JM de los Ríos" 1985-2001

1.1 Incidence

Solid tumors are approximately the 70% of cases of cancer in the children, and the other 30% are leukemias. In the group of solid tumors, soft tissue tumors rank third in frequency with 15.59%, only surpassed by lymphomas 21.71% and central nervous system tumors 21.60% (5) Table N° 2.

Incidence of soft tissue tumors in children and adolescents is not uniform across all ages. It is greater in children younger than 10 years with 73.92% and, children less of 5 years old, account for nearly half (48.57%) the cases of soft tissue tumors (Table N° 3).

Age groups	Porcentaje
Under 1 year of age	27 (9.64%)
1 to 4 years	109 (38.92%)
5 to 9 years	71 (25.35%)
10 to 15 years	69 (24.64%)
16 to 18 years	4 (1.42%)

Table 3. Soft tissue tumors. Distribution by age groups. Children's Hospital "J.M. de los Ríos" 1985-2001 (5)

1.2 Definition

Soft tissue have been defined as nonepithelial extraskeletal tissue of the body, exclusive the reticuloendothelial system, glia and supporting tissue of various parenchymal organs (6); it is represented by voluntary muscle, fat, fibrous tissue and vessels serving these tissues. The soft tissue tumors are a heterogeneous group of tumors that derived from embryonic mesenchymal cells; they are histopatholólogically classified, according to adult tissue that resembles, and may be benign or malignant. Malignant soft tissue tumors are called sarcomas, and there are three main groups: - rhabdomyosarcoma, - non-rhabdomyosarcoma soft tissue sarcoma, and - Ewing's sarcoma.

2. Rhadomyosarcoma (RMS)

2.1 Definition e incidence

Rhabdomyosarcoma is the most common malignant soft tissue tumor in childhood and adolescense; and represents 60% of cases in under 18 years of age. It is originate from embryonic mesenchymal cells, with potential to differentiate into skeletal muscle cells, and is characterized by a tendency to exhibit histologic and molecular features of skeletal myogenesis. These tumors may arise anywhere in the body, even in sites where skeletal muscle is not normally found (7), and at diagnosis, the more frequent location of the tumor was: head and neck, genitourinary and limbs (8).

2.2 Age distribution

The incidence of rhabdomyosarcoma in childhood and adolescence is 60%, and is higher in the first decade of life with 82.73%. Approximately, 50 percent of the cases of rhabdomyosarcoma (48.80%) are diagnosed in children under 5 years old (1-4 years old) (5), and, represent 75% of soft tissue tumors in this age group tumors. (Table No. 4).

Age groups	soft tissue tumors	Rhabdomyosarcomas
Under 1 year of age	27	12 (44.44%)
1 to 4 years	109	82 (75.22%)
5 to 9 years	71	45 (63.38%)
10 to 15 years	69	27 (39.13%)
16 to 18 years	4	2 (50%)
Total	280	168 (60%)

Table 4. Relation rhabdomyosarcoma/soft tissue tumor. Distribution by age groups. Children's Hospital "J.M. de los Ríos" 1985-2001 (5)

2.3 Histopathologic classification

According to the histopathological and prognosis features, the rhadomyosarcomas are classified in the following varieties (8). Table N°5:

Histopathologic varieties	Prognosis
Botryoid embryonal rhabdomyosarcoma Spindle cell rhabdomyosarcoma	Superior prognosis
Embryonal rhabdomyosarcoma	Intermediate prognosis
Alveolar rhabdomyosarcoma Undifferentiated sarcoma Rhabdomyosarcoma with diffuse anaplasia	Poor prognosis

Table 5. International Prognostic Classification of Pediatric Rhabdomyosarcoma

The incidence of the different varieties of rhabdomyosarcoma, in descending order, is the following (9): Embryonic (64%), Alveolar (21%), undifferenciated (8%), botryoides (6%), pleomorphic (1%).

2.4 Etiology, pathogenesis and cytogenetics

Most rhabdomyosarcomas occur sporadically without predisposing factors, and only one third of patients have recognizable genetic anomalies (7, 9). The cause of the rhabdomyosarcomas remains unknown; but now we know, that certain genetic alterations are associated with the development of this tumor. Alveolar RMS has a characteristic translocation between the long arm of chromosome 2 and the long arm of chromosome 13. This translocation has been cloned molecularly, and shown to involve the juxtaposition of the PAX3 gene, which thought to regulate transcription during early neuromuscular development (7). The embryonal rhabdomyosarcoma, has loss of heterozygosity (LOH) at the 11p15 locus (10).

The Li-Fraumeni syndrome, a well-defined family cancer, that includes rhabdomyosarcoma and other soft tissue sarcomas has been associated with germline mutations of the p53 gene. Rhabdomyosarcoma has been observed in association with Beckwith-Wiedemann syndrome, a fetal overgrowth syndrome associated with abnormalities on 11p15.

The history of cancer in the family is an important, reported in 45.76% of cases. (11).

2.5 Histopathological varieties

There are 4 types of rhabdomyosarcoma in children, clearly defined by Imbach (9), which we reproduce it textually.

2.5.1 Embryonal

- Frequency: 53–64% of all rhabdomyosarcomas in childhood
- Location: orbit, head and neck, abdomen, genitourinary tract
- Microscopically resemblance to embryonic muscle tissue; mainly primitive round cells, some spindle cells with central nucleus and eosinophilic cytoplasm; cross striations characteristic of skeletal muscle in about 30% of cases.
- **Subtype: Sarcoma botryoides** (6% of all rhabdomyosarcomas in children); in vagina, bladder, uterus; microscopically as embryonal type with polypoid mass and presence of a dense subepithelial cell layer.

- **Subtype Spindle cell rhabdomyosarcoma**, is a variety of embryonal rhabdomyosarcoma composed of tight bundles of spindle cells and resembling smooth muscle and fibrous neoplasms (8). It is usually located paratesticular or head and neck, and is difficult to differentiate from congenital fibrosarcoma. Compared to other rhabdomyosarcomas, this has a good prognosis. (spindle cell subtype does not appear in the classification of Imbach (9), so we add it)

2.5.2 Alveolar

- Frequency: 21% of all rhabdomyosarcomas in children
- Location: mainly extremities
- Histology: round cells with eosinophilic cytoplasm, occasionally with vacuoles; multinucleated giant cells; rarely cross-striations; groups of tumor cells separated by fibrotic septation (alveolar structure)

2.5.3 Pleomorphic

- Frequency: 1% of all rhabdomyosarcoma in children
- Occurrence: mainly in adulthood
- Histology: undifferentiated muscle tissue; spindle cells with variable eosinophilic cytoplasm and pleomorphic nuclei, frequently mitotic cells, often cross-striations, structured in rows and bundles.

2.5.4 Undifferentiated subtype

- Frequency: 8% without muscle-specific gene proteins.

The histopathological types found in order of decreasing frequency, in Children's Hospital "J.M. de los Ríos", are shown in Table N°6 (10):

histopathological types	number of cases (%)
Embryonal rhabdomyosarcoma	39 (66.10%)
Embryonal rhabdomyosarcoma botryoides subtype	6 (10.16%)
Embryonal rhabdomyosarcoma spindle cell subtype	1 (1.69%)
Alveolar rhabdomyosarcoma	11 (18.64%)
Non typeable	2 (3.38%)
Total	59 (100%)

Table 6. Rhabdomyosarcoma, Rhabdomyosarcoma histopathological types, Children's Hospital "J.M. de los Ríos" 1997-2005 (10)

The histologic variants embryonal and alveolar are the two more common.

2.6 Location

The most common sites of primary tumor are: head and neck, including the orbit; genitourinary tract including the prostate, testis, vulva, cérvix and uterus; and extremities. (Table N° 7); and less frequent are: trunk, retroperitoneum, perianal and anal (7, 9, 10, 12).

Location	number of cases (%)
Head and neck	20 (33.89%)
Genitourinary	14 (23.72%)
Extremities	13 (22.03%)
Pelvic floor	7 (11.86%)
Trunk	4 (6.77%)
Perianal and anal	1 (1.69%)

Table 7. Rhabdomyosarcoma, Location of primary tumor, Children's Hospital "J.M. de los Ríos" 1997-2005 (10)

The age and location of the tumor are associated with histological varieties certain of rhabdomyosarcoma. Head and neck tumors are more common in children younger than eight years of age and when arising in the orbit are almost always of the embryonal variety, while extremity tumors are more common in adolescents and are typically of the alveolar subtype. The variant botryoides of bladder or vagina, occurs almost exclusively in infants (7).

2.7 Clinical presentation

The clinical manifestations of rhabdomyosarcoma depends on the age at diagnosis, location of primary tumor, and the presence or absence of metastasis.

2.7.1 Head and neck

The primary tumor is usually located in: orbit, head and neck superficial, and parameningeal. Clinical symptoms will depend on the location of the tumor and usually present with a painless, enlarging mass that can obstruct a sinus, grow into the nasal cavity, cause proptosis, or simulate chronic otitis media (12) and clinical symptoms include nasal discharge or obstruction of the airways, otorrhea, and rapid proptosis. The more deep-seated tumors, signs and symptoms may result from compression of nerves, blocked vessels, or both; cranial nerve palsy or other neurological deficits indicates the extent of the tumor at the base of the skull or the central nervous system. (13). The parameningeal localization is the most frequent and a poorer prognosis; usually located in pterygoid infratemporal fossa, nasopharyngeal cavity, paranasal sinuses and middle ear and mastoid, and these four locations include the 91.52% of cases (14).

2.7.2 Genitourinary tract

The embryonal type is the commonest in this regiǿn, and arise in the bladder, prostate, vagina, uterus, vulva, paratesticular regions. Children with bladder rhadomyosarcoma are usually under 4 years of age, and may present with hematuria, urinary obstruction and rarely extrusion of tumor tissue. The bladder tumors usually grow intra-luminally, in the region of the trigone and have a polypoidal appearance on gross or endoscopic examination. Prostatic tumors can occur in relatively older children and usually present as large pelvic masses with or without urethral strangury and/ or constipation. Within the category of genitourinary rhabdomyosarcoma, tumors located in the vulva, vagina and paratesticular are a good prognosis; whereas those located in the bladder and prostate have the worst prognosis.

2.7.3 Extremities

Rhabdomyosarcomas are located in the extremities present clinically as painless masses. As soon as the suspected tumor, this diagnosis should be confirmed through an MRI, and to establish the histopathological diagnosis of the lesion should be performed an open biopsy, or with needle. If frozen sections suggest that the lesion is malignant, tissue samples must be sent for chromosome analysis.

2.8 Staging classification, treatment and prognosis

To plan appropriate treatment, it is necessary to determine the degree of progression of the disease. The clinical classification grouping (15), classifies the extent of the disease into four groups.

IRS clinical grouping classification (stage)

Group I: Localized disease, completely resected, no microscopic residual

Regional nodes not involved—lymph node biopsy or dissection is required except for head and neck lesions

A. Confined to muscle or organ of origin, completed resected

B. Infiltrating beyond site of origin, completely resected

Notation: This includes both gross inspection and microscopic confirmation of complete resection. Any nodes that may be inadvertently taken with the specimen must be negative. If the latter should be involved microscopically, then the patient is placed in group IIB or group IIC (see below).

Group II: Total gross resection with evidence of regional spread, completely resected

A. Grossly resected tumor with microscopic residual disease

Surgeon believes that all the tumor has been removed, but the pathologist finds tumor at the margin of resection, and additional resection to achieve a clean margin is not feasible. No evidence of gross residual tumor; no evidence of regional node involvement; once radiotherapy and/or chemotherapy have been started, re-exploration and removal of the area of microscopic residual does not change the patient's group.

B. Regional disease with involved nodes, completely resected with no microscopic residual

Notation: Complete resection with microscopic confirmation of no residual disease makes this different from group IIA and group IIC. Additionally, in contrast to group IIA, regional nodes (which are completely resected, however) are involved, but the most distal node is histologically negative.

C. Regional disease with involved nodes, grossly resected, but with evidence of microscopic residual and/or histologic involvement of the most distal regional node (from the primary site) in the dissection

Notation: The presence of microscopic residual disease makes this group different from group IIB, and nodal involvement makes this group different from group IIA.

Group III: Incomplete resection with gross residual disease

A. After biopsy only

B. After gross or major resection of the primary (>50%)

Group IV: Distant metastatic disease present at onset

Lung, liver, bones, bone marrow, brain, and distant muscle and nodes.

Notation: The above excludes regional nodes and adjacent organ infiltration, which places the patient in a more favorablegrouping (as noted above under group II).

The presence of positive cytology in the cerebrospinal fluid, pleural or abdominal fluids, as well as implants on pleural or peritoneal surfaces are regarded as indications for placing the patient in group IV.

The size of the primary tumor is a prognostic factor. Tumors less than or equal to 5 cm are classified in the subgroup a, and tumors larger than 5 cm are classified in subgroup b (16). However, this tumor size has a different meaning according to the body surface. A tumor of 5 cm in a children or an adolescent have not the same meaning a 5 cm tumor in a neonate or an infant, what is proposed, relating the size of the primary tumor with the patient's body surface (17).

Rhabdomyosarcoma is a systemic disease, with high probability of spread to lymph nodes, bone marrow, bone, soft tissue distance, and pleural or peritoneal spaces adjacent to the primary site; and have propensity to spread to the lung parenchyma. Therefore, the diagnostic study to determine the extent of the disease includes: obtaining a chest radiograph and lateral, computed tomography (CT) scan of the chest, bone marrow aspiration, biopsy, total body bone scan and cerebrospinal fluid samples from patients with orbital tumors parameningeal or other (eg, tumors of the nasopharynx, paranasal sinuses, pterygoid fossa / infratemporal, and the region middle-ear/mastoid). Patients with rhabdomyosarcomas are classified on the basis de their low, intermediate, or high risk for treatment failure (18). Treatment is then tailored to the appropriate risk level. It is standard practice to repeat imaging studies at 2- to 4-month intervals during and after therapy and to obtain blood samples and chemistries before each course of multiple-agent chemotherapy. (12).

At the present time, more than 70% of children and adolescents with rhabdomyosarcoma are cured with combined modality treatment (chemotherapy, radiation and surgery) (19), but the results will be different depending on the clinical group, histological type, anatomic location and age at presentation of disease, factors that determine the prognosis of the disease and levels of risk of treatment failure.

- The low-risk patients are those with rhabdomyosarcomas of the embryonal variety, in any anatomical location, which have been surgically resected (stages 1-3), or irresectables but in favorable anatomical sites. Favorable anatomic locations are considered nonparameningeal head and neck sites (oropharynx, scalp, parotid, neck, larynx, cheeks, eyelids, hypopharynx), and genitourinary system excluding the bladder and prostate. Their survival rate is over 90% when treated with vincristine and dactinomycin or vincristine, dactinomycin and cyclophosphamide with or without radiotherapy.
- The intermédiate-risk patients are those with unresectable tumors of the embrional variety, in unfavorable locations, ó that are metastatic at the time of diagnosis in patients younger than 10 years old; and all those with non metastatic rhabdomyosarcomas of the alveolar variety. The survival of this group is about 50%-75% and investigated the effectiveness of new drugs such as topotecan. Rhabdomyosarcomas of the alveolar variety, stages I-III, require complementary treatment with radiotherapy
- The high-risk patients are those with metastatic at the time of diagnosis and the survival of this group is only 25%

3. Nonrhabdomyosarcomas soft tissue tumors

3.1 Definition e incidence

Nonrhabdomyosarcomas soft tissue tumors are a heterogeneous group of mesenchymal cell neoplasms, most of which are typified with the named for the mature tissue that the tumor most resembles and represent 4.23% of solid tumors (5) and 27.14% of soft tissue tumors in patients under 18 years Fig N° 1

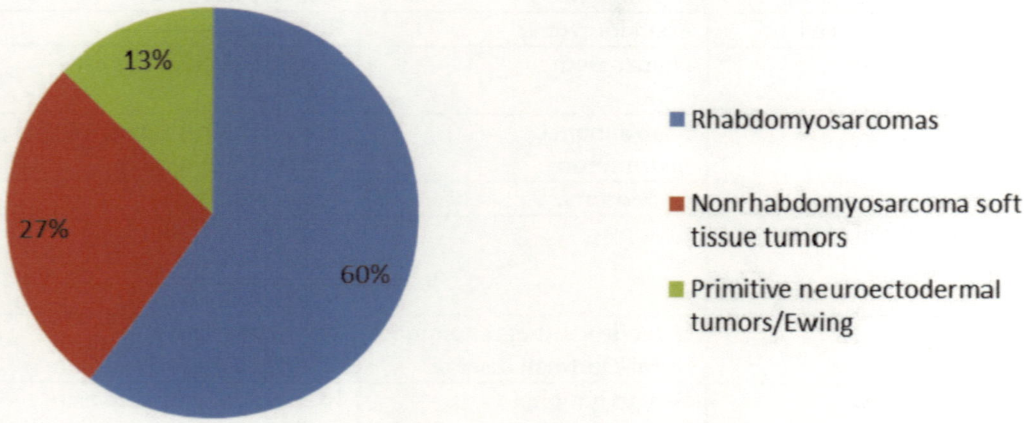

Fig. 1. Soft tissue tumors 280 cases, Children Hospital "JM de los Rios" 1985-2001.

There are differences in soft tissue sarcomas in children and adults in terms of histological types and frequency; differences which have therapeutic implications (20). In Children are more frequent the malignant tumors of the peripheral nerve sheath and fibrosarcoma (5), while adults are more frequent Kaposi's sarcoma, leiomyosarcoma and malignant fibrous histiocytoma (20).

3.2 Age distribution

The distribution of the different varieties of norhabdomyosarcomas soft tissue tumors varies with age; myofibromas and fibrosarcoma are more common in infants, whereas the synovial sarcoma and malignant peripheral nerve sheath tumor is more common in older children and adolescents (12). It is necessary to highlight the characteristics of soft tissue tumors in the first year of life. Approximately 20% of soft tissue tumors that occur in children under 20 years are presented in the first year of age, and of these just over half presented in the first three months of life. 85% of soft tissue tumors present in the first year of life are classified as benign or borderline lesions and the remaining 15% are malignant. The benign and borderline lesions most common are: infantile hemangioendothelioma, lymphangiomas, myofibromas, fibrous histiocytoma, and congenital or infantile fibrosarcoma and represent 68.71% of this group, while embryonal rhabdomyosarcoma and primitive neuroectodermal tumor are the most common malignant lesions, and represent for 62.96% of this group (21).

3.3 Histopathologic classification

Soft tissue tumors are grouped for classification according to cell type that most resembles. Table N° 8.

Cell Type	Benign Tumor	Malignant Tumor
Fibroblast, including myofibroblast	Fibroma, myxoma	Fibrosarcoma, malignant fibrous histiocytoma
Adipocyte	Lipoma	Liposarcoma
Smooth muscle cell	Leiomyoma	Leiomyosarcoma
Skeletal muscle cell	Rhabdomyoma	Rhabdomyosarcoma
Endothelial cell	Hemangioma	Angiosarocoma, Kaposi sarcoma
Schwann cell	Schwannoma, neurofibroma	Some malignant peripheral nerve sheath tumors
Cartilage cell	Chondroma	Chondrosarcoma
Interstitial cell of Cajal of intestines		Gastrointestinal stromal tumors, a spectrum from benign to malignant
Histiocyte	Juvenile xanthogranuloma Rosai-Dorfman disease?	Histiocytic sarcoma (True histiocytic lymphoma)
Lymphoid cells	Benign lymphoid hyperplasia	Extranodal lymphomas in soft tissues
No known normal cell or benign counterparts		Ewing family tumors Synovial sarcoma Epithelioid sarcoma Alveolar soft part sarcoma

[a]Intermediate categories between benign and malignant tumors are excluded for simplicity.

Table 8. Simplified Chart of the Major Types of Primary Soft Tissue Tumors Grouped According to the Cell Types that They Resemblea (22)

3.4 Etiology, pathogenesis and cytogenetics

The cause of the soft tissue sarcomas remains unknown, but in nonrhabdomyosarcomas soft tissue tumors have identified genetic alterations. In the fibrosarcoma, a characteristic translocation t (12; 15) (p13; q25) with an ETV6-NTRK3 gene fusion, and gains of chromosomes 8, 11, 17 and 20 (23). Synovial sarcoma has and a specific chromosomal translocation t(X;18)(p11;q11) (23).

3.5 Location

The anatomical location of primary tumor in descending order of frequency is: head and neck, trunk and extremities. However this varies depending on the histologic type of tumor. The most frequent primary tumor site was: in fibrosarcoma, the limbs in 66% (24); in myofibromas, head, neck, and trunk in 69% (25); in sinovial sarcoma, the limbs nears joints and tendons in the 77.96% (26).

3.6 Clinical presentation

The most common clinical presentation is a painless mass, although the involvement of adjacent structures can cause pain and other symptoms (27)

3.7 Staging classification, treatment and prognosis

Non rhabdomiosarcomas soft tissue tumors can be benign or malignant and malignant are called sarcomas. The histopathologic features determine the prognosis and treatment follow (28, 29) and hence the classification of degrees. Table Nº 9

Grade 1
Myxoid and well-differentiated liposarcoma
Well-differentiated or infantile (≤4 years old) fibrosarcoma
Well-differentiated or infantile (≤4 years old) hemangiopericytoma
Well-differentiated malignant peripheral nerve sheath tumor
Angiomatoid malignant fibrous histiocytomab
Deep-seated dermatofibrosarcoma protuberans
Myxoid chondrosarcoma
Grade 2
≤15% of the surface area shows necrosis
The mitotic count is <5 mitotic figures per 10 high-power fields using a 340 objective
Nuclear atypia is not marked
The tumor is not markedly cellular
Grade 3
Pleomorphic or round-cell liposarcoma
Mesenchymal chondrosarcoma
Extraskeletal osteogenic sarcoma
Malignant triton tumor
Alveolar soft part sarcoma
Any other sarcoma not in grade 1 with >15% necrosis and/or ‡5 mitotic figures per10 high-power fields using a 340 objective

Table 9. The Pediatric Oncology Group Grading System for Nonrhabdomyosarcomatous Soft Tissue Sarcomas of Children

The proper classification of non rhabdomyosarcomas soft tissue tumors is not easy and raises diagnostic problems that require additional methods such as immunohistochemistry, genetic studies, and consultation by experts (30). Myofibromas are benign lesions with difficulty diagnostic because they may be mistaken for malign lesions with hemangiopericytoma-like findings (31).

The evalucación diagnosed, requires magnetic resonance imaging and computed tomography to determine the extent of the disease and a plan for surgery (32).

Treatment and prognosis depends on the extent of disease and histological type of injury, poor prognostic factors are: high histologic grade, intra-abdominal primary tumor, and microscopic residual disease after initial resection (32, 33). Radiation therapy is useful in tumors whose location does not allow excision and all tumors larger than 5 cm. or that could not be completely resected. Sarcomas in children are more sensitive to chemotherapy report answer 40 to 60% using multiple drugs, hence its use in all tumors larger than 5 cm, of axial location, with histological high grade, or with metastatic disease.

4. References

[1] Mota-Salazar A, Trejo-Padilla E, Millán M, Flores-Bello I, Benedetto A, Caballero F. Tumores malignos en niños. Estudio clínico-patológico de 174 casos en el Hospital de Niños "J.M. de los Ríos", Caracas. Memorias del VII Congreso Venezolano de Cirugía 1963. XVII (4): 523-530.

[2] Mota-Salazar A. Cáncer en el niño. Tribuna Médica 1975. XLIII (10): A5-A10.

[3] Trejo-Padilla E, Barba-Flores J, Bello-Ordaz E, Andrade H, De La Silvia MC. Tumores malignos en el niño. Correlación clínico-patológica de 116 casos del quinquenio 1972-1976. (Reviewing unpublished)

[4] Pereira G A, Martínez Siso M, Machado AC, Moschella F, Casale E, Santos S, Mora E, Arcamone G. Tumores sólidos en niños. Experiencia del S.A. Hospital de Niños "J.M. de los Ríos". Caracas Rev Venez Oncol 1997. 9 (3): 64-75.

[5] Pereira GA, Santos S, Mota F. Tumores sólidos en niños y adolescentes. Registro hospitalario de Cáncer (1985-2001). Rev Venez Oncol 2003. 15(3): 161-169.

[6] Weiss SW, Goldblum JR. Enzinger and Weiss's Soft Tissue Tumors. 4th ed. St Louis, MO: Mosby; 2001.

[7] Wesler LH, Helman LJ. Pediatric Soft Tissue Sarcomas CA Cancer J Clin 1994; 44 (4): 211 - 247.

[8] Prasad V, Sayed K, Ramji F, Parham DM. Rhabdomyomas and Rhabdomyosarcomas. In: Miettinen M, editor. Modern Soft Tissue Pathology: Tumors and non-neoplastic conditions. Cambridge University Press., New York 2010: 545-573

[9] Imbach P. Soft tissue sarcoma. In: Imbach P, KühneTh, Arceci R, editors. Pediatric Oncology. A comprehensive guide. Springer-Verlag Berlin Heidelberg New York 1999, 2004: 137-157.

[10] Dagher R, Helman L. Rhabdomyosarcoma: An Overview. The Oncologist 1999; 4: 34-44.

[11] Arcamone G, Gimenez C, Pereira A, et al. Rhabdomiosarcoma en niños. Rev Venez Oncol 2007; 19(1): 63-70.

[12] Beverly Raney R, Andrassy RJ, Blakely M, Fanning TV, Maor MH, and Stewart J. Soft-Tissue Tumors In: Pediatric Oncology. Ka Wah Chan, MB, BS and R. Beverly Raney, Jr., MD., Editors. Aman U. Buzdar, MD Ralph S. Freedman, MD, PhD Series Editors. M. D. ANDERSON CANCER CARE S E R I E S. 2005 Springer Science+Business Media, Inc.

[13] Agarwala S. Pediatric Rhabdomyosarcoma and NonRhabdomyosarcoma soft tissue sarcoma. J Indian Assoc Pediatr Surg 2006; 11(1): 15-23.

[14] Defachelles AS, Rey A, Oberlin O, Spooner D, and. Stevens MCG. Treatment of Nonmetastatic Cranial Parameningeal Rhabdomyosarcoma in Children Younger Than 3 Years Old: Results From International Society of Pediatric Oncology Studies MMT 89 and 95. Journal of Clinical Oncology 2009; 27(8): 1310-1315.

[15] Maurer HM, Beltangady M, Gehan EA, Crist W, Hammond D, Hays D, et al. The Intergroup Rhabdomyosarcoma Study I: A final report. Cancer 1988; 61:209-20.

[16] Crist WC, Anderson JR, Meza JL, Fryer Ch, Berverly Raney R, Ruymann FB, Breneman J, Qualman J, Wiener E, Wharam M, Lobe T, Webber B, Maurer HM, and Donaldson SS. Intergroup rhabdomyosarcoma study-IV: Results for patients with nonmetastatic disease. Journal of Clinical Oncology 2001, 19(12): 3091-3102.

[17] Ferrari A, Miceli R, Meazza C, Zaffignani E, Gronchi A, Piva L, Collini P, Podda M, Massimino M, Luksch R, Cefalo G, Terenziani M, Spreafico F, Polastri D, Fossati-Bellani F, Casanova M, and Mariani L. Soft Tissue Sarcomas of Childhood and Adolescence: The Prognostic Role of Tumor Size in Relation to Patient Body Size. Journal of Clinical Oncology 2009, 27(3): 371-376.

[18] McCarville, M. Beth, Spunt, Sheri L., Pappo, Alberto S. Rhabdomyosarcoma in Pediatric Patients: The Good, the Bad, and the Unusual.Am. J. Roentgenol. 2001, 176: 1563-1569.

[19] Breitfeld P, Meyer WH. Rhabdomyosarcoma: New windows of opportunity. The oncologist 2005; 10:518-527.

[20] Spunt SL, Pappo AS. Childhood Nonrhabdomyosarcoma Soft Tissue Sarcomas Are Not Adult-Type Tumors. J Clin Oncol. 2006 20;24(24):4042-3

[21] Coffin ChM, Dehner LP. Soft tissue tumors in first year of life: A report of 190 cases. Pediatric Pathology 1990; 10:509-526.

[22] Miettinen M. Overview of soft tissue tumors. In Miettinen M, Editor. Modern soft tissue pathology: tumors and non-neoplastic conditions. Cambridge University Press, New York 2010: 1-10.

[23] Cheryl M. Coffin, MD, Amy Lowichik, MD, PhD, and Holly Zhou, MD. Treatment Effects in Pediatric Soft Tissue and Bone Tumors. Practical Considerations for the Pathologist. Am J Clin Pathol 2005;123:75-90

[24] Daniel Orbach D, et al. Infantile Fibrosarcoma: Management Based on the European Experience. Journal of clinical oncology 2010 28(2) 318-323

[25] Chung EB, Enzinger FM. Infantile myofibromatosis. Cancer 1981; 48:1807-1818.

[26] McCarville MB; et al. Synovial Sarcoma in Pediatric Patients *AJR* 2002; 179:797-801

[27] Spunt SL, Skapen SX, Coffin Ch M. Pediatric nonrhabdomyosarcoma soft tissue sarcomas. The Oncologist 2008; 13:668-678.

[28] Parham DM, Webber BL, Jenkins JJ, 3rd, Cantor AB, Maurer HM. Nonrhabdomyosarcomatous soft tissue sarcomas of childhood: formulation of a simplified system for grading. Mod Pathol. 1995;8:705-710.

[29] Khoury JD, Coffin CM, Spunt SL, Anderson JR, Meyer WH, Parham DM. Grading of nonrhabdomyosarcoma soft tissue sarcoma in children and adolescents: a comparison of parameters used for the Fédération Nationale des Centers de Lutte Contre le Cancer and Pediatric Oncology Group Systems. Cancer. 2010 May 1; 116 (9):2266-74.

[30] Arbiser ZK, Folpe AL, and Weiss SW, MD. Consultative (Expert) Second Opinions in Soft Tissue Pathology Analysis of Problem-Prone Diagnostic Situations Am J Clin Pathol 2001;116: 473-476

[31] Trejo-Scorza E, Viña-Ramírez MI, Oviedo-Ayala N, ernández-Faraco AA, Alvarado-Sanavria JM y Paz-Ivanov S. Miofibroma congénito. Un hemangiopericitoma verdadero. Un caso neonatal con estudio inmunohistoquímico y ultraestructural. Invest Clin 2007; 48(4): 515 – 527

[32] Merchant MS, Mackall CL. Current approach to pediatric soft tissue sarcomas. The Oncologist 2009;14: 1139-1153

[33] Spunt SL et al. Prognostic Factors for Children and Adolescents With Surgically Resected Nonrhabdomyosarcoma Soft Tissue Sarcoma: An Analysis of 121 Patients Treated at St Jude Children's Research Hospital. Journal of Clinical Oncology 2002;20(15): 3225-3235

7

Head and Neck Soft Tissue Sarcoma

Rogelio Gonzalez - Gonzalez, Ronell Bologna - Molina,
Omar Tremillo - Maldonado, Ramon Gil Carreon - Burciaga
and Marcelo Gomez Palacio - Gastelúm
Departamento de Investigacion, Escuela de Odontologia,
Universidad Juarez del Estado de Durango
Mexico

1. Introduction

Soft tissue sarcomas are a group of heterogeneous tumors that have their origin primarily in the embryonic mesoderm; more than 50 histological subtypes and diverse clinical behaviors have been identified. Soft tissue sarcomas can range from relatively slow growth, causing little destructive growth, to being locally aggressive, regionally destructive and having a great potential for systemic metastases [Greene et al, 2002; Pelliteri et al, 2003]. The approximate incidence for this kind of neoplasia is 3-4.5/100,000 [Zahm et al, 1997], representing approximately 1% of all malignant adult neoplasias. Soft tissue sarcomas are rare in the head and neck and have an approximate frequency of 5-15% of all adult sarcomas and less than 1% of all head and neck neoplasias [Patel et al, 2001; Pandey et al, 2003; Colville et al, 2005]. The age at presentation is variable with a mean of 50 to 55 years (minimum is 3 months and the maximum is 89 years old) and the male/female ratio is approximately 2:1, which varies depending on the review series. The symptoms depend on location, but the most frequently reported symptoms are the following: headache, nasal obstruction, dysphagia, hoarseness and dyspnea. However, the majority of patients are asymptomatic [Farhood et al]. The most frequently reported involved sites include the following: the face, neck, scalp, nasopharynx, maxillary antrum, cranial base and parotid gland. However, frequencies at each site differ depending on the published series [Colville et al, 2005; Bentz et al, 2004; de Bree et al, 2006]. The histological varieties are diverse, but the most frequent are malignant fibrous histiocytoma (MFH) and fibrosarcoma [de Bree et al, 2006]. In Mexico, a total of 27 cases were reported by the National Institute of Cancerology (INCan) from 1982-1993, and the most frequent histological types were rhabdomyosarcoma and malignant peripheral nerve sheath tumors [Barrera et al, 1997]. The General Hospital of Mexico reported a total of 29 head and neck sarcomas cases 1993 to 1997, and the most frequent histological types were neurogenic sarcomas and leiomyosarcomas [Lazos et al, 1999]. The natural history of head and neck sarcomas is similar to that of sarcomas in other parts of the body; however, because of their location, they present a greater surgical difficulty, and residual disease is often left behind thus reducing the patient's life expectancy [Barrera et al, 1997]. Despite this variety of histologic subtypes, soft tissue sarcomas have some clinical and pathologic features in common. The current American Joint Committee on Cancer (AJCC) and International Union Against Cancer (UICC) staging

criteria for soft tissue sarcomas are universal for almost all histologic subtypes and rely on the histologic grade, tumor size and depth and the presence of distant or nodal metastases. Therefore, the particular subtype seems to be of less importance [de Bree et al, 2006]. The main prognostic factor for soft tissue sarcomas is histological grade and tumor size. Staging is performed according to the AJCC, which has four clinical stages ranging from I to IV [Mendenhall et al, 2005]. Regarding the evolution of the disease, head and neck sarcomas frequently present metastases, most commonly lung metastases, and the initial management therefore includes a chest X-ray or a computed tomography scan. The absence of metastatic lesions excludes the possibility of a systemic disease [Mendenhall et al, 2005]. In children, head and neck sarcomas respond appropriately when treated with chemotherapy and radiation therapy. In adults, the main treatment modality is surgical, although multidisciplinary treatment is also important because these kinds of tumors frequently invade or are in close proximity to vital structures. As a result, surgical resection could be incomplete, making it necessary to locally control the disease by means of adjuvant therapies [Le QT et al, 1997].
The purpose of this chapter is a review of frequency, clinical features, histopathology, molecular biology, metastasis and treatment of soft tissue sarcomas of the head and neck.

2. Angiosarcoma of head and neck

Angiosarcoma is a malignant neoplasm that frequently occurs in the skin and subcutis or in a visceral location and very rarely affects the oral cavity [Loudon JA et al, 2000, Oliver AJ et al, 1991]. Clinically, angiosarcoma appears as a poorly demarcated nodular tumor that is red-blue to purplish in color [Toth BB, et al, 1981]. Angiosarcomas of the head and neck most commonly involve the scalp, and only 4–5% of them form in the pharynx, oral cavity or maxillary sinus [Loudon JA et al, 2000, Lanigan DT, et al 1989]. They may represent either primary or metastatic lesions. In a recent review of the literature, only 23 cases were reported to involve the head and neck, with the exception of the scalp, at an age of presentation ranging from 1 day to 68 years [Abdullah BH et al, 2000, Loudon JA et al, 2000]. Angiosarcomas predominantly affect elderly men and may be present in any region of the body, but they usually occur in the skin or superficial soft tissues (head and neck) in the post-radiotherapy area. The prognosis is poor because of frequent local recurrence and metastatic spread to the lymph nodes, bones (vertebrae) and lungs [Forton Glen EJ et al, 2005]. Primary angiosarcoma of the non-irradiated parotid gland is extremely rare. There are only a few articles in literature that discuss patients with angiosarcoma, but most of these angiosarcomas affected the irradiated region or originated in the skin and secondarily affected the parotid gland. All angiosarcomas tend to be aggressive, and they are often multicentered. These tumors have a high local recurrence rate and metastasize because of their intrinsic biological properties and because they are often misdiagnosed, which leads to a poor prognosis and high mortality rate. This malignant vascular tumor is clinically aggressive, difficult to treat, and has a reported five-year survival rate of less than 20%. Advanced stage at presentation and lack of extensive excision are associated with higher recurrence, distant metastasis rates, and worsened survival [Mahdhaoui A et al, 2004]. About 30% of oral metastases are the first sign of an undiscovered malignancy at a distant site. Angiosarcomas represent 1% of all soft tissue sarcomas. Their clinical outcomes are poor due to a rapid growth and high risk of metastatic extension. The median overall survival of all clinical types of angiosarcomas ranges between 15 and 30 months [Penel N et al, 2003, Favia G et al, 2002]. Angiosarcoma can occur in pre-existing benign or intermediate vascular lesions; there are several case reports of angiosarcomas arising spontaneously from hemangiomas or vascular malformations. The mechanism of malignant transformation in benign vascular tumors is unclear because there are few case reports [Hunt SJ et al, 2004]. A history of trauma may be an etiological factor in angiosarcomas, but most authors think that a traumatic event only alerts the patient to a lesion that already existed. Other factors that have been implicated include hormonal influences from anabolic steroids, synthetic estrogens or pregnancy, exposure to environmental toxins, such as thorium dioxide, vinyl chloride, thorotrast (used for angiography in the past), or insecticides. Immunohistochemical analysis is an important adjunctive diagnostic approach for angiosarcoma [Koch M et al, 2008]. The tumors are usually positive for factor VIII-related antigen, vimentin, CD31, CD34 and UEA-1. Among these factors, CD31 is positive in almost 80– 90% of angiosarcomas, with relatively good specificity and excellent sensitivity [Morgan MB et al, 2004]. The microscopic appearance of angiosarcoma varies from epithelioid to spindled areas, with the former being more common. Various prognostic factors have been reported, including older age, tumor size larger than 5 cm, high grade, positive margin and lymphedema field location [Skubitz KM et al, 2005]. A prospective clinical study with a larger sample size is needed to determine the prognostic factors in angiosarcoma patients. Early diagnosis is important for early treatment. A medical history should be obtained, and a thorough physical examination should be performed. Magnetic resonance imaging (MRI) and contrast-enhanced computed tomography (CT) are nonspecific for diagnosis, but they may be used to define the extent of the primary tumor and evaluate distant metastasis. The diagnosis of angiosarcoma can only be established by microscopic examination. The macroscopic and microscopic appearance of this tumor can lead to a misdiagnosis of pyogenic granuloma. The differential clinical diagnoses should include pyogenic granuloma, giant cell granuloma, Kaposi sarcoma, hemangioma, and malignant melanoma [Mullick SS et al, 1997]. Likewise, the differential microscopic diagnoses should include hemangioma, hemangiopericytoma, papillary endothelial hyperplasia, angiolymphoid hyperplasia with eosinophilia, Kaposi sarcoma, malignant melanoma, metastatic renal cell carcinoma, and pyogenic granuloma [Mullick SS et al, 1997]. Treatment of angiosarcomas is greatly complicated by the diffuse infiltration typical of these tumors. Various interventions have been attempted to stem the disease process. In a recent detailed treatment analysis, surgery in combination with radiation therapy affords the most favorable opportunity for angiosarcoma control [Mark RJ et al, 1996]. The prognosis for patients with angiosarcoma is generally considered to be rather poor, although tumor size (and hence stage), site, and the histopathologic grade may influence survival. Investigations indicate that one-half of patients die within 15 months of diagnosis, with only approximately 12% surviving 5 years or longer. However, those patients presenting with lesions less than 10 cm in diameter respond better to therapy [Mentzel T et al, 1998].

Recurrence after local treatment manifests primarily in local failure, yet distant metastasis is not insignificant in the post-treatment failure group [Mark RJ et al, 1996]. These factors, both for local and distant spread, are reflective of the highly aggressive nature of this illness and serve to explain the poor survival statistics.

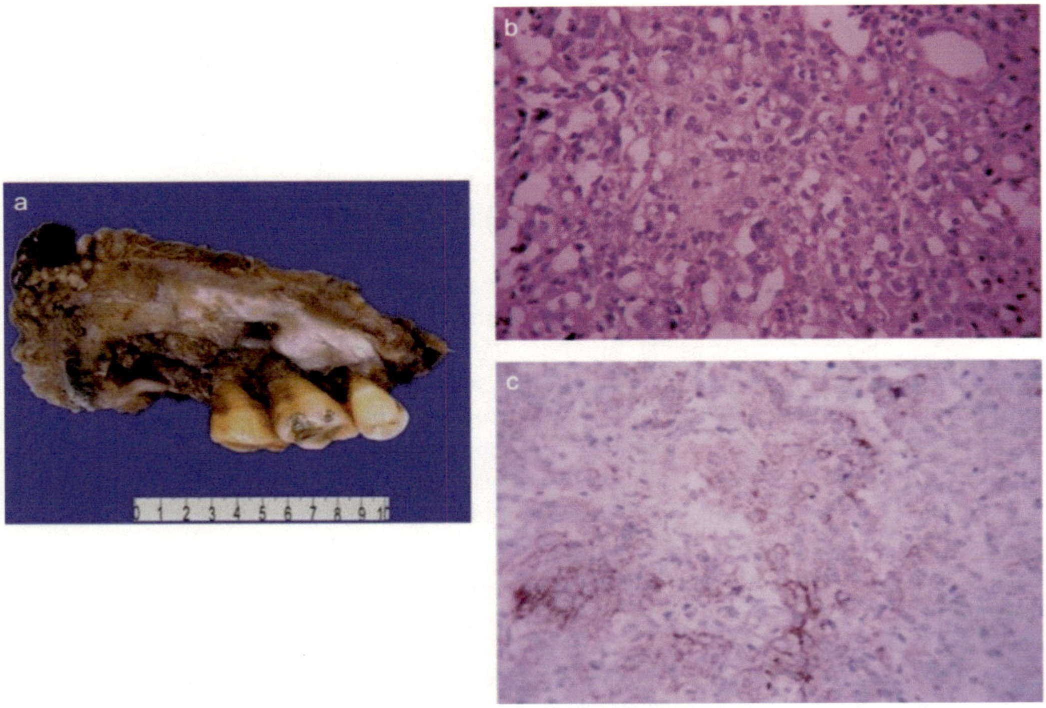

Fig. 1. a) Angiosarcoma of the maxilla in an elderly woman, b) Epithelioid angiosarcoma of oral mucosal maxillar region, 40X, c) Inmunostain for factor VIII shows intense staining of most angiosarcoma cells, 40X.

3. Fibrosarcoma of head and neck

Fibrosarcoma is defined as a malignant spindle cell tumor that shows a herringbone or interlacing fasicular pattern without the expression of other connective tissue cell markers [Sapp JP et al, 2004]. Fibrosarcoma can arise in soft tissues or within bones. Intraossesous fibrosarcomas may develop enosteally or possibly periosteally, affecting the bone by spreading from adjacent soft tissue. Fibrosarcomas can occur in any location, but the bone extremities are the main affected sites; occurrence in the maxilla is rare, with an incidence ranging from 0-6.1% of all primary fibrosarcomas of the bone. The mandible is the most common site for fibrosarcomas [Soares et al 2006, Pereira CM et al, 2005]. The clinical behavior of fibrosarcoma is characterized by a high local recurrence rate and a low incidence of locoregional lymph node and/or distant hematogenous metastases. However, hematogenus metastases may involve the lungs, mediastinum, abdominal cavity and bone [Conley J et al, 1967]. Local recurrence poses a serious and complex problem, particularly with occurrence of mediastinum infiltration, local destruction, airway compression, esophageal compression and extension. Radiation therapy is generally considered only in cases for which resection is impossible; chemotherapy is only used for palliative treatment. Prognosis is directly related to adequate, complete resection, which obviously requires early detection before the extensive involvement of soft tissue [Lukinmaa P et al, 1988].

The histological appearance of fibrosarcoma does not allow a distinction between a tumor of the bone from one arising in soft tissue [Chen Y et al, 2007]. Histologically, the degree of differentiation is variable, from being comparable to a benign fibroma to a highly anaplastic tumor, thus presenting a diagnostic dilemma to histopathologists. Fibrosarcoma can be graded as either a low or high grade of malignancy. Low-grade fibrosarcoma shows spindle cells arranged in fascicles with low to moderate cellularity and a herringbone appearance.
This type of fibrosarcoma has a mild degree of nuclear pleomorphism and rare mitosis, with a collagenous stroma. High-grade lesions show an intense nuclear pleomorphism, greater cellularity and atypical mitosis. The nuclei can be spindle shaped, oval or round. The histological appearance of high-grade fibrosarcoma may be similar to other tumors, such as malignant fibrous histiocytoma, liposarcoma or synovial sarcoma. The positive immunostaining for vimentin, together with negative staining for muscular immunomarkers, helps to diagnose fibrosarcoma [Wadhwan V et al, 2010].

3.1 Sclerosing epithelioid fibrosarcoma of head and neck

Sclerosing epithelioid fibrosarcoma was originally described in 1995 by Meis-Kindblom et al [Meis-Kindblom JM et al, 1995], as an uncommon low-grade variant of fibrosarcoma that is found mainly in the deep soft tissue of the extremities. It is characterized by distinctive epithelioid cytomorphology associated with extensive stromal hyalinization. Tumors with definitive intraosseous origin are uncommon, despite the fact that sclerosing epithelioid fibrosarcoma has a predilection for bone invasion [Antonescu CR et al, 2001]. Histologically, it is characterized by a multinodular proliferation of sheets, nests, or cords of uniform round to oval epithelioid cells with distinctive cell borders. The cytoplasm of the tumor cells is pale eosinophilic to clear, and the nuclei are rounded, although in some areas where the tumor cells are tightly packed together, nuclear angulation may be evident. These cells are embedded in a densely hyalinized stroma. Areas of myxoid degeneration, cystic change, foci of metaplastic bone, hyaline cartilage, and calcification are additional features that may be present [Eyden BP et al, 1998]. Immunohistochemically, the tumor cells of sclerosing epithelioid fibrosarcoma do not display definitive evidence of differentiation along a specific lineage. Most examples are immunoreactive with vimentin, but variable staining for EMA, S100, AE1/AE3, Bcl-2, CD34 and CD99 has been reported [Antonescu et al, 2001, Donner LR et al, 2000].

3.2 Ameloblastic fibrosarcoma

Ameloblastic fibrosarcoma, first described by Heath in 1887, is an extremely rare malignant odontogenic tumor. It is composed of a benign odontogenic epithelium and a malignant ectomesenchymal component. It is regarded as the malignant counterpart of the ameloblastic fibroma. Ameloblastic fibrosarcoma normally presents as a painful swelling and intraosseous mass (2-6 cm), with occasional ulceration in the posterior regions of the mandible and/or maxilla. The posterior mandibular area is the most commonly affected site; the disease is more likely to occur in males than females (1.6:1). Ameloblastic fibrosarcoma occurs in a wide age range, from 3 to 83 years (mean age, 27.3 years). Only one case of peripheral presentation has been reported. The histopathology of ameloblastic fibrosarcoma is characterized by a consistent appearance in which a malignant ectomesenchymal component is mixed with a benign epithelial odontogenic component; the malignant ectomesechymal component consistently takes up more than 70% of the tumor area compared with 30% by the odontogenic epithelium. Ameloblastic fibrosarcoma resembles a malignant connective tissue. The World Health Organization distinguishes odontogenic sarcomas devoid of dental hard tissue ameloblastic fibrosarcoma from those displaying focal evidence of dentinoid (ameloblastic fibrodentinosarcoma) or dentinoid plus enameloid (ameloblastic fibro-odontosarcoma) but acknowledges that the presence or absence of dental hard tissue in an odontogenic sarcoma is of no prognostic significance. This sacorma has an unknown etiology, with some cases representing malignant transformation of a preexistent ameloblastic fibrosarcoma. Although approximately two-thirds of ameloblastic fibrosarcomas seemed to have arisen de novo, several authors have demonstrated that ameloblastic fibroma to be the precursor of ameloblastic fibrosarcoma, i.e., malignant transformation. This neoplasm has a higly localized behavior with low potential for distant metastasis. The treatment of choice is the radical extensive surgery, usually necessitating partial or total mandibulectomy. The prognosis of ameloblastic fibrosarcoma seems better than that for other fibrosarcomas of the orofacial region [Carlos R et al, 2005, Reichart PA et al, 2004]

4. Malignant fibrous histiocytoma of head and neck

Malignant fibrous histiocytoma (MFH) was first described by Ozzelo et al, in 1963 [Pezzi CM et al, 1992] and by O'Brien and Stout in 1964 [Sabesan T et al, 2006]. It was widely accepted as a clinicopathological entity after the description of cases by Kempson and Kyriakos in 1972 [Barnes L et al, 1988]. The etiology is unknown, and the histiogenesis remains controversial. Several hypotheses have been suggested, including an origin from true histiocytes, fibroblasts, both fibroblasts and histiocytes, or from primitive mesenchymal cells. [Ogawa A et al, 2005].

Malignant fibrous histiocytoma is now recognized as one of the most common soft tissue sarcomas in adults. In addition to occurring in soft tissue, it can also occur as a primary intraosseous tumor in bones. It affects, in order of frequency, the lower extremity, the upper extremity, the retroperitonoum and abdominal cavity, and lastly, the head and neck, where it accounts for 1–3% of all cases [Gibbs JF et al, 2001]. Therefore, it is relatively uncommon in the head and neck region. Surgery is the most reliable treatment for MFH, but the five year survival rate for MFH in the head and neck is low compared with MFH in the extremities and trunk. In the head and neck, MFH has been observed in the nasal sinus, salivary gland, oral cavity, mandible, larynx, auricula and eyelid, and Barnes et al [Barnes L et al, 1988], reported that MFH onset occurs most commonly in the accessory nasal sinuses, followed by the salivary glands. In a study of 11 sarcomas of the parotid gland, histological classification showed that three of the lesions were MFH and two cases each of neurosarcoma, rhabdomyosarcoma, fibrosarcoma, and osteosarcoma. A single case of MFH in the buccal region was also reported [Ogawa A et al, 2005]. In the literature, in cases of MFH in the head and neck, the onset age ranged from 16 years old in a patient with MFH in the mandible to 85 years old in a patient with MFH in the eyelid, and the mean age of 12 patients with head and neck MFH was reported to be 55 years old [Khong JJ et al, 2005, Barnes L et al, 1988, Narvaez JA et al, 1996]. The occurrence of MFH in membranous bones is unusual. Involvement of the mandible accounts for only 3% of all MFH of the bone. MFH of the head and neck that extend into bony structures are associated with a much more aggressive clinical course than those that are restricted to soft tissues [Rinaldo A et al, 2004, Iguchi Y et al, 2002] The occurrence of MFH in the head and neck region was primarily in middle-aged adults (mean age, 45 years), with men affected more frequently than women. The sinonasal tract is the most common site of origin, followed by the soft tissue of the face and neck, the oral cavity, and the craniofacial region [Park SW et al, 2009]. The signs and symptoms of MFH of the maxilla include swelling of the cheek, facial pain, nasal obstruction and rhinorrhea. The rarer symptoms include infraorbital nerve paresthesia, visual disturbance, and ocular proptosis. In cases of MFH of the mandible, Kanazawa et al [Kanazawa H et al, 2003]. reported in their review that those lesions are usually first noticed due to swelling, paresthesia, and loosening of teeth. A history of antecedent trauma in about 20% of the cases suggests that some of these tumors may represent an initial proliferative response to the trauma [Senel FC et al, 2006]. Although radical tumor resection with adequate tumor-free margins is essential, from the anatomic point of view, it is often difficult to perform in the head and neck region [Kearney MM et al, 1980]. Park et al [Park SW et al, 2009]. reported in a review that CT and MRI features of MFH of the head and neck have also been nonspecific. On CT scans, MFH is usually seen as a large lobulated soft-tissue mass, which is isoattenuated to muscle. Sato et al [Sato T et al, 2001] . reported that lesions of the maxilla sometimes present radiographically as fairly well-demarcated bone margins, with uniform density or no necrotic areas, and with a clear separation from surrounding soft tissues in CT images, which lead to a misdiagnosis of low-grade malignant tumors or benign tumors. On the MRI, MFH is seen as a heterogeneous hyperintense pattern on T2-weighted images, with an isointensity that is almost the same as that of the muscles on T1-weighted images [Park SW et al, 2009]. Intraosseous MFH has a tendency to indicate a poor prognosis. However, in the maxillary area, it is difficult to differentiate intraosseous MFHs from extraosseous MFHs and to definitively determine the origin when these MFHs were large in size and had aggressive bone involvement [Yamaguchi S et al, 2004]. Also, survival rates of MFH of the maxilla are difficult to evaluate due to the small number of documented cases Chan YW et al, 2004]. With regard to sinonasal MFH, the five year disease-free survival rate and the five year overall survival rate are only 21.5% and 25.1%, respectively [Wang CP et al, 2009]. Anavi et al [Anavi Y et al, 1989]. reported in their review of mandibular MFH that the overall survival estimate at five years was 46% regardless of the type of treatment. Clinical stage, histological grade of malignancy, and local recurrences were the most important prognostic factors for MFH in the bone. Huvos et al [Huvos AG et al, 1985]. suggested that metastatic spread in patients with MFH primarily in the bone was not to the regional lymph nodes, but rather a hematogenous dissemination predominantly to the lungs. The reported frequency of nodal metastases for head and neck MFH varies between 0% and 15%. Prognosis differs according to the morphologic subtypes of MFH [Park SW et al, 2009], Derbel F et al [Derberl F et al, 2010], reported a case of MFH in the neck with metastases to liver. Metastases from MFH in liver are rare, representing 1% of reported metastasis of MFH [Derbel F et al, 2010]. Metastasis occurs in 42% of cases. Lung (82%) and lymph nodes (32%) metastases are most frequent [Derbel et al, 2010]. Factors that influence the rate of metastasis included depth, size and the inflammatory component of the tumour [Derbel F et al, 2010].

The myxoid type has a higher rate of local recurrence, with recurrence in approximately 50–60% of patients and with an overall risk of subsequent metastases at 20–35% [Marotta D et, al, 2009, Mentzel T et al, 2002]. Histologically, the tumor contains both fibroblast-like and histiocyte-like cells in varying proportions, with spindle and round cells exhibiting a storiform arrangement. These tumors have been divided into four morphologic subtypes that depend on the predominant cellular components: storiform – pleomorphic (50–60%), myxoid (25%), giant cell (5–10%), and inflammatory (about 5%). The myxoid variant has been reported to have better prognosis when compared with the storiform-pleomorphic type [Park SW et al, 2009]. In the treatment of MFH of the region, adjuvant chemotherapy is considered for high-grade tumors because these tumors may present subclinical or microscopic metastases at the time of diagnosis [Pereira CM et al, 2005]. The effectiveness of surgery in combination with radiotherapy and/or chemotherapy has not been well established. Three-drug regimens with high-dose MTX, CDDP and DOX or four-drug regimens with high-dose IFO, high-dose MTX, CDDP, and DOX used in patients with osteosarcoma have been evaluated.

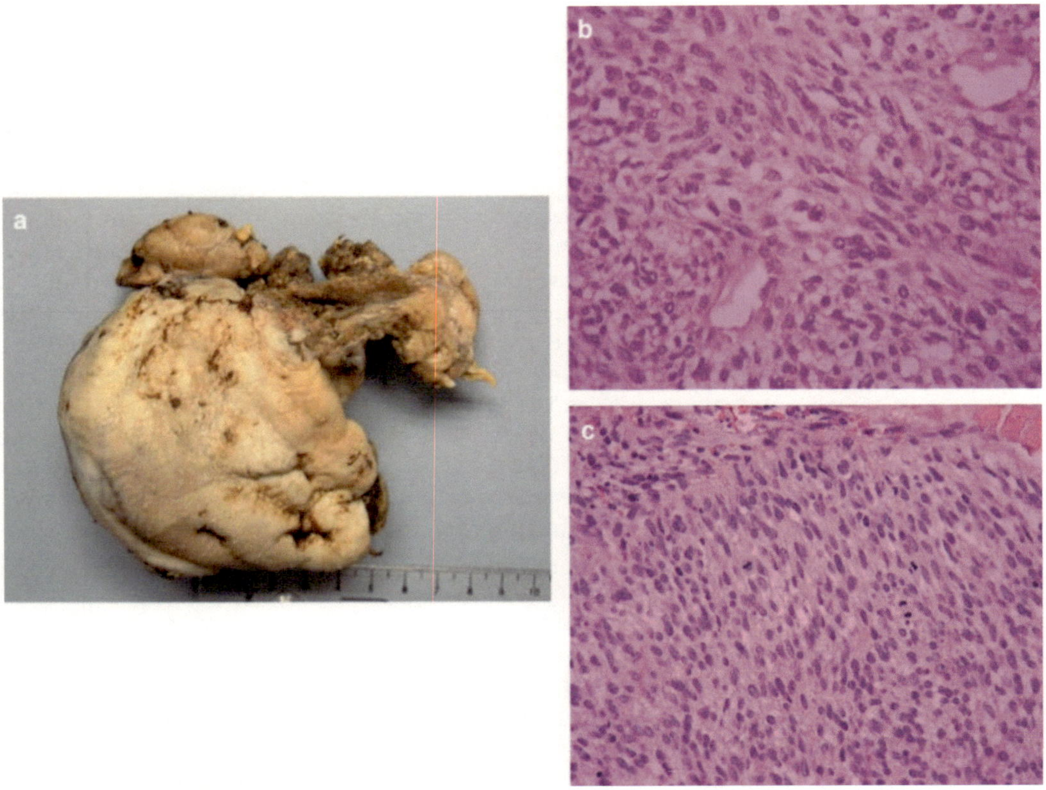

Fig. 2. a) Malignant fibrous histiocytoma of the dorsum tongue , b) Gross appearance of intramuscular malignant fibrous histiocytoma involving tongue, c) Malignant fibrous histiocytoma with fascicular pattern degree nuclear atypia and mitotic activity.

The regimen of neoadjuvant chemotherapy with three or four drugs has been tested in a randomized study of MFH in the bone [Hugate RR et al, 2008]. Few studies estimate the survival benefits of chemotherapy with IFO, CDDP and DOX for osteosarcoma [Zalupski MM et al, 2004]. Further research is needed to determine if adjuvant chemotherapy with the three-drug combination of IFO, CDDP and DOX would be effective for MFH of the jaws. Radiotherapy alone may be reserved for inoperable patients and patients with high surgical risk or those with regional or systemic metastases. Incomplete excision may lead to a high rate of recurrence. High rates local recurrence of MFH in the bone are due to the fact that this tumor infiltrates skeletal muscle fibers and fascial planes [Enjoji M et al, 1980]. Complete excision has been achieved under frozen section control, and all margins were free of tumor. The prognosis depends on the size and site of the tumor and its malignant potential in terms of metastasis. The lungs are the most common site of metastasis. Post-radiation sarcomas have been reported to have poor prognosis [LinkTM et al, 1998]. One patient, however, has been reported to have long-term disease- free survival despite earlier exposure to radiation. Overall, the five year survival for mandibular malignant fibrous histioctyoma has been reported to be 46%, irrespective of the treatment type [Anavi et al, 1989].

5. Leiomyosarcoma of head and neck

Leiomyosarcoma is a malignant tumor derived from smooth muscle that accounts for 5–6% of all soft tissue sarcomas. Leiomyosarcoma usually occurs in the soft tissues of the extremities and trunk; only 3% of leiomyosarcomas are in the head and neck. In the head and neck region, most leiomyosarcomas occur in the nasal cavity and paranasal sinuses, mouth, and larynx [Marioni G et al, 2000]. The signs and symptoms of leiomyosarcoma involving the head and neck region depend on the site and the size of the tumor. Hoarseness, stridor, dyspnea and dysphagia are the most common complaints of the laryngeal and the parapharyngeal tumors. While the initial symptom in a patient with laryngeal leiomyosarcoma in one report was dysphonia, the main symptom in a second patient with parapharyngeal leiomyosarcoma was dysphagia due to the mechanic compression of the cervical esophagus. The scarcity of the smooth muscle in the head and neck region may be the probable reason for the rarity of leiomyosarcoma. Because blood vessels are the only structures in the larynx and parapharyngeal region with smooth muscles, leiomyosarcoma may develop from the smooth muscle in the tunica media of vessel walls. Aberrant mesenchymal differentiation and metastasis are the other possible modes of origin [Freije JE et al, 1992, Chen JM et al, 1991]. Leiomyosarcoma that originate in the head and neck region are very rare. Leiomyosarcoma of the hypopharynx has been reported only four times in the English medical literature. The rarity of a leiomyosarcoma in the hypopharynx can be attributed to the limited smooth muscle tissue in the hypopharynx. A possible candidate for the origin of leiomyosarcoma in the hypopharynx is the smooth muscle surrounding blood vessels. Among the four cases presented in these previous reports, two were located in the posterior wall of the hypopharynx, one in the pyriform sinus, and one in the postcricoid. The age at onset was 39–65 years (mean age, 55.4 years).

The lack of any distinguishing clinical features and the rarity of these lesions often result in their being mistaken for the more common lesions affecting the oral cavity, and correct diagnosis is made only following definitive histological examination [Freedman AM et al, 1989, Cocks H et al, 1999]. The sites of the tumors in this series are similar to the regional variation within the oral cavity noted in the literature, with the maxilla being the most commonly involved site followed by the mandible, tongue, cheek and floor of mouth, in descending frequency. The cause of this apparent variation is unknown and different from benign leiomyomas, which occur more frequently in the lips, tongue, cheeks and palate. Almost 65% of reported tumors are in the maxilla or mandible, and they often involve the jaw bones [Dry SM et al, 2000, Kratochvil FJ et al 1982, Montgomery E et al, 2002]. In cases of head and neck leiomyosarcoma, the success of initial surgical management is an important prognostic factor because complete surgical excision is associated with low local recurrence and longer survival. Resection with microscopically tumor-free margins is of paramount importance for long-term survival. Adjuvant radiation treatment or chemotherapy appears to be ineffective in achieving local control when there is residual tumor postoperatively [Dry SM et al, 2000]. However, gemcitabine has been one of the few agents that shows activity in these tumors, with an observed response rate of 20.5%. Hensley et al [Hensley ML et al, 2002], combined gemcitabine with docetaxel and reported a response rate of 53% in 34 patients, some of whom had failed doxorubicin therapy. The cause of leiomyosarcoma remains uncertain, although cases may be associated with trauma, oestrogenic stimulation, and ion involvement. Other publications suggest that the prognosis of oral leiomyosarcoma that affects the tongue is good if clear excision can be achieved. In the previous eight cases reported in which follow-up ranged from one to five years, there has been no evidence of recurrence [Bass B et al, 1986]. This suggests that primary leiomyosarcoma has a better prognosis if it arises within the tongue than elsewhere in the body. The recurrence rate for tumors that arise from and are limited to the dermis is reported to be between 14% and 42% [Farman AG et al, 1977]. Histopathologically displayed a prominent spindle cell component, with the cells arranged in intersecting fascicles, containing characteristic `cigar-shaped' nuclei. These features are typical for leiomyosarcoma. Nevertheless, similar findings may occur in a wide number of diferent neoplasms, such as fibrobrosarcoma, myofibrosarcoma, synovial sarcoma, solitary fibrous tumor, malignant peripheral nerve sheath tumors (MPNSTs), spindle cell rhabdomyosarcoma, spindle cell liposarcoma, spindle cell carcinoma and other spindle cell neoplasms [Izumi et al, 1995]. The arrangement of neoplastic fascicles in perpendicular, intersecting bundles, the peculiar `cigar-shaped' nuclear morphology, the occurrence of paranuclear vacuolization and intracytoplasmic PAS-positive granularity are indicative, but not exclusive, of leiomyosarcomatous diferentiation. In addition, the diagnosis of spindle cell carcinoma should always be ruled out when a spindle cell neoplasm occurs in a visceral location. In most instances, immunohistochemistry may provide useful clues to the diagnosis; muscle-specific markers for smooth muscle actin and vimentin are most frequently detectable, but myofibroblastic tumor cells, rhabdomyosarcoma and, inconstantly, spindle cell carcinomas may display a similar immunoprofile. Cytokeratin and EMA negativity, as in the case reported herein, rules out the diagnosis of spindle cell carcinoma as well as that of synovial sarcoma, the latter being vimentin and CD99 positive.

Desmin immunoreactivity is not detectable in myofibroblasts, neither normal or neoplastic, but is encountered in other myogenic neoplasms, such as rhabdomyosarcoma [Muzio L et al, 2000]. Although numerous prognostic factors, including size, site, grade and TNM stage, have been identified for leiomyosarcoma arising in other sites, there are no reliable prognostic factors in the case of primary oral leiomyosarcoma. The TNM classification of soft-tissue tumors is not directly applicable to oral leiomyosarcoma, especially in terms of the T stage, and the histological grade of the tumor has rarely been reported in oral leiomyosarcoma. It is important to identify factors of prognostic significance in this patient group. The estimated five year survival for the whole group is 55%. Tumors that demonstrated bony involvement (maxilla/mandible) and metastasis were associated with poorer prognosis. Increasing age and male gender showed a trend toward worse prognosis, although this was not statistically significant. Interestingly, neither the increased size of the tumor nor recurrence was associated with poor survival, unlike tumors occurring at other sites [Miyajima K et al 2002, Weiss SW et al, 2001, Dry SM et al, 2000, Nikitakis NG et al, 2002].

6. Liposarcoma of head and neck

Liposarcoma is the second most common soft tissue sarcoma in adults. Its occurrence in the head and neck region is reported to be very rare. The majority of liposarcomas occur in middle-aged adults; however, very uncommon cases of liposarcoma can be generated in infancy and early childhood [Hicks J et al, 2001]. The occurrence of liposarcoma in the head and neck region is rare, comprising 5.6–9% of all cases [Enzinger FM et al, 2001]. Liposarcoma of the oral cavity is even less frequent, making up about 10% of all cases in the head and neck. In a 1995 literature review, Golledge et al [Golledge J et al, 1995]. found that liposarcoma of the head and neck was poorly addressed and that its incidence is rare, representing approximately 4-5% of liposarcomas (50 reported cases). Most cases originated in the neck (28%), followed by the head (scalp and face, 26%), larynx (20%), pharynx (18%), and mouth (8%) [Golledge J et al, 1995].

Since the publication of that review, liposarcomas of the head and neck have gained more attention; however, most of the subsequent reports have addressed the primary liposarcomas of the head and neck. Fifteen cases of liposarcoma metastases to the head and neck region have been previously reported. The associated primary tumors from these reports occurred most fequently in the thigh and retroperitoneum and equally between men and women, showing no deviance from the normal trends found in liposarcoma. The average age of the patients was 53 years old. Most of the head and neck metastases were to the orbit, thyroid, and dura mater in 31%, 25%, and 19% of the cases, respectively. Other metastatic foci included the gingival mucosa, submandibular region, and scalp [McElderry et al, 2008]. Although head and neck liposarcomas are rare, specialists should be aware of the natural history, prognosis and treatment. As with liposarcomas elsewhere in the body, most cases present in adults, and there is a male predominance. Factors considered to be important in the etiology of liposarcomas include genetics, trauma and irradiation. Usually, the tumor appears firm, relatively fixed to adjacent tissues, encapsulated, and to be growing steadily but not rapidly. Patients do not usually have regional lymph node or distant metastasis at presentation [Feles RA et al, 1993, Freedman AM et al, 1989]. Radiological investigations are necessary in most cases to determine precise size, localization, limits, extensions of the tumor and its relations with neurovascular structures. It is also necessary for detecting distant metastases [Enzinger FM et al, 2001].. Liposarcoma originates from primitive mesenchymal cells rather than mature fat cells. Thus, liposarcoma seldom originates from normal fat tissue or lipoma. Furthermore, in contrast to lipoma, which ordinarily arises in the subcutaneous, submucous, or subserous tissue, liposarcoma rarely arises in such tissues, but rather in the perimuscular or perifascial structures of spindle cell liposarcoma. The next major type is the myxoid type, which is composed of three main tissue components: proliferating lipoblasts at varying stages of differentiation, a delicate plexiform capillary pattern, and a myxoid matrix containing abundant nonsulfated glycosaminoglycans. A subset of myxoid liposarcomas shows histological progression to hypercellular or round cell morphology, which is associated with poor prognosis [Christopher DM et al, 2002]. The most infrequent type is pleomorphic liposarcoma, which contains huge lipoblastic multinucleated cells by which it distinguishes itself from other pleomorphic sarcomas, such as malignant fibrohistiocytoma.The dedifferentiated type was added to these criteria recently and is composed of a well-differentiated area and a poorly differentiated area in parts of the same neoplasm, recurrent tumor or metastatic lesion. The prognosis of this tumor depends on the tumor subtype; well-differentiated and myxoid liposarcomas are considered to be low-grade malignancies, whereas the pleomorphic and round cell types are regarded to be high-grade. Golledge et al [Golledge J et al, 1995]. reported 5-year survival rates of 100% for well-differentiated, 73% for myxoid, 42% for pleomorphic, and 0% for round cell liposarcomas in 76 cases in the head and neck area. The best choice for treatment is complete surgical excision, where a wide or radical excision with sufficient margins is possible. McCulloch et al [McCulloch et al, 1992]. reported an 80% rate of local or distant recurrence in patients with incomplete surgical excision compared with a rate of only 17% when complete excision was accomplished.

Liposarcoma appears to have a clear capsule and is easy to separate, but it often infiltrates the surrounding structures microscopically, so occasionally, incomplete resection occurs. In contrast to its characteristic high recurrence, lymph node metastasis is quite rare, so neck lymph node dissection is considered unnecessary [Weing BM et al, 1995]. Cases of distant metastasis, which result from hematogenous metastasis, are occasionally reported, and the most common metastatic sites are the lung, intra-abdominal area, bone, skull and liver [Wong CK et al, 1997]. In the head and neck area, the majority of metastasized cases appear to be round cell or pleomorphic liposarcomas. Radiotherapy, particularly postoperative radiation, is considered useful and might delay or prevent local recurrence.

7. Rhabdomyosarcoma of head and neck

Rhabdomyosarcomas (RMS) account for 40% of all sarcomas found in the head and neck region, and they are a morphologically and clinically heterogeneous family of malignant soft tissue tumors of a myogenic lineage [Abali H et al, 2003]. Alveolar rhabdomyosarcoma (ARMS) and embryonal rhabdomyosarcoma (ERMS) represent the two main histologic patterns and must be differentiated from other small round cell tumors. RMS is the most common soft tissue sarcoma in the pediatric population, comprising approximately 5% of all childhood cancers and nearly 50% of soft tissue sarcomas arising in children 0 to 14 years of age [Ferlito A et al, 1999]. By contrast, RMS is remarkably uncommon in older adults, representing merely 2-5% of all malignant soft tissue tumors, with the majority being the pleomorphic subtype [Sivanandan R et al, 2004]. Head and neck tumors are divided into three major groups based on anatomic location and propensity for invasion of the central nervous system: orbital, parameningeal, and nonparameningeal. Parameningeal tumors carry the worst prognosis. Orbital RMS represents 75% of those tumors in the head and neck and is associated with the best prognosis. Oral rhabdomyosarcomas are classified within the non-orbital, nonparameningeal group of tumors, which present a better prognosis and tend not to invade the central nervous system. The five-year survival rate is approximately 85% for this RMS subtype. RMS is more aggressive in adults compared with children. Poor prognosis in adults is thought to be due to a combination of advanced tumor stage, unfavorable histology, a decreased tolerance to treatment and other unknown biological factors [Franca CM et al, 2006, Bras J et al 1987, Pavithran K et al, 1997]. Alveolar rhabdomyosarcoma is known to be rare in adults aged over 45 years and to be commonly located in the extremities; the clinical features of the case presented were exceptional. As a result of the lack of characteristic histopathologic features, the final diagnosis of alveolar rhabdomyosarcoma is difficult to establish. The histochemical findings suggested differentiation from other small anaplastic round cell tumors, such as undifferentiated carcinoma, neuroblastoma, neuroepithelioma, Ewing's sarcoma, and malignant lymphoma. The immunohistochemical character of the tumor cells increases the diagnostic accuracy;

positivity for vimentin, MSA, and desmins confirm the diagnosis. Rhabdomyosarcoma is a malignant neoplasm consisting of undifferentiated mesodermal tissue that expresses myogenic differentiation. Histopathologic diagnosis is based on conventional light microscopy and confirmed by immunhistochemistry. Antibodies against desmin, muscle-specific actin, and myoglobulin are most widely used for diagnostic purposes. The three major morphologic categories of rhabdomyosarcomas are embryonal, alveolar, and pleomophic. The embryonal subtype is the most common, accounting for 70–75% of all rhabdomyosarcomas, followed by the alveolar (20–25%) and pleomorphic differentiations (5%). While the embryonal and alveolar subtypes are most commonly seen in children - therefore termed juvenile - the pleomorphic subtype occurs almost exclusively in adults. Rhabdomyosarcomas are generally seen in children, usually consisting of the embryonal type, which represents the most frequent form of soft tissue sarcomas at this age. The pleomorphic subtype is one of the most malignant sarcomas. In a publication in 1998, Akyol [Akyol MU et al, 1998] reviewed the 13 documented cases of laryngeal pleomorphic rhabdomyosarcoma. Radiotherapy as the primary treatment has been reported with varying success, while adjunctive radiation therapy is given whenever a tumor is not completely surgically removed. Randomized trials on adult sarcoma in general found that

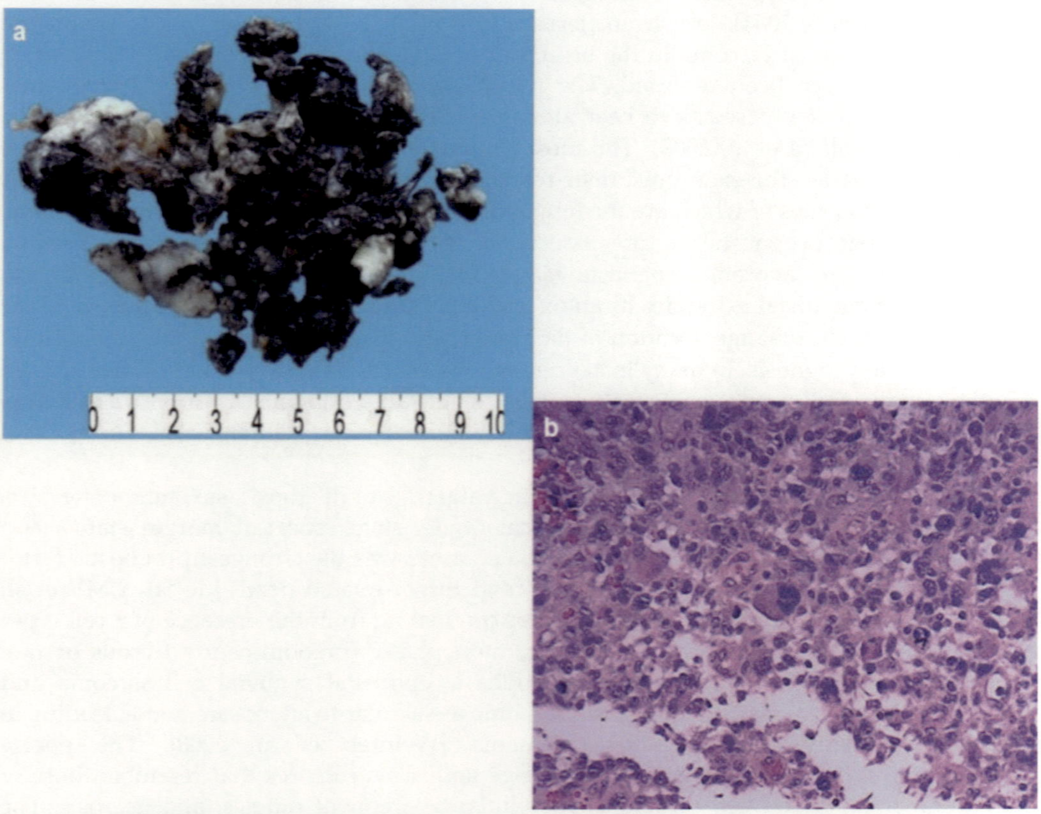

Fig. 3. a) Rhabdomyosarcoma of larynx showing a multinodular white and brown mass, b) Pleomorphic Rabdomiosarcoma with large cells containing deeply eosinophilic rhabdomyosarcoma

the addition of radiation resulted in significant improvement in local control over surgery alone. However, rhabdomyosarcomas in adults are not as radiosensitive as those in children [Haerr RW et al, 1987, Little DJ et al, 2002].

8. Synovial sarcoma of head and neck

Synovial sarcoma is a malignant soft tissue neoplasm that occurs most frequently in the extremities of young adults, near large joints [Enzinger FM et al, 2001]. The most common site is around the knee. As opposed to most other soft tissue sarcomas, these lesions are occasionally painful [Devita TJ et al, 2001]. Synovial sarcoma is more common in males than in females, although there is no evidence of a race difference. This sarcoma represents 5.6-10% of all soft tissue sarcomas. The tumor usually occurs in close association with tendon sheaths, bursae, and joint capsules, primarily in the paraarticular regions of the extremities. The origin of synovial sarcoma remains unknown, but the neoplasm is thought to arise from primitive undifferentiated pluripotential mesenchymal cells unrelated to synovial tissue [Grayson et al, 1998]. Although 85% of synovial sarcomas arise in the extremities, sites in the head and neck, trunk, abdomen, pelvis, mediastinum and lung are rarely involved. Approximately 3.7% of patients of all ages with synovial sarcoma have it in the head and neck [Ferrari A et al,2004]. Jernstrom [Jernstrom P et al, 1994] was the first to report the occurrence of synovial sarcoma in the head and neck region in 1954, and since then, more than 100 cases have been reported. The parapharyngeal region is the most frequently affected site, and few cases have been documented to arise within the orofacial region [Almeida - Lawall M et al, 2009]. The most important and accurate prognostic factors in synovial sarcoma are the extent of tumor resection and the presence of metastatic disease, the most common sites of which are the lung and regional lymph node [Rangheard AS et al, 2001]. The other prognostic factors associated with synovial sarcoma are conflicting. Previously reported favorable prognostic factors include age below 20-25 years, tumor size smaller than 5 cm, distal extremity location, and biphasic histological type. However, some studies have shown that age, location of the tumor, and histology type are not significantly associated with prognosis. In many instances, synovial sarcomas are so poorly differentiated that they do not show any specific features sufficient to suggest their true origin, and hence, they may be confused with other poorly differentiated sarcomas [Limon J et al, Turc - Carel et al, 1986].

The following factors have potential prognostic value: age at diagnosis, sex, tumor site, size, histology, mitotic count, necrosis, histological grade, stage, surgical margin status, and fusion type. The presence of poorly differentiated areas was the strongest prognostic factor associated with local recurrence, metastases, and tumor-related death [de Silva MV et al, Guillou J et al, 2004]. Three histologic subtypes originating from the presence of 2 cell types exist along a continuous spectrum: biphasic, monophasic (predominantly fibrous or rare epithelial), and poorly differentiated. Monophasic epithelial synovial cell sarcoma and gland-predominant biphasic synovial cell sarcoma are similar to adenocarcinoma, leading to potential misidentification as adenocarcinoma [Weinreb et al, 2008]. The poorly differentiated type poses a diagnostic challenge and has structures that resemble those of high-grade small round cell tumors: high cellularity, frequent mitosis, and necrosis. The common diagnosis of synovial cell sarcoma is the biphasic pattern or monophasic fibrous type but can also be easily confused with spindle cell carcinoma, myofibromatosis, leiomyosarcoma, primitive neuroectodermal tumors, malignant peripheral nerve sheath tumors, and malignant fibrous histiocytoma. A panel of antibodies in an immunohistochemistry assay must be assessed together with other observations. Several investigations showed that the epithelial component of biphasic synovial sarcomas stains for cytokeratin in almost 90% of cases and that EMA is also frequently expressed. The spindle cells in some, but not all, tumors express cytokeratin or EMA focally and less intensely than epithelial cells. In monophasic synovial sarcoma, the expression of these epithelial markers is less evident, necessitating the examination of many sections from different sites. Reactivity for vimentin is observed in epithelial elements in about 15-30% of biphasic tumors; in spindle cells, it is observed in about 80-90% of both biphasic synovial sarcomas and monophasic synovial sarcomas and a wide variety of epithelial neoplasms express vimentin, making its reactivity less significant in the diagnosis of synovial sarcoma. The S-100 protein may be detectable in 30% of these tumors, causing confusion with malignant peripheral nerve-sheath tumors. In addition, bcl-2 protein was reported in 75-100% of Sinovial sarcomas, typically in a strong and diffuse fashion, especially in spindle cells [Fletcher et al, 2002, Kempson et al, 2001]. CD99 can be detected in 60% to 70% of cases. Nevertheless, these findings are of little diagnostic value because bcl-2 and CD99 are also expressed in a variety of distinct neoplasms. Chromosomal studies showed a balanced reciprocal translocation t (X;18)(p11.2;q11.2) in more than 90% of all synovial sarcoma subtypes in all anatomic sites, including the oral cavity. The translocation results in the fusion of SYT or SSXT from chromosome 18 to either SSX1, SSX2, or SSX4 genes from the X-chromosome [Almeida – Lawall M et al., 2009, Kempson RL et al, 2001].

9. Malignant Peripheral Nerve Sheath Tumors of head and neck

Malignant Peripheral Nerve Sheath Tumors (MPNSTs) are rare neoplasms with an estimated incidence of 0.1 per 100,000 per year in the general population. They account for approximately 5-10% of all soft tissue sarcomas and have a strong association with neurofibromatosis type 1 (NF-1), also known as von Recklinghausen's neurofibromatosis [Hajdu SI, 1993]. MPNSTs have been defined as any malignant tumor that arises from or differentiates toward cells of the peripheral nerve sheath, with the exception of tumors that originate from the epineurium or the peripheral nerve vasculature [Wong WW et al, 1998]. Various misleading synonyms, including the terms neurofibrosarcoma, neurogenic sarcoma, malignant neurilemmoma and malignant schwannoma, have previously all been applied to this neoplasm and are merely a reflection of the controversial clinicopathologic classification of this rare tumor [Wanebo JE, 1993]. MPNSTs of the head and neck, in particular, represent exceptional neoplasms; MPNSTs are one of the most aggressive malignant tumors and have the highest local recurrence rate of any sarcoma, and they have a marked propensity for dissemination and metastatic spread [Stark AM. 2001]. Despite multimodal therapy, including radical surgical resection and adjuvant radiochemotherapy, the prognosis of MPNSTs is said to remain dismal, particularly in the head and neck. However, prognostic factors and treatment modalities have not been consistently identified [Anghileri M et al, 2006]. Up to 30-50% of all MPNSTs are found in association with NF-1, with a reported incidence of MPNSTs in this subgroup ranging from 2-29% [al - Otieschan AA et al, 1998] MPNSTs can affect all age groups but usually present in adult life between 20 and 50 years of age, with no established predilection for sex or race. However, the mean age of patients with NF-1-associated MPNSTs is approximately a decade younger [Nagayama I et al, 1993]. The most common sites of involvement are the extremities, trunk, chest, and retroperitoneum. While benign peripheral nerve sheath tumors, such as benign schwannoma and neurofibroma, have a propensity for the head and neck, fewer than 10% of MPNSTs affect this anatomic region. The majority of MPNSTs arise either de novo or from pre-existing neurofibromas, with an estimated incidence of malignant transformation ranging 3-30%. Only very rare examples of MPNSTs arise in the schwannoma, ganglioneuroma or phaeochromocytoma, and they arise from all cranial nerves except the optic and olfactory nerves, which have no nerve sheath [Shingh B et al, 2001]. CT and MRI scans delineate the extent of the disease and the involvement of vital structures and allow staging. MPNSTs infiltrate local tissues extensively and spread preferentially, as with other sarcomas, via the bloodstream to the liver, lungs and bone rather than the lymphatic system.

Regional lymph node involvement occurs in less than 1% of deep-seated disease [Ducatman BS et al, 2006] and is even rarer in the superficial form, but no studies have described the statistics. Punjabi described an MPNST in the left parotid that metastased to the contralateral parotid and auditory canal with intra-cranial extension, but it is unclear whether the right parotid was the site of the metastasis or was secondarily invaded. Histological diagnosis has become more stringent because of similarities with other spindle cell malignancies, e.g., leiomyosarcomas, malignant fibrous histiocytomas and neurotropic malignant melanoma. In the past, it was necessary to demonstrate the origin from a nerve; however, cutaneous nerves are generally too small to be grossly identified, and hence, electron microscopy and immunochemistry are used to show ultrastructural evidence of Schwann cell differentiation with the absence of premelanosomes and absence of epidermal melanocyte proliferation. There are no specific immunohistological markers, and therefore, to make a diagnosis, a panel of antibodies and immunoreactivity with at least two of the following antibodies is required: S100, Leu7, myelin basic protein, glial fibrillary acid protein and PGP 9.5. [Wick MR et al, 1990]. Surgery is the main treatment for MPNSTs, which require radical resection and additional frozen sectioning of the proximal nerve to ensure clear margins, although reviews do not suggest a margin of excision. Because lymph node involvement is very unusual, elective neck dissection is not recommended. Adjuvant high-dose radiotherapy is used, particularly after incomplete resection or where radical excision is impossible, and chemotherapy remains controversial. The superficial form of the disease after primary surgery has a local recurrence rate of 78%, metastatic spread rate of 22% and a 4-year survival rate of 66%. Unfortunately, Dabski's series was small, and only half the lesions were located in the head and neck region [Dabski C et al, 1990]. The five-year survival of all patients with MPNSTs of the head and neck ranges from 15 to 34%, with 50% of the cases developing local recurrences and 33% metastases, particularly to the lung [Punjabi et al, 1996, Hujala K et al, 1993]. MPNSTs have been described in English in the literature, and most of these cases presented with a complex karyotype with triploid or tetraploid clones. The most frequent structural aberrations found in MPNST involve chromosomes 7, 9, 13, and 17, whereas the most frequent numerical chromosomal abnormalities include trisomy 7 and 2 and monosomy X and 17. Breakpoints at 12q24, as a part of a complex karyotype, were previously described in six cases of MPNSTs and in two cases of Xq22. Breakpoints at 2q35 or 4q31 have not been described for MPNSTs. Moreover, of the previously described cases of MPNSTs, only eight displayed a diploid karyotype, and six displayed a simple karyotype with unbalanced chromosomal aberrations 47,XY, 7/45,X,

Y; the literature also revealed another gene, PTPN11, which encodes the non-receptor protein tyrosine phosphatase SHP-2. This gene was mapped to the chromosome 5 region on 12q24.1, the same region involved in the second translocation of our patient. Noonan syndrome is an autosomal dominant disorder characterized by dysmorphic body features, heart disease, mental retardation, and bleeding diatheses. Interestingly, a child with Noonan syndrome and malignant schwannoma of the left forearm has been reported. These findings initially raised our suspicion, and we have further tested the possibility that the patient carried concealed characteristics of Noonan syndrome [Rao UN et al, 1996, Tartaglia M et al, 2001, Noonan JA et al, 1968, Kaplan et al, 1968].

9.1 Malignant Triton Tumor (MTT) of head and neck

MTT was first described by Masson in 1932. It is a rare subtype of MPNSTs in which the malignant schwannoma has rhabdomyoblastic differentiation, a so-called mosaic tumor with both a muscular and a neurogene component. One third of these tumors arise in the head and neck region, and at least one third of these are associated with neurofibromatosis type 1. In sporadic cases, the mean age at debut is 38 years, while cases associated with neurofibromatosis are, on average, 12 years younger [Kim ST et al, 2001, Barnes L. 2004]. The MTT is named after the Triton salamander, which is capable of regenerating limbs consisting of both muscle and nerve tissue after the cut end of the sciatic nerve is implanted into the soft tissue of its back. The MTT pathogenesis is not known. One hypothesis is that malignant schwan cells differentiate into rhabdomyoblasts. Another hypothesis is that both cell lines arise from less differentiated neural crest cells with both ectodermal and mesodermal potential. Although MTT can occur as a sporadic tumor, approximately half to two thirds of cases occur in association with neurofibromatosis type 1 (NF1), usually affecting individuals in their third or fourth decade of life. MTT is generally considered a high-grade malignant neoplasm with a poor outcome [Yakulis et al, 1996]. Previous studies [Daimaru Y et al, 1984, Victoria L et al, 1999], reviewed the treatment and outcome of 27 MTTs arising in the head and neck and commented that there may be a subset of MTTs that occurr in this region as low-grade malignancies with favorable long-term prognosis. The primary involvement of the oral cavity is extremely rare. MTTs occur predominantly in the trunk, head and neck, and lower extremities [Enzinger FM, 2001]. Among all reported cases, approximately one third appear to arise in the head and neck region. In a recent detailed review of the literature, Victoria et al [Victoria L et al, 1999] summarized the anatomic distribution of head and neck cases. The data showed that 12 of the 27 cases described were found to arise in the structures of the neck or upper thorax.

Taken together with a recent report describing MTT of the maxilla, it can be concluded that intraoral presentation of MTT is rare. The hallmark of this tumor is the presence of rhabdomyoblasts scattered throughout the stroma indistinguishably from ordinary MPNST. The number of rhabdomyoblasts varies greatly from tumor to tumor and even from area to area in the same tumor. Chromosome analysis of MTTs showed a complex hyperdiploid karyotype with multiple unbalanced translocations, large markers, and ring formations. Although some of the markers were highly variable, other markers were reasonably stable and were seen in the majority of the abnormal metaphases. Haddadin et al [Haddadin et al, 2003], compared the chromosomal breakpoints in MTT, MPNST, and rhabdomyosarcoma to identify common regions of involvement. These included 7p22, 7q36, 11p15, 12p13, 13p11.2, 17q11.2, and 19q13.1.

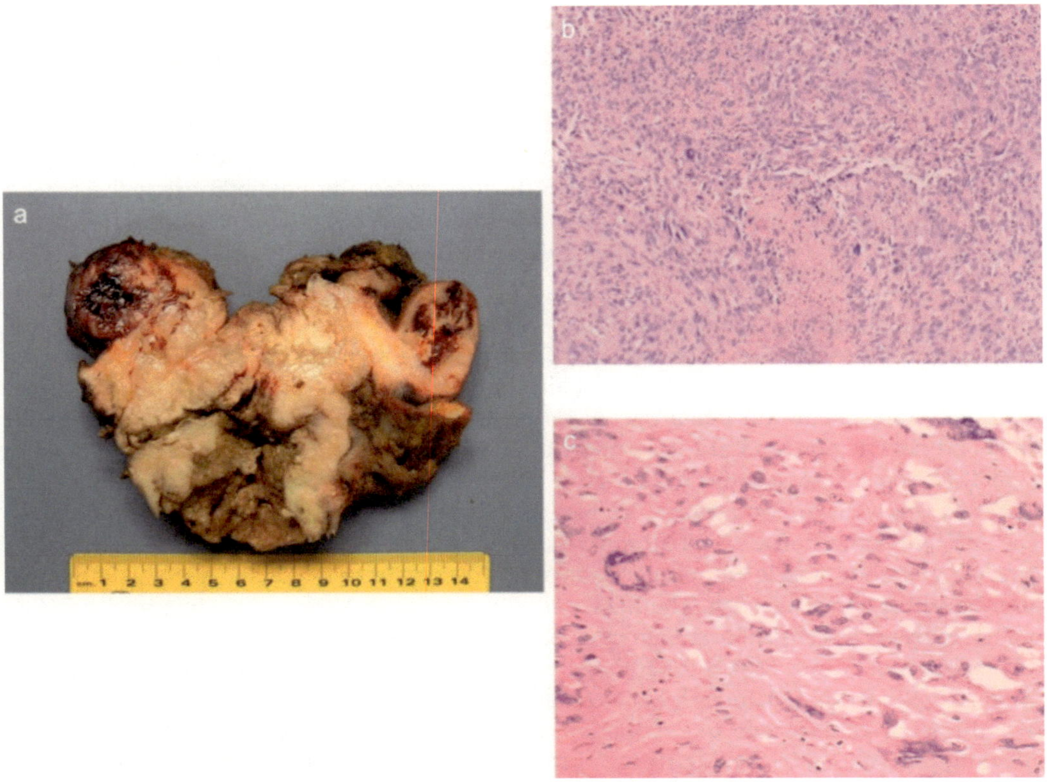

Fig. 4. a) Malignant Triton Tumor high-grade located in the neck with extensive areas of necrosis and hemorrhage, b) Malignant peripheral nerve sheath tumor with rhabdomyoblastic differentiation 40X, c) Rounded or enlongated rhabdomyoblasts throughout the tumor, 40X.

10. Conclusions

Head and neck soft tissue sarcomas are rare and represent 1-5% of all corporal neoplasias. The cause of the majority of sarcomas is yet unknown; however, it is thought that a number of environmental and genetic factors are closely linked to the development of these types of neoplasias. The survival range depends on the histological grade and the clinical stage. At five years, survival is approximately 60–70%, and with local control, it becomes 60–80%. The survival range depends on the histological grade and the clinical stage. Approximately 10–30% of patients presented with distant metastases within the first two years. In general, young patients with low-grade, small and superficial sarcomas have a better prognosis than high-grade sarcomas. Patients with sarcomas greater than 5 cm in clinical stage III or IV with positive surgical margins, can die from progression and metastases. To determine how a neoplasm is likely to behave, with or without treatment, it is necessary to know certain facts about the disease. The management of soft tissue sarcomas of the head and neck is particularly challenging and depends upon some prognostic factors. The assessment of prognostic factors, which correlate baseline clinical and experimental covariables to outcomes, is one of the major objectives of clinical research.

11. References

Abali H, Aksoy S, Sungur A, Yalcin S (2003) Laryngeal involvement of rhabdomyosarcoma in an adult. World J Surg Oncol; 1:17.

Abdullah BH, Yahya HI, Talabani NA, Alash NI, Mirza KB. (2000) Gingival and cutaneous angiosarcoma. J Oral Pathol Med; 29 410 - 2.

Abeloff (2008) Abeloff: Clinical Oncology, 4th ed. Copyright Churchill Livingstone.

Akyol MU, Sozeri B, Kucukali T, Ogretmenoglu O. (1998) Laryngeal pleomorphic rhabdomyosarcoma. Eur Arch Otorhinolaryngol; 255:307–10.

al-Otieschan AA, Saleem M, Manohar MB, Larson S, Atallah A: (1998) Malignant schwannoma of the parapharyngeal space. J Laryngol Otol 112: 883-87.

Almeida – Lawall M, Mosqueda – Taylor A, Bologna – Molina R, Dominguez – Malagon H, Cano – Valdez AM, Luna – Ortiz K, Werneck da Cumba I (2009). Synovial sarcoma of the tongue: case report and review of the literature J Oral Maxillofac Surg; 67:914-920.

Anavi Y, Herman GE, Graybill S. (1989) Malignant fibrous histiocytoma of the mandible. Oral Surg Oral Med Oral Pathol; 68:436–43.

Anghileri M, Miceli R, Fiore M, Mariani L, Ferrari A, Mussi C, Lozza L, Collini P, Olmi P, Casali PG, Pilotti S, Gronchi A (2006). Malignant peripheral nerve sheath tumours: prognostic factors and survival in a series of patients treated at a single institution. Cancer 07: 1065 – 74.

Antonescu CR, Rosenblum MK, Pereira P, et al. (2001) Sclerosing epithelioid fibrosarcoma: a study of 16 cases and confirmation of a clinicopathologically distinct tumor. Am J Surg Pathol; 25:699–709.

Barnes L, Kanbour A. (1988) Malignant fibrous histiocytoma of the head and neck A report of 12 cases. Arch Otolaryngol Head Neck Surg; 114:1149–56.

Barnes L. (2001) Surgical pathology of the head and neck, 2nd ed., vol. 2, Marcel Dekker, Springer Link.

Barrera FJL, López GCM, Gómez GE, Meneses GA (1997). Sarcomas de cabeza y cuello en adultos. Rev Inst Nal Cancerol Méx; 43: 184-88.

Bass B, Archard H, Sussman R, Stern M, Saunders V. (1986) Case 62: expansile radiolucent lesion of the mandible. J Oral Maxillofacial Surg: 44: 799–803.

Bentz BG, Singh B, Woodruff J, Brennan M, Shah JP, Kraus D (2004). Head and neck soft tissue sarcomas: a multivariate analysis of outcomes. Ann Surg Oncol; 11: 619-28.

Bras J., Batsakis J.G., Luna M.A., (1987) Rhabdomyosarcoma of the oral soft tissues. Oral Surg Oral Med Oral Pathol; 64 585–96.

Carlos R, Altini M, Takeda Y (2005). Odontogenic Sarcomas, pathology and genetics of tumours of the head and neck. In: Barnes L, Eveson JW, Recihart P, Sidransky D, editors. WHO Classification of tumours. Pathology and genetics. Tumours of head and neck. Lyon: IARC Press.

Chan YW, Guo YC, Tsai TL, Tsay SH, Lin CZ. (2004) Malignant fibrous histiocytoma of the maxillary sinus presenting as toothache. J Chin Med Assoc; 67:104–7.

Chen JM, Novick WH, Logan CA. (1991) Leiomyosarcoma of the larynx. J Otolaryngol;20:345–8.

Chen Y, Wang JM, Li JT. (2007). Ameloblastic fibroma: A review of published studies with special reference to its nature and biological behavior. Oral Oncology; 43:960-9.

Cocks H, Quraishi M, Morgan D, Bradley P. (1999) Leiomyosarcoma of the larynx. Otolaryngol Head Neck Surg; 121:643–6.

Colville RJ, Charlton F, Kelly CG, Nicoll JJ, McLean NR (2005). Multidisciplinary management of head and neck sarcomas. Head Neck; 27: 814-24.

Conley J, Stout A, Healey W.(1967) Clinicopathologic analysis of eighty four patients with an original diagnosis of fibrosarcoma of the head and neck. Am J Surg 114: 564–569.

Dabski C, Reiman Jr HM, Muller SA (1990). Neurofibrosarcoma of skin and subcutaneous tissues. Mayo Clin Proc; 65: 164 - 72.

Daimaru Y, Hashimoto H, Enjoji M. (1984) Malignant "triton" tumors: a clinicopathologic and immunohistochemical study of nine cases. Hum Pathol;15:768-78.

de Bree R, van der Valk P, Kuik DJ, van Dies PJ, Doornaert P, Buter J, Eerenstein SE, Langendijk JA, van der Waal I, Leemans CR (2006). Prognostic factors in adult soft tissue sarcomas of the head and neck: A single-centre experience. Oral Oncology; 42: 703-9.

de Silva M.V., McMahon A.D., Reid R., (2004) Prognostic factors associated with local recurrence, metastases, and tumorrelated death in patients with synovial sarcoma, Am. J. Clin. Oncol; 27:113 -121.

Derbel F, Hajji H, Mitmet A, Hadj -Hamida MB, Mazhoud J, Youssef S, Ben – Ali A, Khochtali H, Chaouch A, Mokni M, Jemni H, Hadj-Hamida BR (2010). Liver metastasis of malignant fibrous histiocytoma: A case report. Arab J Gastroenterol; 11:113-15.

Devita TJ Jr, Hellman S, Rosenberg SA. (2001) Cancer principles and practice of oncology. 7th ed. New York: Lippincott Williams and Wilkins.

Donner LR, Clawson K, Dobin SM. (2000) Sclerosing epithelioid fibrosarcoma: a cytogenetic, immunohistochemical, and ultrastructural study of an unusual histological variant. Cancer Genet Cytogenet; 119:127–31.

Donner LR, Clawson K, Dobin SM. (2000) Sclerosing epithelioid fibrosarcoma: a cytogenetic, immunohistochemical, and ultrastructural study of an unusual histological variant. Cancer Genet Cytogenet; 119:127–31.

Dry SM, Jorgensen JL, Fletcher CDM. (2000) Leiomyosarcomas of the oral cavity: an unusual topographic subset easily mistaken for nonmesenchymal tumours. Histopathology: 36: 210–220.

Dry SM, Jorgensen JL, Fletcher CDM. (2000) Leiomyosarcomas of the oral cavity: an unusual topographic subset easily mistaken for nonmesenchymal tumours. Histopathology; 36: 210–220.

Ducatman BS, Scheithauer BW, Piepgras DG, Reiman HM, Ilstrup DM. (2006) Malignant peripheral nerve sheath tumours: a clinicopathologic study of 120 cases. Cancer; 1986:57.

Eeles RA, Ficher C, A'Hern RP, Robinson M, Rhys-Evans P, Henk JM, et al. Head and neck sarcomas: prognostic factors and implications for treatment. Br J Cancer 1993; 68:201–7.

Enjoji M, HashimotoH, TsuneyoshiM, Iwasaki H. (1980) Malignant fibrous histiocytoma. A clinico pathologic study of 130 cases. Acta Pathol Jpn; 30:727–41.

Enzinger FM, Weiss SW. Liposarcoma. In: Weiss SW, Goldblum JR, editors. (2001) Soft tissue tumors. 4th ed. St. Louis: Mosby.

Enzinger FM, Weiss SW. Soft tissue tumors. Foruth edition. St Louis: Mosby, 2001.

Farman AG, Kay S. (1977) Oral leiomyosarcoma: report of a case and review of the literature pertaining to smooth muscle tumours of the oral cavity. Oral Surg; 43: 402–409.

Favia G, Lomuzio L, Serpico R, Mariorano E. (2002) Angiosarcoma of the head and neck with intraoral presentation. A clinicopathologic study of four cases. Oral Oncol; 38:757 - 62.

Ferlito A, Rinaldo A, Marioni G. (1999) Laryngeal malignant neoplasms in children and adolescents. Int J Pediatr Otorhinolaryngol; 49:1–14.

Ferrari A, Gronchi A., Casanova M., Meazza C., Gandola L., P. Collini, et al (2004). Synovial sarcoma: a retrospective analysis of 271 patients of all ages treated at a single institution, Cancer; 101:627 - 634.

Fletcher CDM, Unni KK, Mertens F: (2002)World Health Organization Classification of Tumours. Pathology and Genetics of Tumours of Soft Tissues and Bone. Lyon, IARC Press.

Forton - Glen EJ, Van Parys G, Hertveldt K. (2005) Primary angiosarcoma of the non-irradiated parotid gland: a most uncommon, highly malignant tumor. Eur Arch Oto Rhino Laryngology; 262:173 - 7.

Franca CM, Caran EM, Alves MTS (2006) Rhabdomyosarcoma of the oral tissues two new cases and literature review. Medicina Oral, Patologia Oral y Cirugia Bucal; 11:E136 - 40.

Freedman AM, Reiman HM, Woods JE. (1989) Soft-tissue sarcomas of the head and neck. Am J Surg;158:367–72.

Freedman AM, Reiman HM, Woods JE. Soft tissue sarcomas of the head and neck. Am J Surg 1989;158:367–72.

Freije JE, Gluckman JL, Biddinger PW,Wiot G. (1992) Muscle tumors in the parapharyngeal space. Head Neck;14:49–54.

Gibbs JF, Huang PP, Lee RJ, McGrath B, Brooks J, McKinley B et al. (2001). Malignant fibrous histiocytoma: an institutional review. Cancer Invest; 19:23–7.

Golledge J, Fisher C, Rhys-Evans PH. Head and neck liposarcoma. Cancer 1995; 76:1051-8.

Grayson W, Nayler SJ, Jena GP.(1998) Synovial sarcoma of the parotid gland. A case report with clinicopathological analysis and review of the literature. S Afr J Surg; 36:32-5.

Greene FL, Page DL, Flemming FD (2002). American Joint Committee on cancer: cancer staging manual. 6th ed. New York (NY); Springer: 221–6.

Guillou, J. Benhattar, F. Bonichon, G. Gallagher, P. Terrier, E. Stauffer, et al (2004). Histologic grade, but not SYT-SSX fusion type, is an important prognostic factor in patients with synovial sarcoma: a multicenter, retrospective analysis, J. Clin. Oncol; 22:4040 - 50.

Haddadin MH, Hawkins AL, Morsberger LA, Depew D, Epstein JI, Griffin CA (2003). Cyotgenetic study of malignant triton tumor: case report. Cancer Genet Cytogenet; 144:100-5.

Haerr RW, Turalba CI, el-Mahdi AM, Brown KL. (1987) Alveolar rhabdomyosarcoma of the larynx: case report and literature review. Laryngoscope; 97:339–44.

Hajdu SI (1993). Peripheral nerve sheath tumours. Histogenesis, classification, and prognosis. Cancer 72: 3549 - 52.

Hensley ML, Maki R, Venkatraman E, Geeler G, Lovegren M, Aghajanian C, et al. (2002) Gemcitabine and docetaxel in patients with unresectable leiomyosarcoma: results of a phase II trial. J Clin Oncol;20(12):2824–31.

Hicks J, Dilley A, Patel D, Barrish J, Zhu SH, Brandt M (2001). Lipoblastoma and lipoblastomatosis in infancy and childhood: histopathologic, ultrastructural, and cytogenetic features. Ultrastruct Pathol; 25:321–33.

Hoffmann DF, Everts EC, Smith JD, Kyriakopoulos DD, Kessler S (1988). Malignant nerve sheath tumours of the head and neck. Otolaryngol Head Neck Surg 99: 309-314.

Hujala K, Martikainen P, Minn H, Grenman R (1993). Malignant nerve sheath tumours of the head and neck: four case studies and review of the literature. Eur Arch Otorhinolaryngol; 250:379 - 82.

Hunt SJ, Santa Cruz DJ. (2004) Vascular tumors of the skin: a selective review. Semin Diagn Pathol; 21: 166–218.

Huvos AG, Heilweil M, Bretsky SS. (1985) The pathology of malignant fibrous histiocytoma of bone. A study of 130 patients. Am J Surg Pathol; 9:853–71.

Iguchi Y, Takahashi H, Yao K, Nakayama M, Nagai H, Okamoto M. (2002) Malignant fibrous histiocytoma of the nasal cavity and paranasal sinuses: review of the last 30 years. Acta Oto Laryngol; 122:75–8.

Izumi K, Maeda T, Cheng J, Saku T. (1995) Primary leiomyosarcoma of the maxilla with regional lymph node metastasis. Report of a case and review of the literature. Oral Surg Oral Med Oral Pathol Oral Radiol Endod; 80:310 - 9.

Jernstrom P: (1954) Synovial sarcoma of the pharynx: Report of a case. Am J Clin Pathol; 24:957.

Kanazawa H, Watanabe T, Kasamatsu A. (2003) Primary malignant fibrous histiocytoma of the mandible: review of literature and report of a case. J Oral Maxillofac Surg; 61:1224–7.

Kaplan MS, Opitz JM, Gosset FR (1968). Noonan's syndrome. A case with elevated serum alkaline phosphatase levels and malignant schwannoma of the left forearm. Am J Dis Child; 116:359–66.

Kaplan MS, Opitz JM, Gosset FR (1968). Noonan's syndrome. A case with elevated serum alkaline phosphatase levels and malignant schwannoma of the left forearm. Am J Dis Child; 116:359–66.

Kearney MM, Soule EH, Ivins JC. (1980) Malignant fibrous histiocytoma: a retrospective study of 167 cases. Cancer; 45:167–78.

Kempson RL, Fletcher CDM, Evans HL, Hendrickson MR, Sibley RK: (2001) Atlas of Tumor Pathology. Tumors of the Soft Tissues. Bethesda, Armed Forces Institute of Pathology.

Khong JJ, Chen CS, James CL, Huilgol SC, O'Donnell BA, Sullivan TJ, et al. (2005) Malignant fibrous histiocytoma of the eyelid: differential diagnosis and management. Ophthal Plast Reconstr Surg; 21: 103–8.

Kim ST, Kim CW, Han GC, Park C, Jang IH, Cha HE, et al (2001). Malignant Triton Tumor of the nasal cavity. Head Neck;23:1075–8.

Koch M, Nielsen GP, Yoon SS. (2008) Malignant tumors of blood vessels: angiosarcomas, hemangioendotheliomas, and hemangioperictyomas. J Surg Oncol; 97: 321–329.

Kratochvil FJ, MacGregor SD, Budnick SD, Hewan-Lowe K, Allsup HW. (1982) Leiomyosarcoma of the maxilla. Report of a case and review of the literature. Oral Surg Oral Med Oral Pathol; 54:647-55.

Lanigan DT, Hey JH, Lee L. (1989) Angiosarcoma of the maxilla and maxillary sinus: report of a case and review of the literature. J Oral Maxillofac Surg; 47:747–53.

Lazos OM, Ávila TA, Hernández GM. Sarcomas de cabeza y cuello (1999). Estudio clinicopatológico de 29 casos. Rev Med Hosp Gen Mex; 62: 176-82.

Le QT, Fu KK, Kroll S, Fitts L, Massullo V, Ferrell L, Kaplan MJ, Phillips TL (1997). Prognostic Factors in adult soft tissue sarcomas of the head and neck. Int J Radiat Oncol Biol Phys; 37: 975-84.

Limon J, Dalcin P, Sandberg AA. (1986) Cytogenetic findings in a primary leiomyosarcoma of the prostate. Cancer Genet Cytogenet;22:159–67.

Link TM, Haeussler MD, Poppek S, Woertler K, Blasius S, Lindner N ,et al. (1998) Malignant fibrous histiocytoma of bone: conventional X-ray and MR imaging features. Skeletal Radiol; 27:552–8.

Little DJ, Ballo MT, Zagars GK, Pisters PWT, Patel SR, El-Naggar AK, Garden AS, Benjamin RS. (2002) Adult rhabdomyosarcoma. Outcome following multimodality treatment. Cancer; 2:377–88.

Loudon JA, Billy ML, DeYoung BR, Allen CM. (2000) Angiosarcoma of the mandible: a case report and review of the literature. Oral Surg Oral Med Oral Pathol Oral Radiol Endod; 89:471–6.

Magrini E, Pragliola A, Fantasia D, Calabrese G, Gaiba A, Farnedi A, et al (2003). Acquisition of i(8q) as an early event in Malignant Triton Tumors. Cancer Genet Cytogenet;154:150–5. Cancer Genetics and Cytogenetics 144 100 105.

Mahdhaoui A, Bouraoui H, Chenivor M, Trimech B, Mesghani M. (2004) Right atrium angiosarcoma disclosed by alveolar hemorrhage. Rev Med Sci; 12:115 - 6.

Marioni G, Bertino G, Mariuzzi L, Bergamin-Bracale AM, Lombardo M, Beltrami CA. (2000) Laryngeal leiomyosarcoma. J Laryngol Otol ;114:398–401.

Mark RJ, Poen JC, Tran LM, Fu YS, Juillard GF. (1996) Angiosarcoma. A report of 67 patients and a review of the literature. Cancer; 77: 2400 - 6.

Mark RJ, Poen JC, Tran LM, Fu YS, Juillard GF. (1996) Angiosarcoma. A report of 67 patients and a review of the literature. Cancer; 77: 2400 - 6.

Marotta D, Angeloni M, Salgarello M, Ricciardella ML, Chalidis B, Maccauro G. (2009) Surgical treatment of a giant tibial high-grade mixofibrosarcoma with preservation of limb function: a case report. Int Semin Surg Oncol; 17: 16.

McCulloch TM, Makielski KH, McNutt MA (1992). Head and neck liposarcoma. A histopathologic reevaluation of reported cases. Arch Otolaryngol Head Neck Surg;118:1045–9.

McElderry J, McKenney JK, Stack BC. (2008), High - grade liposarcoma metastasic to the gingival mucosa: case report and literature review. Am J Otol; 29: 130-34.

Meis-Kindblom JM, Kindblom LG, Enzinger FM. (1995) Sclerosing epithelioid fibrosarcoma. A variant of fibrosarcoma simulating carcinoma. Am J Surg Pathol; 19:979–93.

Mendenhall WM, Mendenhall CM, Werning JW, Riggs CE, Mendenhall NP (2005). Adult head and neck soft tissue sarcomas. Head Neck; 27: 916-22.

Mentzel T, Kutzner H, Wollina U. (1998) Cutaneous angiosarcoma of the face: clinicopathologic and immunohistochemical study of a case resembling rosacea clinically. J Am Acad Dermatol; 38:837 - 40.

Mentzel T, van den Berg E, Molenaar WM. (2002) Myxofibrosarcoma, pathology and genetics of tumors of soft tissue and bone. In: Fletcher C, Unni KK, Mertens F, editors. WHO Classification of tumours. Pathology and genetics. Tumours of soft tissue and bone. Lyon: IARC Press.

Miyajima K, Oda Y, Oshiro Y, Tamiya S, Kinukawa N,Masuda K, Tsuneyoshi M. (2002) Clinicopathological prognostic factors in soft tissue leiomyosarcoma: a multivariate analysis. Histopathology; 40: 353–359.

Montgomery E, Goldblum JR, Fisher C. (2002) Leiomyosarcoma of the head and neck: a clinicopathological study. Histopathology; 40: 518–525.

Morgan MB, Swann M, Somach S, Eng W, Smoller B. (2004) Cutaneous angiosarcoma: a case series with prognostic correlation. J Am Acad Dermatol; 50: 864–867.

Mullick SS, Mody DR, Schwarz MR. (1997) Angiosarcoma at unusual sites, a report of two cases with aspiration cytology and diagnostic pitfalls. Acta Cytol; 41:839 - 44.

Muzio L, Favia G, Mignogna MD, Piattelli A, Maiorano E. (2000) Primary intraoral leiomyosarcoma of the tongue: an immunohistochemical study and review of the literature. Oral Oncology; 36 519-524.

Nagayama I, Nishimura T, Furukawa M (1993) Malignant schwannoma arising in a paranasal sinus. J Laryngol Otol 107: 146 – 148.

Narvaez JA, Muntane A, Narvaez J, Martin F, Monfort JL, Pons LC. (1996) Malignant fibrous histiocytoma of the mandible. Skeletal Radiol; 25:96–9.

Nikitakis NG, Lopes MA, Bailey JS, Blanchaert RH, Ord RA, Saul JJ. (2002) Oral leiomyosarcoma: review of the literature and report of two cases with assessment of the prognostic and diagnostic significance of immunohistochemical and molecular markers. Oral Oncol: 38: 201–208.

Noonan JA (1968) Hypertelorism with Turner phenotype. A new syndrome with associated congenital heart disease. Am J Dis Child; 116:373–80.

Ogawa A, Kawashima K. (2005) Rigid reconstruction of the cheek by free skull bone grafting: a case report. J Jpn Soc Plast Reconstr Surg; 25:454–8.

Oliver AJ, Gibbons SD, Radden BG, Busmanis I, Cook RM. (1991) Primary angiosarcoma of the oral cavity. Br J Oral Maxillofac Surg; 29:38–41.

Pandey M, Chandramohan K, Thomas G, Mathew A, Sebastian P, Somanathan T, Abrham EK, Rajan B, Krishnan Nair M (2003). Soft tissue sarcoma of the head and neck in adults. Int J Oral Maxillofac Surg; 32: 43-8.

Park SW, Kim HJ, Lee JH, Ko YH. (2009) Malignant fibrous histiocytoma of the head and neck: CT and MR imaging findings. Am J Neuroradiol 2009; 30:71–6.

Park SW, Kim HJ, Lee JH, Ko YH. (2009) Malignant fibrous histiocytoma of the head and neck: CT and MR imaging findings. Am J Neuroradiol 2009; 30:71–6.

Patel SG, Shaha AR, Shah JP (2001). Soft tissue sarcomas of the head and neck: an update. Am J Otolaryngol; 22: 2–18.

Pavithran K, Doval DC, Mukherjee G, Kannan V, Kumaraswamy SV, Bapsy PP (1997). Rhabdomyosarcoma of the oral cavity, Acta Oncol; 36: 819–821.

Pellitteri PK, Ferlito A, Bradley PJ, Shaha AR, Rinaldo A (2003). Management of sarcomas of the head and neck in adults. Oral Oncol; 39: 2–12.

Penel N, Depadt G, Vilain M-O, Vanseymortier L, et al. (2003) Fre´quence des ge´nopathies et des ante´ce´dents carcinologiques chez 493 adultes atteints de sarcomes visce´raux ou des tissues mous. Bull Cancer;90(10):887–95.

Pereira CM Jr, Jorge J Jr, Hipolito OD, Kowalski LP, Lopes MA.(2005) Primary intraosseous fibrosarcoma of jaw. Int J Oral Maxillofac Surg; 34:579-81.

Pereira CM, Jorge J, Di Hipolito O, Kowalski LP, Lopes MA. (2005) Primary intraosseous fibrosarcoma of jaw. Int J Oral Maxillofac Surg; 34:579–81.

Pezzi CM, Rawlings Jr MS, Esgro JJ, Pollock RE, Romsdahl MM. (1992) Prognostic factors in 277 patients with malignant fibrous histiocytoma. Cancer; 69:2098–103.

Punjabi AP, Haug RH, Chung-Park Moon JA, Likavek M. J (1996). Oral Maxillofac Surg; 54:765 - 9.

Rangheard AS, Vanel D, Viala J, Schwaab G, Casiraghi O, Sigal R. (2001)Synovial sarcomas of the head and neck: CT and MR imaging findings of eight patients. AJNR Am J Neuroradiol; 22:851-7.

Rao UN, Surti U, Hoffner L, Yaw K (1996) Cytogenetic and histologic correlation of peripheral nerve sheath tumors of soft tissue. Cancer Genet Cytogenet; 88:17–25.

Reichart PA, Philipsen HP, Hans P (2004). Odontogenic Tumours. Quintessence Publishing Co Ltd, UK.

Rinaldo A, Shaha AR, Pellitteri PK, Bradley PJ, Ferlito A. (2004) Management of malignant sublingual salivary gland tumors. Oral Oncol; 40:2–5.

Sabesan T, Xuexi W, Yongfa Q, Pingzhang T, Ilankovan V. (2006) Malignant fibrous histiocytoma: outcome of tumors in the head and neck compared with those in the trunk and extremities. Br J Oral Maxillofac Surg; 44:209–12.

Sapp JP, Eversole LR, Wysocki GP, editors.(2004) Contemporary oral and maxillofacial pathology. St. Louis: Mosby.

Senel FC, Bektas D, Caylan R, Onder E, Gunhano O. (2006) Malignant fibrous histiocytoma of the mandible. Dentomaxillofac Radiol; 35:125–8.

Singh B, GogineniSK, Sacks PG, Shaha AR, Shah JP, Stoffel A, Rao PH (2001). Molecular cytogenetic characterization of head and neck squamous cell carcinoma and refinement of 3q amplification. Cancer Res; 61:4506–13.

Sivanandan R, Kong CS, Kaplan MJ, Fee Jr WE, Thu-Le Q, Goffinet DR. (2004) Laryngeal embryonal rhabdomyosarcoma. Arch tolaryngol Head and Neck surg; 130:1217–22.

Skubitz KM, Haddad PA. (2005) Paclitaxel and pegylated-liposomal doxorubicin are both active in angiosarcoma. Cancer; 104: 361–366.

Soares AB, Lins LHS, Mazedo AP, Neto JSP, Vargas PA.(2006) Fibrosarcoma originating in the mandible. Med Oral Patol Oral Cir Bucal; 11: E 243-6.

Stark AM, Buhl R, Hugo HH, Mehdorn HM (2001). Malignant peripheral nerve sheath tumours e report of 8 cases and review of the literature. Acta Neurochir (Wien) 143: 357 - 364.

Tartaglia M, Mehler EL, Goldberg R, Zampino G, Brunner HG, Kremer H, van der Burgt I, Crosby AH, Ion A, Jeffery S, Kalidas K, Patton MA, Kucherlapati RS, Gelb BD (2001). Mutations in PTPN11, encoding the protein tyrosine phosphatase SHP-2, cause Noonan syndrome. Nat Genet; 29:465–8.

Toth BB, Fleming TJ, Lomba JA, Martin JW. (1981) Angiosarcoma metastatic to the maxillary tuberosity gingiva. Oral Surg Oral Med Oral Pathol; 52:71–4.

Turc-Carel C, Pietrzak E, Kakati S, Kinniburgh AJ, Sandberg AA.(1987)The human int-1 gene is located at chromosome region 12q12-12q13 and is not rearranged in myxoid liposarcoma with t(12;16)(q13;p11). Oncogene Res;1:397–405.

Victoria L, McCulloch TM, Callaghan EJ, Bauman NM. (1999). Malignant Triton Tumor of the head and neck: a case report and review of the literature. Head Neck;21:663–70.

Wadhwan V, Chaudhary MS, Gawande M. (2010) Fibrosarcoma of the oral cavity. Indian J Dent Res; 21:295-8.

Wang CP, Chang YL, Ting LL, Yang TL, Ko JY, Lou PJ. (2009) Malignant fibrous histiocytoma of the sinonasal tract. Head Neck; 31:85–93.

Weiss SW, (2001) 4th ed: Enzinger and Weiss's soft tissue tumours 4th edn. St Louis: CV Mosby.

Weiss SW, Goldblum JR. (2001) Malignant soft tissue, in Weiss SW, Goldblum JR (eds): Enzinger and Weiss's Soft Tissue Tumors. St Louis, Mosby.

Wenig BM, Heffner DK. Liposarcomas of the larynx and hypopharynx: a clincopathologic study of eight new cases and a review of the literature. Laryngoscope 1995;105:747–56.

Wick MR (1990). Malignant peripheral nerve sheath tumours of the skin. Mayo Clin Proc; 65:279 - 82.

Wong CK, Edwards AT, Rees BI. Liposarcoma: a review of current diagnosis and management. Br J Hosp Med 1997;58: 589–91.

Wong WW, Hirose T, Scheithauer BW, Schild SE, Gunderson L (1998). Malignant peripheral nerve sheath tumour: analysis of treatment outcome. Int J Radiat Oncol Biol Phys 42: 351 - 360.

Yakulis R, Manack L, Murphy AI Jr. (1996) Postradiation malignant triton tumor: a case report and review of the literature. Arch Pathol Lab Med;120:541-8.

Zahm SH, Fraumeni JFJr (1997). The epidemiology of soft tissue sarcoma. Semin Oncol; 24: 504-14.

8

Dermatofibrosarcoma Protuberans – Special Challenges of Management in Resources Constrained Countries

Titus Osita Chukwuanukwu and Stanley Anyanwu
Nnamdi Azikiwe University
Teaching Hospital
Nigeria

1. Introduction

Dermatofibrosarcoma protuberans (DFSP) is best described as a fibroblastic neoplasm. It is a low to moderate grade type of soft tissue sarcoma (STS) arising from cells of mesenchymal origin in the dermal layer of the skin[1-4]. This entity was first described in 1924 by Darier and Ferrand5. Though DFSP is a low grade malignancy, fibrosarcomatous variant can be very aggressive especially when provoked by inadequate excision. It is a rare type of skin cancer that can grow deeply into the skin to invade the fat, muscle, and bone. DFSP is a locally aggressive tumour and rarely metastasizes. This gives it a higher survival rate when adequately excised[1-7].

In developing countries however, late presentation to hospitals are very common. Patients here seek help first from unqualified persons and only come to the specialists late into their illness. This has led to poor outcomes in many cases.

2. Epidemiology

DFSP comprises 0.01% of all malignant tumours and 2 - 6% of all soft tissue sarcomas[1,2,3]. STS constitute overall less than 1% of human adult solid malignant tumour[7] but can be life threatening and sometimes difficult to diagnose and very challenging to treat. It has no sex predilection nor specified age incidence but is commoner between the ages of 20 and 50 years[6-8]. It is stated to be commoner in blacks with an estimated incidence of 0.8 to 5 per/million persons per year in America[6,8].

3. Aetiology

The exact cause of Soft Tissue Sarcomas and Dermatofibrosarcoma Protuberans is not well known. Predisposing factors include genetic mutation of the P 53 gene, exposure to ionising radiations, post burn and other scars and exposure to certain carcinogens have been documented. Of particular note is its recurrent nature especially following inadequate excision either in margin or depth. High rate recurrence is noted in developing countries like Nigeria[3].

4. Pathology

DFSP are skin cancers that arise from the dermal fibroblasts. Recent evidences by immunohistochemical tests however suggest that they may arise from the dendritic cells in the skin

It grows in a finger like manner into the surrounding tissues leading to uneven penetration. This is a major cause of recurrence as some malignant cells may have projected far beyond the macroscopic margin at the time of initial resection.

DFSP is highly cellular and comprises spindle cells arranged in a radial fashion most characteristic at the periphery of the tumor. It displays immunoreactivity to CD34. Haematogenous spread to the lungs is the commonest route of metastasis, regional lymph nodes are rarely involved[7].

The variants of DFSP include the Bednar tumour, myxiod DFSP, atrophic type and the fibrosarcomatous variant which is very aggressive.

There is no staging system yet developed specific for DFSP but it is currently staged in accordance with the American Musculoskeletal Tumour society staging system taking into account tumour grade and compartmentalization[6].

5. Clinical presentation

The usual pattern is an initial painless slow growing tumour. It may remain indolent for many years and sometimes grow to a very large size (more than 5cm in diameter over a few years). It may ulcerate but more commonly the patient intervenes one way or the other. Inadequate excision lead to recurrence of larger tumour and sometimes very slow healing ulcer. In the developing countries, they usually present with very large often fungating recurrent tumours. Other symptoms then depend on local effects and its site of location.

Metastasis is a late event and is commonest to the lung[1,2,6,7,10]. Later to liver, lymph nodes, peritoneum (for abdominal wall tumours) and nearby structures. Progression depends on the histological variant, grade, stage, size, how deeply seated the tumour is and presence or absence of other tumours and patients genetic predisposition. The immune status may also play a role as a rare recurrence of the fibrosarcomatous variant has been reported to occur in pregnancy[11].

Rate of recurrence depends on the adequacy of resection margin and other management modalities employed. A DFSP has been reported to occur at the surgical scar of an earlier excised tumour after many years[12].

Pain is as a result of pressure. When infected, there may be fever, anorexia and Weight loss. Overall, patient presents with large tumours without much constitutional symptoms/sign.

6. Investigations

Biopsy of all suspicious lesions is mandatory. Histological and immunochemistry studies are done. The investigative tool of choice is the magnetic resonance imaging (MRI). This is capable of delineating tissues planes thereby detecting extent of invasion of surrounding tissues including muscles and fat. This diagnostic tool is usually not available in developing countries. CT scan and contrast enhanced studies aid the diagnosis. X Rays of the affected parts and chest for metastasis to the lungs are also indicated in many cases. Biopsy of all suspicious tissues is recommended and for all lesions more than 5cm in diameter, an incision biopsy should precede definitive resection for adequate planning to avoid the danger of inadequate excision. Other investigations are done to determine the extent of local spread, distant metastasis and effects of the tumour on the patient generally.

7. Treatment

Surgery is the main stay of treatment. Wide local excision with histologically negative margins is the cornerstone of treatment[3,6]. For tumour less than 5cm in diameter a 3cm margin is recommended and for lesions greater than 5cm and recurrent lesions resection margin should be 5cm. The underlying tissue is also excised beyond the normal plane. The margins are examined to ensure they are tumour-free. Adjuvant radiotherapy increases tumour clearance and decreases rate of recurrence. Resection of tumours close to neurovascular bundle, bone and other vital structures may not obey these rules and adjuvant radiotherapy and chemotherapy will then be absolutely indicated. It is usually difficult to identify the margin of the tumour macroscopically as the finger like projections into muscle, fascia, fat resemble normal tissue. Fibrosis from previous surgeries may also make adequate excision difficult. Radiotherapy and chemotherapy may be used pre-operatively to downsize the tumour and make it more resectable or post-operatively to manage residual tumours and metastasis.

Mohs micrographic surgery is presently employed (where available) and hold great promise for complete tumour excision[7]. Very large defects may be created after tumour excision which requires the services of a plastic reconstructive surgeon. When the limb is involved, limb sparing surgeries are first attempted where feasible otherwise amputation may be resorted to. Reconstructive procedures include local rotation and advancement flaps, regional flaps, pedicle and free tissue transfers. Prosthetic mesh has been used for reconstructing full thickness abdominal /chest wall defects[3,31,14].

A multidisciplinary approach by healthcare team with experience in management of STS is recommended for proper treatment of DFSP.

8. Follow up

Follow up of the patient is for life. Tumours have been known to recur many years after adequate excision. Any suspicious lesion around the area of an initial excision including the scars is subjected to full investigations and expert care.

9. Prognosis

Prognosis depends on both tumour and patient factors as well as availability of investigative and support services. Size is an important prognostic variable and so affects the quality of

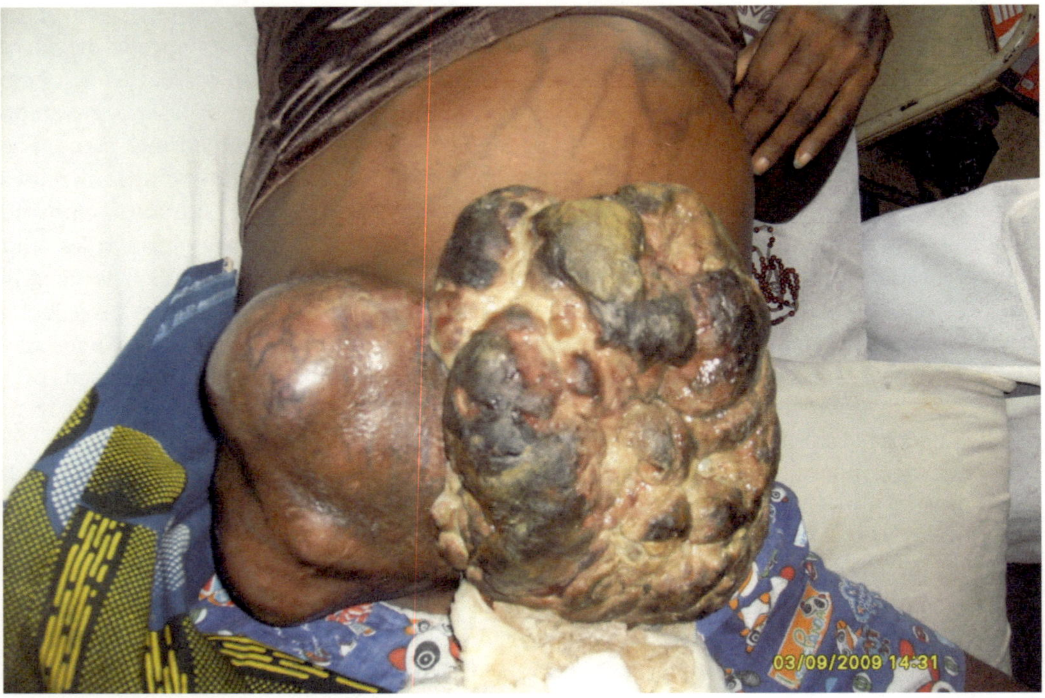

Fig. 1. Recurrence in pregnancy after 3rd excision, now very aggressive and fatal.resection.

In developed countries, the prognosis has improved remarkably but in the developing world however, prognosis remain poor due to a variety of factors. These include poverty, ignorance, late presentation with very large often fungating and metastatic lesions, low infrastructure and low availability of expertise.

10. References

[1] LeBoit P.E., Burg G., weedon D., sarasain A. 9Eds): World Health Organisation Classification of tumours. Pathology and Genetics of Skin Tumour. IARC Press: Lyon 2006.

[2] Fletcher C.D.M., Rydholm A., Singer S., Sundaram M., Coindre J.M: In Fletcher C.D.M., Unni K.K., Mertens F. (Eds): World Health Organisation classification of Tumours. Pathology and Genetics of Tumours of soft Tissue and Bone. IARC Press Lyon 2002. 13-18.

[3] Chukwuanukwu T.O.G., Anyanwu S.N.C. Giant Fibrosarcoma Protuberans of Abdominal Wall Management Problems in Resources - Constrained Country. Nig. J. Clin Prac. Sept 2009 12 (3); 338-340.

[4] Adigun I.A., Rahman G.A. A review of soft tissue sarcoma: Nig. J. Med. 16 (2); 94-101.

[5] Darier J, Ferrand M: Dermatofibromes progressifs et recidivants ou fibrosarcomes de la peau. Ann Dermatol Syphiliga 1924; 5:545-562.

[6] Kenny R.J, Cheney R., Stull M. A., Kraybill W. Soft Tissue Sarcomas; Current Management and Future Directions. Surg Clin N. AM 89 (2009) 235-247.

[7] Burkhardt BR, Soule EH, Winkelmann RK, Ivans JC: Dermatofibrosarcoma protuberans: study of fifty-six cases. Am J Surg 1966;111:634-644.

[8] Derek D, Vincent C, Lori I, Timothy M.J., Vernon K.S., Low recurrence rate after Surgery for Dermetofibrosarcoma protuberans. A multidisciplinary approach from a single institution. Cancer 2004; 100: 1008.16.

[9] Stojanovic A, Hoos A, Karpoff HM, Leung DH, Antonescu CR, Brennan MF, Lewis JJ. Soft tissue tumours of the Abdominal wall; Analysis of disease patterns and treatment. Arch Surg. 2001; 136: 70-79.

[10] Canale ST. Campbell's operative Orthopaedics. 10th ed. Philadelphia P.A: Mosby; 2003:864.

[11] Cakir B., Misirlioglu A., Gideroglu K., Akoz T: Giant fibrosarcoma arising in doumatofibnrosarcoma protuberance on the scalp during pregnancy. Dermatol Surg; 2003 Mar; 29 (3): 297-299.

[12] Kshirsugar A.Y., Kanetkar S.R., Nikam Y.P., Vasisth G.O: Recurrent dermatofibrosarcoma proliberans over auterior abdominal wall. J. Cutan Aesthet Surg; 2010; 3(3): 167-169.

[13] Kao CC, Rand RP, Stridde BC, Marchioro TL. Techniques in the composite reconstruction of extensive thoracoabdominal tumour resections. J. AM Coll. Surg. 1995. 180 (2).146-149.

[14] Servant JM., Arnault E., Revol M., Damino A. Reconstruction of large thoraco-abdominal defects using two-stage free tissue transfers and prosthetic materials. J Plast Reconstr. Aesthet. Surg. 2006; 59(4): 360-365.

9

Clinical and Molecular Biology of Angiosarcoma

N.J. Andersen[1], R.E. Froman[1], B.E. Kitchell[2] and N.S. Duesbery[1]
[1]*Laboratory of Cancer and Developmental Cell Biology, Van Andel Research Institute Grand Rapids,*
[2]*College of Veterinary Medicine, Michigan State University East Lansing, Michigan, USA*

1. Introduction

'Skepticism is a healthy response to diagnosis of any tumor as angiosarcoma.' (Lane, 1952)
Angiosarcoma (AS) is an aggressive malignancy of vascular tissue or vessel forming cells (Requena & Sangueza 1998). AS is rare in humans, making up 1-2 % of soft-tissue sarcomas (Young et al. 2010) and having an estimated incidence of 0.2/100,000 persons per year. Although AS can present anywhere in the body, in humans they typically arise in the skin or superficial soft tissues. It is most frequently noted on the face and scalp of elderly men where their persistent growth causes ulceration and infection, as well as on breasts, and extremities (Brennan et al. 2001; Fayette et al. 2007; Glazebrook et al. 2008). Less frequently AS arises in liver, heart, and spleen (Young et al. 2010). The literature is replete with retrospective analyses and case studies on AS but the rarity of patients diagnosed with this disease makes it difficult to perform more than a superficial investigation on the biology and clinical behavior of AS. However, the occurrence of AS is not restricted to humans and there are several alternative animal models with the potential to inform human studies. We have written this review to collect, compare, and contrast diverse reports on the biology and treatment of AS in humans and alternative animal models. Our objective is to establish a comparative framework to focus further discussion and scientific enquiry.

2. Types of AS

While there is general agreement angiosarcomas arise from endothelial cells, its causes are uncertain. There appears to be no single cause of AS in humans; rather, a variety of factors have been reported to contribute to risk of disease. Broadly speaking the causes of this disease may be classified as environmental, familial, and iatrogenic.

2.1 Environmental AS

Chronic exposure to any of several environmental risk factors has been linked with AS. Each of these directly or indirectly induce genetic mutations and alter gene expression. Vinyl chloride was first identified as an AS inducing compound when it was noticed that industrial plastic and synthetic rubber manufacturers as well as beauty salon personnel had an elevated incidence of AS. Exposure to vinyl chloride was the only common element identified in both populations (Creech & Johnson 1974; Infante et al. 2009; Sahmel et al. 2009). Vinyl chloride was used for the production of industrial resins and as a hairspray propellant. Interestingly, vinyl chloride increases the rate of hepatic AS because vinyl chloride is a carcinogen that is predominantly directed towards hepatic endothelial cells. The metabolism of vinyl chloride produces reactive metabolites that form pro-mutagenic DNA adducts (reviewed by Bolt (2005)).

Chronic exposure to arsenic in pesticides or in a traditional medicinal tonic (Fowler's solution) has also been linked to hepatic AS (Centeno et al. 2002; Falk et al. 1993). The precise mechanism(s) of arsenic carcinogenesis is uncertain, although it appears to act in an epigenetic fashion rather than as a classical mutagen, causing pleiotropic cellular effects that promote tumorigenesis (reviewed by Flora (2011)).

No link between AS and UV exposure has been documented. However, there are published case reports of xeroderma pigmentosum patients developing cutaneous AS. Xeroderma pigmentosum is a rare autosomal recessive disease causing defects in nucleotide excision repair; the patients are sensitive to UV radiation and are at higher risk for developing skin cancers (de Boer & Hoeijmakers 2000; Kraemer et al. 1987). Whereas cutaneous AS normally develops in older patients with a mean onset of 63 years (Aust et al. 1997), cutaneous AS in xeroderma pigmentosum patients appears to have an earlier onset, ranging from 13 to 40 years with a mean of 19.2 years (Arlett et al. 2006; Arora et al. 2008; Ludolph-Hauser et al. 2000; Marcon et al. 2004; van Geel & den Bakker 2009). Further work is needed to establish whether there is a role for UV as a causative agent of cutaneous AS.

2.2 Iatrogenic AS

There are several examples of AS being induced as a consequence of prior medical treatment. Exposure to Thorotrast® (colloidal thorium-232 dioxide) has been linked to hepatic AS. Thorotrast® was used in the United States from the 1930's through the 1960's as a radiographic contrast compound to visualize blood vessels. Upon injection, Thorotrast is absorbed by bones, liver, spleen, and lymph nodes where it has a high bioavailability and releases alpha particles for imaging. While useful as an imaging agent, Thorotrast® was found to have unanticipated toxicities. Because it has a long biological half-life, patients were exposed to high levels of ionizing radiation for extended (lifelong) periods (Autenrieth & Lange 1979; Kiyosawa et al. 1989). Thorotrast® exposure has also been associated with increased risk of other cancers including hepatic ductal carcinoma and leukemia (Johnson et al. 1977; Looney 1960).

Radiotherapy is an infrequent but well-recognized risk factor for AS (Botros et al. 2009; Fury et al. 2005; Miura et al. 2003). A study of 274,572 breast cancer patients in the SEER Cancer Incidence Public-Use Database (Yap et al. 2002) found that incidence of a subsequent sarcoma while low, was modestly elevated in patients receiving breast irradiation compared to patients not receiving such therapy (87/82,296 [0.0011%] versus 176/192,276 [0.0009%] respectively). Further, whereas AS accounted for approximately 6% of subsequent sarcomas in unirradiated patients, it represented almost 60% of cases within a previously irradiated field (Yap et al. 2002). It seems radiation therapy not only increases the incidence of secondary malignancies but also changes the spectrum of tumors associated with treatment. These results were consistent with a prior study using the same SEER database that showed increased incidence of AS in irradiated breast cancer patients versus unirradiated patients (Huang & Mackillop 2001).

However, a recent retrospective study of Finnish cancer patients showed different results (Virtanen et al. 2007). Surveying more than 300,000 cancer patient records accrued over a 50-year period, Virtanen et al. (2007) failed to identify a statistically significant association of AS with prior radiation treatment. These results agree with an earlier Swedish study of 122,991 women with breast cancer that showed no statistically significant correlation between radiation therapy and angiosarcoma, although they did observe a correlation with lymphedema (Karlsson et al. 1998). The Finnish research team did note a five-fold increase in AS among women with breast or gynecologic cancers when compared with the rest of the population. However, while the SEER-based studies focused on the incidence of subsequent sarcoma within the irradiated field of women with breast cancer, the Finnish study examined incidence irrespective of radiation field within a mixed population of men and women treated for several tumor diagnoses. Thus, the latter studies may have failed to demonstrate a statistically significant association between AS and radiotherapy because they were underpowered.

Chronic lymphedema is another risk factor for AS. The most well known form is Stewart-Treves syndrome, in which lymphedema presents in the adjacent arm after radical mastectomy (Stewart & Treves 1948). Although rare, AS is also associated with other chronic lymphedema disorders such as Milroy disease and elephantiasis (Hallel-Halevy et al. 1999; Offori et al. 1993). It is not immediately apparent why failure of lymph node drainage should promote AS. One possibility is that edema restricts perfusion and induces an ischemic response involving endothelial proliferation. If this were the case one might expect to see increased incidence of AS in association with peripheral arterial disease. However, such an association has not been reported. Alternatively, edema-mediated changes may create a permissive microenvironment allowing phenotypic expression of an otherwise masked trait that promotes endothelial proliferation.

2.3 Familial AS

Although patients with Von Hippel-Lindau disease show increased incidence of cranial hemangioblastoma (Kaelin 2007), no highly penetrant, causal mutation for AS in humans has been reported. This should not be interpreted as an indication that hereditary factors do not influence the risk of developing AS, but that the incidence of AS is so low that identifying such genetic factors may be exceedingly difficult. However, indirect evidence supports a role for hereditary factors in the onset or progression of AS. The incidence of all vascular tumors appears to be increased in offspring whose parents were diagnosed with kidney cancer, nervous system hemangioma, or hemangioblastoma, and AS of the trunk and extremities has been associated with maternal breast cancer (Ji & Hemminki 2007). Moreover, there is strong evidence for breed and strain-specific predisposition of AS in mice and dogs (see below).

3. Clinical features

3.1 Presentation

The presentation of AS is tied to the site of occurrence. In cutaneous AS, tumor may begin as a bruise-like bluish coloration or a red nodular rash (Lane 1952; Morgan et al. 2004). It can also present as purplish multicentric lesions as seen in Stewart-Treves syndrome (Stewart & Treves 1948). Unfortunately due to the innocuous appearance of the initial dermal lesion, a large percentage of patients initially disregard the lesion and as a consequence have systemic disease at the time of ultimate diagnosis (Morgan et al. 2004). For visceral and cardiac disease, AS most often presents as organ failure. Cardiac AS patients commonly have atrial fibrillation, malaise, and resting tachycardia (Ge et al. 2011; Matzke et al.). Splenic AS presents with splenomegaly (enlarged spleen) or abdominal pain and fatigue from splenic rupture (Falk et al. 1993); these patients may also have cytopenia, leukocytosis, and thrombocytosis. Hepatic AS patients initially present with jaundice and may also experience abdominal pain and fatigue (Mahony et al. 1982; Valenzuela et al. 2009).

3.2 Diagnostic pathology

There are two subtypes of angiosarcoma defined by pathology. Angiosarcoma is classically defined by a growth of spindle-shaped endothelial cells (Figure 1). In 1982, Weiss and Enzinger described a new subtype, epithelioid AS, with large rounded or polygonal cells that have an epithelial-like morphology (Weiss & Enzinger 1982). In reality, most tumors have a mixture of both spindle and round endothelial cells (Morgan et al. 2004). Angiosarcoma tumors classically consist of sheets of endothelial cells with multiple irregular anastomosing channels. These channels can be perfused and blood-filled or void and can be lined with a single or multiple layers of atypical endothelial cells (Koch et al. 2008; Ohsawa et al. 1995; Yang et al. 2010). Areas of hemorrhage and necrosis are also common in AS (Armah et al. 2007; Ge et al. 2011; Gong et al. 2011; Neuhauser et al. 2000; Ohsawa et al. 1995; Yang et al. 2010). Low grade lesions display irregular vascular channels lined with atypical endothelial cells in single or multiple layers (Koch et al. 2008). High-grade lesions are comprised of sheets of undifferentiated, pleomorphic cells which can make them difficult to distinguish from carcinomas (Koch et al. 2008). High grade lesions also have large areas of hemorrhage. There is no clinical or survival advantage between low- and high-grade lesions. Definitive diagnosis is made by biopsy and immunohistochemistry with antibodies against the endothelial marker CD31 and Factor VIII-related antigen. Staining with antibodies against von Willebrand's factor II and CD34 may also be used to confirm a diagnosis of AS (Ohsawa et al. 1995).

3.3 Differential diagnosis

Cutaneous AS can initially be misdiagnosed as bruising, multiple different skin infections, and even insect bites. It is the duration and spreading of the lesion that prompts concern. Cutaneous AS is similar in appearance to another endothelial derived malignancy, Kaposi sarcoma. Kaposi sarcoma is a virus-induced cancer (Chang et al. 1994; Kemeny et al. 1996). Both Kaposi sarcoma and AS can be multicentric skin lesions with spindle cell pathology (Morgan et al. 2004; Nickoloff & Griffiths 1989). To further complicate the diagnosis, a percentage of Kaposi cells are CD31 positive and up to half of AS cells are positive for the endothelial lymph factor podoplanin by immunohistochemistry. However, only Kaposi sarcoma are positive for the presence of Kaposi's sarcoma causative virus (Human Herpes Virus 8) by immunohistochemistry using antibodies against Latency nuclear antigen-1 (LANA-1) or by amplifying viral DNA by PCR (reviewed in (Mesri et al. 2010; Schmid & Zietz 2005)). Cutaneous AS may also be confused with irregular growths of superficial vasculature or benign hemangiomas, mostly seen in infants (Lawley et al. 2005). These vascular malformations are commonly referred to as port wine stains or angel kisses. These may be distinguished from visceral AS by immunohistochemistry with antibodies against the Wilms tumor 1 transcription factor (Ge et al. 2011; Lawley et al. 2005).

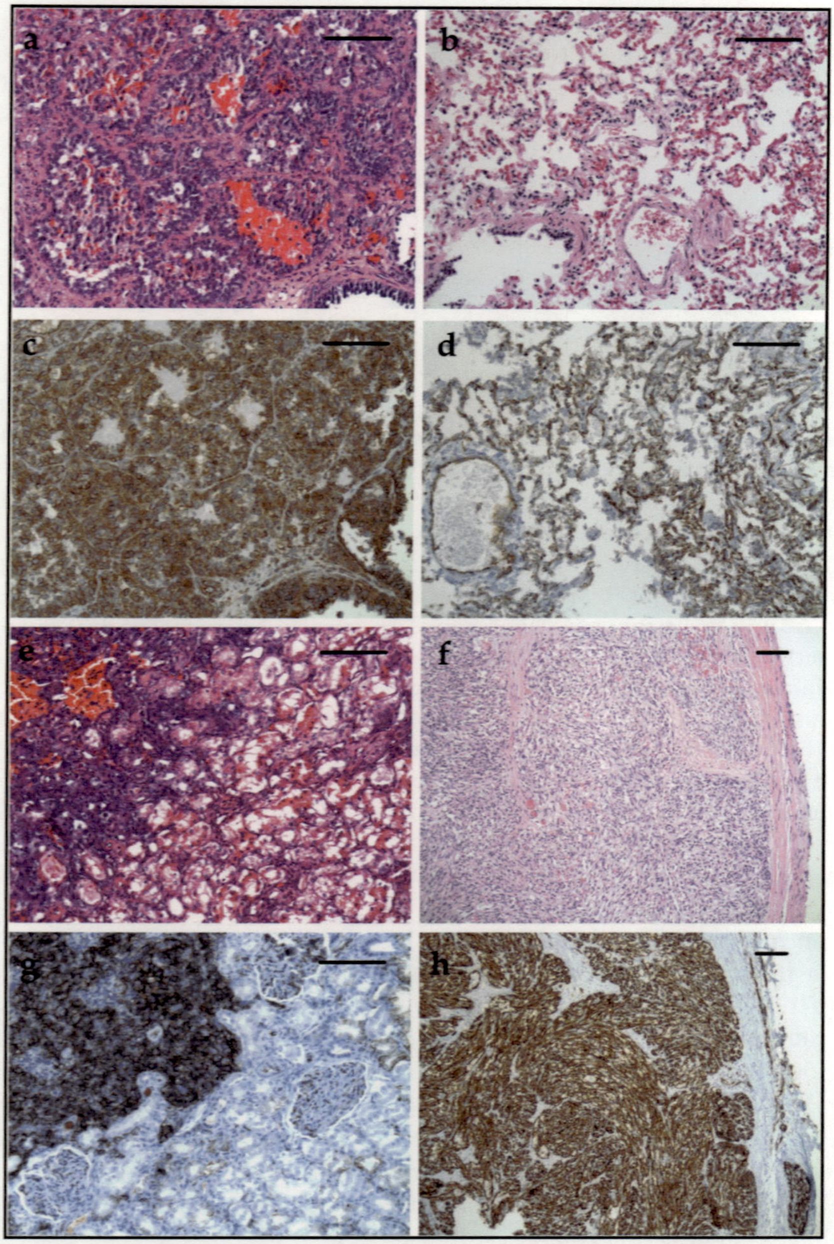

Fig. 1. **Histology of human and canine angiosarcoma.** Stained with Hematoxylin and Eosin (a,b,e,f) or immunostained with antibodies against CD31 (c,d,g,h) both human (a, c) and canine (b, d) splenic angiosarcoma as well as canine kidney angiosarcoma (e, g) show extensive networks of endothelial (CD31 positive) cells with multiple irregular anastomosing channels filled with blood. In contrast this canine cutaneous angiosarcoma (f, h) shows a highly vascular tumor with spindle-shaped CD31-positive endothelial cells. Bars = 100 micrometers.

The main discernible clinical sign of splenic AS is splenomegaly (Neuhauser et al. 2000; Thompson et al. 2005). Any known cause of spleen enlargement is a differential diagnosis for splenic AS. This includes but is not limited to lymphoma or infection (reviewed in (Pozo et al. 2009; Suzuki et al. 2010)). In addition, visceral disease often presents with vague flu-like symptoms such as malaise and abdominal pain (Falk et al. 1993).

Since the epithelioid AS subtype is defined by endothelial cells that have a large, round cell morphology similar to that of epithelial cells, AS may be confused with a carcinoma (Lin et al. 2010; Weiss & Enzinger 1982). However, epitheloid AS cells stain positive for CD31 and Factor VIII on immunohistochemistry (Fletcher et al. 1991; Lin et al. 2010).

3.4 Prognosis and treatment

Over the years AS treatment has changed very little. The usual treatment for primary AS is surgery followed by high-dose radiotherapy either alone or with doxorubicin-based chemotherapy. Even with such interventions survival rates are poor. In addition, there is no current standard of care based on disease subtype or location.

Surgery is the mainstay for the treatment of primary AS. Surgical intervention is limited to local control and is not recommended for widely disseminated disease. Current guidelines call for total surgical resection of the tumor with wide negative margins to reduce re-occurrence (Lahat et al. 2009; Mendenhall et al. 2006). However, the multicentric nature of cutaneous AS and its proximity to vital organs in visceral disease makes achieving complete tumor resection difficult. In a review of head and neck soft tissue sarcomas, positive margins were found in 50% of patients (Farhood et al. 1990).

Survival rates after surgery alone are poor (Holden et al. 1987). While the addition of postoperative radiotherapy improves survival, there are drawbacks to radiation. Effective radiation treatment requires wide radiation fields and often doses of more than 50 Gy to achieve tumor control (Mark et al. 1996; Pawlik et al. 2003). Furthermore, radiotherapy is not recommended for radiation-induced AS (Mark et al. 1996).

Doxorubicin is considered the most efficacious chemotherapy agent for local and metastatic AS but provides minimal tumor control or survival benefit. The response rate to doxorubicin has been reported to be 16 - 36%. In addition, doxorubicin causes long-term damage to the heart at cumulative total doses over 400 mg/m^2 of body surface area (Chlebowski 1979). To reduce cardiotoxicity, doxorubicin can be encased in liposomes, reducing the amount of free doxorubicin (Cattel et al. 2003). Liposomal doxorubicin treatment of soft tissue sarcomas has equivalent activity but fewer adverse effects relative to free doxorubicin, and thus it is included in the current National Comprehensive Cancer Network guidelines for the treatment of soft tissue sarcomas (Judson et al. 2001). However, the lipid envelope increases doxorubicin absorption and retention by the skin. Side effects of liposomal doxorubicin may include dermal rash or sores on the palms and soles of the feet called palmar-plantar erythodysesthesia (Judson et al. 2001; Lorusso et al. 2007). The latter can be severe enough to require a dosage decrease, treatment interruption, or termination of treatment (Lorusso et al. 2007).

Other adjuvant treatments are reported to have had minimal success. The use of taxanes such as paclitaxel to treat AS has increased. In a small study of 9 patients, 8 responded to paclitaxel (Fata et al. 1999). A 32-patient retrospective paclitaxel study documented a 62% response rate with one complete response. A 30-patient prospective study demonstrated a 19% response rate after 6 months with 3 complete responses with surgery and a median overall survival of 7.6 months (Penel et al. 2008). Paclitaxel did show a subtype specificity; the response rate in head and neck AS was 75%, while for other primary tumor locations the response rate was 58%. The median time to progression of head and neck disease was 9.5 months compared with 7 months for AS of other primary sites (Schlemmer et al. 2008). In another study, scalp AS had a progression-free survival of 6.8 months, but only 2.8 months of progression free survival was documented for AS arising below the clavicle (Fury et al. 2005). In comparison to spontaneous tumors that have a median survival expectation of nearly 9 months, radiation induced AS are more resistant to paclitaxel treatment and have a median overall survival of less than 6 months (Penel et al. 2008). Paclitaxel has also been used as a neoadjuvant therapy to decrease primary tumor size prior to surgery for splenic AS (Vakkalanka & Milhem 2010).

4. Etiology

4.1 Cellular origins

The origin of AS tumor cells is still unknown. Angiosarcoma tumors are generally thought to arise from endothelial cells. The majority of cells stain positively for the endothelial cell markers: CD31, CD34, and Factor VIII-antigen. However, up to 70% of CD31 positive AS cells are also positive for the lymph endothelial marker podoplanin (Breiteneder-Geleff et al. 1999). This suggests contributions of both lymph and vascular endothelium in AS. Alternatively, the tumor microenvironment may differentiate a population of undifferentiated endothelial cells to lymph or vascular-like endothelium.

Cancer stem cells or cancer progenitor cells have been documented in a variety of tumors, but the presence of angiosarcoma cancer stem cells is not known. Interestingly, Wnt1 was recently found to be expressed and activated in AS cells. Furthermore, Wnt1 increases endothelial progenitor cell (EPC) proliferation and EPC-dependent angiogenesis (Gherghe et al. 2011). These data suggest a possible role of EPCs in AS tumorigenesis and tumor angiogenesis through a Wnt1 mechanism. As of yet, no study has clearly determined the role of EPCs in tumorigenesis, and the importance of tumor stem cells in AS tumorigenesis is still unknown.

4.2 Molecular biology

Angiosarcoma has no clearly defined causative mutation or chromosomal changes, but genomic abnormalities including chromosomal deletions, amplifications, and rearrangements, have been identified in a variety of these tumors. In general, the karyotypes of AS are complicated and display both clonal and non-clonal chromosomal changes. The breadth and variety of aberrations suggest they may represent chromosomal alterations from unbridled cell proliferation. The importance of these mutations or gene amplifications for tumorigenesis and tumor development is not known. The most common aberrations involve the loss of heterozygosity of chromosome 22 (Gil-Benso et al. 1994; Kindblom et al. 1991; Quezado et al. 1998; Schuborg et al. 1998; Wong et al. 2001; Zu et al. 2001). The genes of both platelet-derived endothelial cell growth factor (PD-ECGF) and the tumor suppressor NF2 mapped to chromosome 22 (Kindblom et al. 1991) but the significance of this observation has not been explored. Losses of the short arm of chromosomes 4 and 7 are also common in AS (Wong et al. 2001). MYC amplification has been found in radiation-induced AS tumors that have an 8q24 gain (Guo et al. 2011).

The loss of tumor suppressor function likely plays an important role in AS development. The tumor suppressor p53 is mutated in a subset of AS tumors. In cardiac AS, mutant p53 is overexpressed and localizes to the nucleus (Hollstein et al. 1994; Soini et al. 1995; Zu et al. 2001). Mutations in p53 codons 141 and 136 were identified in a small cohort of hepatic AS (Soini et al. 1995) and mutations in p53 codons 249 and 255 have been associated with vinyl chloride exposure (Hollstein et al. 1994). Other studies indicate the INK4a-ARF locus is frequently inactivated in liver AS independent of p53 mutations (Weihrauch et al. 2002). Mutations in the PTEN tumor suppressor have also been identified in hepatic AS; an exon 7 mutation codes for a premature stop codon resulting in a nonfunctional protein (Tate et al. 2007).

Activating mutations in key signaling molecules promote AS tumorigenesis. K-Ras2 mutations have been associated with AS (Marion 2005; Przygodzki et al. 1997) and have been detected in hepatic AS after exposure to vinyl chloride (Weihrauch et al. 2002). Ten percent of AS tumors showed activating KDR (VEGFR2) mutations (Antonescu et al. 2009). Also, 25% of a 20 patient study of radiation-induced AS showed a co-amplification of FLT4 (VEGFR3) and MYC (Guo et al. 2011).

Interestingly, vascular endothelial specific cadherin (VE-cadherin) is absent or decreased in AS (Martin-Padura et al. 1995; Tanioka et al. 2001; Zanetta et al. 2005). Loss of VE-cadherin may promote AS growth in several ways. Like other cadherins, VE-cadherin interacts with and retains β-catenin at adherens junctions. Through this mechanism, cadherins indirectly control the free (cytoplasmic) pool of β-catenin. Free β-catenin can be transported to the nucleus to regulate transcription. Thus, loss of VE-cadherin may represent a pathway to induce cancer gene dysregulation. Retention of β-catenin at adherens junctions by VE-cadherin has been inversely correlated with vascular tumor growth and hemorrhage (Zanetta et al. 2005). During angiogenesis, endothelial cells detach and invade surrounding tissue, where they replicate and branch into a vascular network. The loss of VE-cadherin may facilitate angiogenesis. In addition, change in the cadherin profile of cells, or cadherin switching, has been implicated in tumor cell invasion and metastasis (reviewed in Maeda et al. (2005)). Whether cadherin misregulation in AS cells explains the invasive and metastatic nature of AS is not known.

5. Insight from other sources

The rarity of angiosarcoma has restricted the scope of basic and clinical research on this disease. In this section we will discuss experimental models for generating further insight into the biology and treatment of AS, including the study of more common (but related) human tumors, genetically engineered or chemically induced mouse models, and the emerging relevance of studies of naturally occurring AS in companion dogs.

5.1 Related tumors in humans

5.1.1 Kaposi sarcoma

The similarity between Kaposi sarcoma (KS) and AS may provide a foundation for understanding pathways vital for AS tumorigenesis and development. Like AS, KS is an endothelial cell-derived tumor, but Kaposi is derived from lymphatic endothelial cells. Kaposi sarcoma is a vascular tumor characterized histologically by a high degree of angiogenesis and the presence of proliferating spindle cells (Brash & Bale 2001). The spindle cells act in a paracrine fashion, releasing pro-inflammatory and angiogenic factors, including VEGF, which are necessary to promote KS lesions. Kaposi sarcoma is caused by human herpes virus 8 (HHV8 or KSHV; (Ablashi et al. 2002; Chang et al. 1994)). The expression of a single viral gene encoding a constitutively active G-protein coupled receptor (vGPCR) in endothelial cells is sufficient to induce angioproliferative tumors in mice that closely resemble human KS (Montaner et al. 2003). Among other functions, Kaposi sarcoma vGPCR has been demonstrated to activate the mitogen- and stress-activated protein kinases MAPK1/2 and p38 MAPK in a variety of cell lines (Arvanitakis et al. 1997; Bais et al. 1998; Burger et al. 1999; Cannon et al. 2003; Cannon & Cesarman 2004; Sodhi et al. 2000). Significantly, KS vGPCR-induced expression of VEGF depends upon increased activity of both MAPK1/2 and p38 MAPK (Bais et al. 1998; Sodhi et al. 2000). Since these are direct downstream targets of mitogen activated protein kinase kinases (MKKs) (Lewis et al. 1998), MKKs present an attractive potential therapeutic target for treatment of AS. In support of this we have observed that when mouse endothelial cell tumor xenografts expressing vGPCR are treated with a proteolytic inhibitor of MKK tumor growth is blocked and vascularization is decreased (Depeille et al. 2007). MEK inhibitors tested in clinical trials for a variety of tumors, most notably melanoma, have not shown marked efficacy (Lee & Duesbery 2010). However, these drugs target only MEK1 and 2, leaving other MKK signaling pathways intact.

The similarity between Kaposi sarcoma and AS raises interesting questions regarding the etiology and molecular biology of AS. Are there spindle cell equivalents in AS that release cytokines and drive tumor growth? Could AS also have a viral origin? Indeed, several other human cutaneous cancers have viral origins (e.g. Merkel cell carcinoma and polyomavirus, squamous cell carcinoma and HPV) and viruses can cause AS in mouse models (see below). Moreover, similar to iatrogenic KS, cases of AS have been reported to develop in kidney transplant patients taking immune suppressants (e.g. Farag et al. (2005) and references therein). Evidence for a viral origin of AS has been sought through detection of HHV8 viral expression sequences. However, an initial report showing evidence of an HHV8 sequence in a subset of AS (McDonagh et al. 1996) was contradicted by subsequent studies (Lasota & Miettinen 1999). Though it appears HHV8 does not play a role in the origin of AS, we can not yet rule out a viral contribution to AS tumorigenesis.

5.1.2 Hemangioma

Hemangiomas are benign growths arising from vascular endothelial cells. In hemangiomas, endothelial cells form a tortuous network of blood vessels. These lesions are common in newborns as strawberry patches or port wine stains. The causative mechanism of growth is unknown, but serum levels of VEGFA and HIF-1alpha are elevated in children with hemangiomas (Kleinman et al. 2007) suggesting hypoxic signals may be driving AS growth. Hemangiomas have been successfully treated with the beta-blocking agent propranolol (Leaute-Labreze et al. 2008; Sans et al. 2009). While the mechanism of action is not known, Sans et al. (2009) speculate that propranolol inhibits beta-adrenergic receptors expressed in endothelial cells, and in this manner down-regulates MAPK signaling and VEGF release.

5.2 Similar tumors in other species

The incidence of AS has been documented in a variety of species. For discussion purposes we have separated these into 1) genetically engineered or chemically induced AS models and 2) spontaneous or naturally occurring AS.

5.2.1 Induced angiosarcoma

Mice develop AS in response to a viral infection, toxicologic treatment, or genetic manipulation. Study of the common properties or convergent signaling of these diverse agents may reveal a unified mechanism for AS induction.

Viral Infection - Injection of Moloney mouse sarcoma virus (Stoica et al. 1990; Yuen et al. 1991), Harvey Sarcoma virus (Chesterman et al. 1966; Harvey 1964), or Kirsten Sarcoma virus (Pitts et al. 1983) into mice or rats induces the formation of angiomatous lesions resembling angiosarcoma or Kaposi's sarcoma. These viruses encode mutant, oncogenic forms of cellular oncogenes encoding c-Mos, H-Ras, and K-Ras, respectively. Each of these genes stimulates cellular proliferation and oncogenic transformation by activation of the mitogen-activated protein kinase (MAPK) signaling pathway.

Toxicologic treatment - Rodent bioassays have been used to identify several carcinogenic compounds capable of inducing angiosarcoma (reviewed by Cohen et al. (2009)). Some of these compounds react with DNA, acting in a manner similar to vinyl chloride or Thorotrast. Others, such as 2-butoxyethanol, are non-genotoxic and act indirectly through production of reactive oxygen species and cytokines to stimulate endothelial cell proliferation (Corthals et al. 2006; Kamendulis et al. 2010; Klaunig & Kamendulis 2005).

Genetic manipulations - Mice engineered to express knock-in mutations (D1226N or Y1228C) in the activation loop of Met develop a high incidence of angiosarcoma with moderately pleiomorphic endothelial cells, cavernous blood vessels, and palisading epithelioid-like cells (Graveel et al. 2004). Met is a tyrosine kinase receptor for the hepatocyte growth factor/scatter factor and is a potent activator of the MAPK signaling pathway, regulating among other things the epithelial-to-mesenchymal transition and metastatic behavior (Birchmeier et al. 2003). There are several Met antagonists in clinical trials for a variety of tumors (Eder et al. 2009).

As noted above, the loss of tumor suppressor function likely plays an important role in AS development. Not surprisingly then, loss of tumor suppressor function in mice induces AS formation. Heterozygous deletion of p53 causes a broad-based cancer predisposition in which 57% of mice develop a variety of sarcomas including AS (Jacks et al. 1994). The incidence of AS in p53-null mice is dramatically increased from 15% to 53% when mice are crossed to Wrn^{hel} mice harboring homozygous deletions in the helicase domain of the *Wrn* gene (Lebel et al. 2001). Similarly, p53-null mice crossed with mice lacking alleles of Ink4d and/or Ink4c show as high as 75-85% incidence of angiosarcoma (Zindy et al. 2003). The Wrn protein interacts with p53 to promote genomic stability. The Ink4 proteins bind and inactivate cyclin dependent kinases, preventing cell cycle progression and maintaining cells in a quiescent state.

These data show that genomic manipulation resulting in deregulation of cell cycle control and genomic instability in mice readily promotes endothelial cells to switch to a malignant phenotype. Why then do mice develop AS at such high rates in response to a viral infection, toxicologic treatment, or genetic manipulation? The answer may be linked to unidentified hereditary factors since studies of spontaneous tumorigenesis in mice indicate mice are predisposed to develop AS (see below).

5.2.2 Spontaneous tumors

Mice have a substantially higher incidence of spontaneous AS than do humans, but the incidence varies by strain. In a two-year study of approximately 2000 $B6C3F_1$ mice, Haseman et al. (1998) noted that 2.5-2.7% spontaneously developed AS. Although AS arose at many sites, the predominant locations were liver (male/female; 0.7/1.1%), spleen (0.7/1.0%), and uterus (0.4%). Similarly, a second study of $B6C3F_1$ mice (Chandra & Frith 1992) noted 4.5/1.0% (male/female) of mice spontaneously developed AS. In contrast CD-1 and Icr:Ha mice have spontaneous rates of AS around 0.7% and 0.4%, respectively (Chandra & Frith 1992; Eaton et al. 1980). The increased incidence in $B6C3F_1$ mice indicates that certain strains are genetically predisposed to develop AS.

Naturally occurring (spontaneous) AS are not restricted to humans and mice. They have been detected in a variety of animals including rhesus macaques (Mejia et al. 2009; Myers et al. 2001), horses (Schultheiss 2004), cows (Sutton & McLennan 1982), ferrets (Schultheiss 2004), dogs (Hargis et al. 1992), cats (Miller et al. 1992), rats (Schultheiss 2004), and snakes (Tuttle 2006). Any of these animals could potentially serve as a surrogate model system for human disease in an experimental context but dogs seem best suited for this purpose. While sharing many features in common with humans as patients, dogs have a much higher incidence of AS and a more rapid time course of disease progression. The canine model also offers some unique, advantageous features distinguishing it from other animal models and opening novel experimental opportunities. First, because of selective breeding, genetic variation within canine breeds is very low. Second, since each breed is derived from a small group of founders, most tracing back approximately 150 years, many of the genes associated with polygenic traits are fixed, so only a few variable genes determine phenotype. This means that it will be much easier to identify genetic disease determinants in dogs than in humans. Finally, companion dogs share the same environmental exposures as humans and thus may more accurately reflect the human condition. The ability to identify, recruit, and study cancers within a breed of dog offers new avenues of hope for research into clinical oncology and the underlying causes of AS (Gordon et al. 2009; Paoloni & Khanna 2008).

6. Canine AS

In contrast to AS in humans, AS is relatively common in dogs, with an overall incidence of 24/100,000 (Dobson et al. 2002). There is substantial variability in the incidence of canine angiosarcoma (cAS, more commonly referred to as hemangiosarcoma) among breeds, with large breed dogs such as Golden retrievers and German shepherds having a much higher incidence. A health survey of Golden retrievers attributed 62% of all deaths to cancer, with cAS representing 16% of reported cancers (Glickman et al. 1999). Why this tumor is more common in dogs than in humans is uncertain. It is possible that disease-causing genes were over-represented in the founding populations for these dogs. Alternatively, genes promoting susceptibility to cAS may have been co-selected along with artificially selected traits in the directed evolution of these breeds. Regardless, the genetic uniformity within breeds offers a unique and unbiased opportunity to identify genes that cause AS.

6.1 Presentation and diagnosis

cAS may present in virtually any tissue of the body, including bone, kidney, skeletal muscle, liver, lung, aorta, urinary bladder, intestine, oral mucosa, tongue, prostate, vulva/vagina, perineum and the cornea, nictitans or conjunctival tissue of the eye (Bergman 2010; Bulakowski et al. 2008; Hargis et al. 1992; Schultheiss 2004; Withrow & MacEwen 1996). Metastasis can involve any portion of the body, including the central nervous system. While most dogs present with splenic or liver lesions, some breeds show elevated incidence of cutaneous (Whippets, Italian greyhounds) or cardiac (Saluki) cAS (Hargis et al. 1992; Prymak et al. 1988; Schultheiss 2004). This demonstrates that not only do genetic factors influence susceptibility to cAS, but also they determine the location at which the disease will present. From a research perspective, it opens new avenues for discovery of the basic mechanisms of the origin and progression of cancer that could be translated to further our understanding of the etiology, pathophysiology, and treatment of AS in human patients.

Canine AS is the most common malignancy of the spleen in dogs (Spangler & Culbertson 1992). Middle-aged, large (> 20kg) dogs are most prone to splenic cAS. Golden retrievers, German shepherds, and Labrador retrievers are overrepresented, as are other large breeds such as Clumber spaniels. A health survey conducted by the Golden Retriever Club of America/Golden Retriever Foundation reported that 16% of Golden retrievers with cancer die from cAS at an average age of 10 years (Glickman et al. 1999). Mixed breeds are also commonly affected. Dogs with visceral cAS typically present acutely, with profound lethargy, anemia, or sudden collapse. There may be intermittent, nonspecific clinical signs such as inappetance, weight loss and occasional episodes of weakness. Hemoperitoneum most often leads to diagnosis, often on an emergency basis.

Splenic tumor size varies, but the lesions are frequently very large and multinodular, with one to many saccular, blood filled lesions. The tissue is extremely friable, which often leads to spontaneous rupture. It is the acute loss of blood which causes the presenting signs. Dogs may recover from intra-abdominal hemorrhage through resorption of the blood (autotransfusion) and erythrocyte regeneration. However, there will frequently be further hemorrhaging. Anecdotally, more dogs are lost to euthanasia than to spontaneous hemorrhage, as the owners do not wish their dogs to suffer further such episodes.

In contrast to humans, in whom left atrial AS is more frequent (Casha et al. 2002), cardiac cAS most commonly occurs in the right atrium and dogs of the Saluki breed are particularly prone to development of such tumors. Right atrial cAS is also seen in Golden retrievers and German shepherd dogs. Cardiac cAS can be devastating from the outset, with many dogs presenting for cardiac tamponade and signs of right heart failure. The pressure of blood from a ruptured cAS in the right atrium (RA) fills the pericardial sac and leads to extreme respiratory distress, anxiety, and collapse. Alternatively, dogs may simply die acutely from cardiac arrest, and the disease is discovered upon necropsy of what seemed to be an otherwise healthy dog. Many cases are likely never conclusively diagnosed, as necropsy is infrequent in veterinary medicine.

Cardiac cAS are typically red to dark red or purple in color, and ranging from millimeters to centimeters in length. Such tumors are prone to spontaneous hemorrhage, which may lead to pericardial effusion and cardiac tamponade. While no definitive studies have delineated time course for these tumors, anecdotal reports suggest progression may be very rapid. Cardiac cAS can occur with or without splenic involvement and is more likely to present as a solitary lesion in some breeds such as the Saluki. It has not been determined if right atrial involvement is a primary tumor site or reflects a site of metastasis when concurrent visceral disease is present.

As in human AS, cutaneous cAS most often presents as solitary or multiple small dermal masses, which can extend into the subcutis or even into underlying musculature. They are frequently seen on non-haired skin on the ventral abdomen of light-colored dogs (Italian greyhounds, whippets, Dalmatians, pit bulls), especially when those dogs have excess exposure to solar radiation (southern latitudes, tendency towards sunbathing). Cutaneous cAS may also occur on haired skin of darker colored dogs. Solar elastoses has been associated with cutaneous cAS in a large retrospective study involving many dogs from California practices (Hargis et al. 1992). A more recent retrospective study conducted at the University of Colorado did not confirm this finding (Schultheiss 2004), but the patient population for this study may have been comprised of more dogs from northern latitudes. The geographic location of the patients themselves was not annotated in either of these studies.

The small, solitary or multiple dermal lesions of cutaneous cAS are often less than 1 cm in diameter, but may exceed 3 cm (Hargis et al. 1992). Mitotic figures are usually seen in malignant cAS. Conclusive diagnosis is always via histopathology, regardless of tumor location. Several markers can be used (e.g. CD31, factor VIII, Claudin-5, and cardiac troponin) to aid in confirmation of diagnosis (Chun et al. 2010; Jakab et al. 2009; Shaw et al. 2004; Withrow & MacEwen 1996).

6.2 Differential diagnosis

As in human AS, the differential diagnosis of canine AS varies with the location of the disease. Visceral tumors must be distinguished from other neoplasms such as hemangiomas, other sarcomas, lymphoma, leiomyomas, and hematomas (Jakab et al. 2009). Signs of acute anemia, extreme lethargy, or collapse, requires exclusion of immune mediated hemolytic anemia (IMHA), trauma, coagulopathy, toxin exposure and allergic reaction. One retrospective study reported that among anemic dogs presenting with a splenic mass and abdominal bleeding requiring transfusion, 70% had splenic cAS (Hammond & Pesillo-Crosby 2008). Conclusive diagnosis of cAS requires histopathology of the excised tissue.

Cardiac cAS must also be differentiated from other tumors and from idiopathic pericarditis (IP), both of which can cause pericardial effusion. In one retrospective study conducted in the UK, dogs with cardiac masses detected by ultrasound (echo-positive) had significantly shorter survival times than echo-negative dogs (Johnson 2004). Patients with a discernible cardiac mass, ascites, or collapse had a much less favorable prognosis than patients with IP. Another retrospective study reported that dogs with right atrial cAS treated surgically by pericardectomy and chemotherapy had a mean survival time of 164 days, compared to 46 days for dogs treated by pericardectomy alone (Weisse et al. 2005). However, this report also noted that dogs receiving chemotherapy were significantly younger and had significantly lower white blood cell counts than the dogs that did not receive chemotherapy, so case collection bias was a concern.

Cutaneous cAS must be differentiated from other cutaneous tumors, nevi, and cysts. Histopathology is the only conclusive method of diagnosis. Because dogs may suffer from hemangiomas as well as hemangiosarcomas, and because depth of invasion can be a prognostic indicator, it is recommended that all tumors be submitted for histopathologic examination and confirmation of clear surgical margins.

6.3 Prognosis and treatment

The behavior of cAS is also linked to the site of origin, with visceral lesions being more aggressive than cutaneous lesions (Schultheiss 2004). For visceral disease, the high rate of early metastasis and the lack of early clinical signs or hematologic changes lead to late diagnosis and extremely poor prognosis. The average life span upon diagnosis of splenic cAS is less than three months for dogs treated with splenectomy alone (Spangler &

Culbertson 1992). Dogs treated with adjunctive chemotherapy (usually doxorubicin-based protocols) average less than six months survival (Kim et al. 2007; Sorenmo et al. 2004). Owners frequently elect to euthanize the dog at the time of diagnosis or shortly thereafter.

Cardiac cAS is equally grim, with many dogs dying of acute cardiac arrest prior to any overt clinical signs. This sudden death syndrome is seen particularly among Saluki. Dogs may appear clinically normal and sometimes die in their sleep. Others may develop exercise intolerance, weakness, lethargy, and inappetance prior to developing ascites secondary to cardiac tamponade. One retrospective study of 23 cases of right atrial cAS treated surgically, with or without chemotherapy, reported a mean survival time of 175 days or 42 days, respectively (Weisse et al. 2005). Another retrospective study from the UK which evaluated dogs with pericardial effusion reported a mean survival time of 26 days for dogs with echocardiograms revealing a cardiac mass versus 1068 days for those with effusion but no detectable mass. However, in this study, no dogs with detectable masses had treatment beyond pericardiocentesis, and many were euthanized at diagnosis (Johnson 2004).

In stark contrast is the positive prognosis for cutaneous cAS. A majority of dogs with strictly cutaneous cAS survive many years with local recurrent disease (Schultheiss 2004). Schultheiss reported that complete surgical resection of cutaneous cAS was the most important prognostic factor for survival (Schultheiss 2004). A retrospective study of 25 dogs reported that those with cutaneous cAS confined to the dermis had a mean survival time of 780 days, compared with 172 and 307 days for dogs with a primary tumor involving the hypodermis or underlying muscle, respectively (Ward et al. 1994). Confinement to the dermis also was correlated with better outcome, most likely due to complete surgical resection (Schultheiss 2004).

The response of cAS tumors to treatment varies greatly depending on the site of the tumor. Dogs with splenic tumors survive a few months beyond splenectomy but live longer than those that do not have surgery. Survival time is measured in months regardless of treatment, but owners frequently elect splenectomy for palliative care, extension of quality time, and reduction of the worry regarding continued intra-abdominal hemorrhage. The addition of doxorubicin-based chemotherapy protocols may add a few more months of survival. Single agent doxorubicin, administered intravenously every three weeks for up to five cycles is commonly used if chemotherapy is elected. Alternate protocols include doxorubicin plus cyclophosphamide, or doxorubicin, vincristine and cyclosphosphamide. No protocol is superior. Doxorubicin can induce dose-dependent cardiotoxicities in dogs; the total cumulative dose should not exceed 180-240 mg/m^2. A study evaluating the potential use of epirubicin in splenectomized cAS patients reported no cardiac toxicity *(Kim et al. 2007)*. However, gastrointestinal side effects occurred in a majority of the patients, and neutropenia was also common. The expense of this treatment may also preclude this drug from becoming more commonly used, although it may provide an option for dogs with preexisting cardiac disease *(Kim et al. 2007)*.

Cutaneous cAS is generally treated with complete surgical excision. There are minimal long-term consequences apart from the necessity of multiple surgeries often being required. This is not generally due to recurrence of excised tumors; rather, patients tend to develop tumors spontaneously in multiple sites. It is unclear whether these represent new primary tumors or metastatic disease (Hargis et al. 1992; Ward et al. 1994). Multiple surgeries can create a financial hardship for the owner, and may be the cause for dogs to be relinquished to rescue organizations or euthanized.

6.4 Cell and molecular biology

Molecular insight into cAS is limited and focuses primarily on visceral disease, but what is known is consistent with the biology of human AS. Tumor-derived cell lines and cell isolates express endothelial and hematopoietic stem cell markers, suggesting they may arise from pluripotent bone marrow-derived stem cells and/or cells committed to the endothelial lineage (Fosmire et al. 2004; Lamerato-Kozicki et al. 2006; Tamburini BA 2010; Thamm et al. 2006). Cells form branching vascular structures when grown on Matrigel (Thamm et al. 2006), secrete pro-angiogenic factors including VEGF and bFGF , and express elevated levels of Ang-1 and Ang-2 mRNA (Kato et al. 2006). Upon injection into immune-compromised mice, such cells readily form AS-like tumors expressing endothelial markers including CD31, vWF, VEGF-A, bFGF, flt-1, flk-1, FGFR-1, HoxA9, HoxB3, HoxB7, HoxD3, Pbx1, and Meis1 (Kodama et al. 2009). Although mutations in p53 have not been detected, cAS stain positively for nuclear p53 (Yonemaru et al. 2007). As in the human disease, cAS lesions have been found to harbor point mutations or deletions in the C-terminal domain of PTEN (Dickerson et al. 2005).

7. Conclusions

The rarity of angiosarcoma has had a profound impact on its clinical management and research. Most clinicians are unfamiliar with this disease and thus do not have experience to guide management decisions. Much of the literature regarding these rare tumors is comprised of anecdotal case reports or retrospective analyses which are difficult to assimilate and interpret. Thus, we must be especially wary not to assume all AS are equivalent. The varied morphology and presentation of these lesions indicates we may be dealing with not one, but several diseases with unique physiologic or clinical properties and pharmacologic responsiveness. For instance, it has been reported that tumor behavior might depend on the site of origin, with superficial tumors associating with a longer progression-free survival after initial treatment (Fury et al. 2005; Schlemmer et al. 2008). However, it is unclear whether this is caused by intrinsic biologic differences or differences in clinical presentation and prior treatment. Unfortunately, when AS is examined prospectively in clinical trials it is usually included as a limited number of cases within a larger study of various soft-tissue sarcomas. Further progress in our understanding of the biology and treatment of AS depends on the willingness of the medical research and clinical oncology communities to share resources through multi-center collaborations. In the absence of such efforts, alternative strategies are needed to generate meaningful insight into this disease.

Significant insight into the biology of AS has been generated through translational studies of related human tumors and mouse models. Collectively, studies of Kaposi sarcoma and hemangiomas, plus studies conducted in mouse models provide strong support for the hypothesis that MAPK signaling is a key event in the induction of endothelial cell proliferation and AS in mice and humans. This pathway has been invoked to explain the origins of many other tumor types. MAPK signaling pathways are frequently activated in endothelial cells during developmental and pathologic angiogenesis (reviewed in (Depeille et al. 2007)). Further, MAPK signaling is physiologically activated in response to shear stress (Azuma et al. 2000) and in pre-atherosclerotic plaques (Muslin 2008). A key question that needs to be addressed may therefore be not how these events trigger AS, but why they do not trigger AS more frequently. An examination of the role of MAPK phosphatases in endothelial cells and in AS tumorigenesis may be instructive.

However, important questions remain to be asked and answered. What are the key biochemical pathways involved in this disease? Does misregulation of MAPK signaling by phosphatases allow constitutive signaling to promote tumorigenesis? Do genetic mutations contribute to or establish a microenvironment that predisposes scalp, spleen, liver, or heart to develop AS? Why is angiosarcoma infrequent in humans, while it is more prevalent in dogs? Can we identify molecular targets for drug therapies? Can we devise a fundable and meaningful clinical trial to test novel therapies for such a rare disease? Will the use of spontaneous animal tumor models prove useful in informing human clinical trials?
The canine model is of growing interest in this regard since it closely resembles human disease. Studies of spontaneous cAS offer a clear experimental advantage through genome-wide association studies of single nucleotide polymorphisms that provide an unbiased approach to identify the genes contributing to the onset and progression of disease in a compressed time frame. This, combined with the availability of tumor material and the presence of multi-institution consortia such as the Canine Comparative Oncology and Genomics Consortium, the LUPA consortium, the Canine Hereditary Cancer Consortium, and the Canine Oncology Trials Consortium, may facilitate rapid identification and translation of novel therapies through clinical trials that may benefit dogs and humans alike.

8. Acknowledgements

We thank Drs. Jennifer Bromberg-White and Chih-Shia Lee for their critical comments on the manuscript, as well as Ms. Diana Lewis for administrative support and Mr. David Nadziejka for scientific editing of the manuscript. We also acknowledge financial support from the National Institutes of Health/National Cancer Institute (RC2CA148149), the Animal Cancer Foundation, and the Dwight Reed Memorial Foundation.

9. References

Ablashi, D. V., L. G. Chatlynne, J. E. Whitman, Jr. & E. Cesarman (2002). Spectrum of Kaposi's sarcoma-associated herpesvirus, or human herpesvirus 8, diseases. *Clin Microbiol Rev* 15(3): 439-64.

Antonescu, C. R., A. Yoshida, T. Guo, N. E. Chang, L. Zhang, N. P. Agaram, L. X. Qin, M. F. Brennan, S. Singer & R. G. Maki (2009). KDR activating mutations in human angiosarcomas are sensitive to specific kinase inhibitors. *Cancer Res* 69(18): 7175-9.

Arlett, C. F., P. N. Plowman, P. B. Rogers, C. N. Parris, F. Abbaszadeh, M. H. Green, T. J. McMillan, C. Bush, N. Foray & A. R. Lehmann (2006). Clinical and cellular ionizing radiation sensitivity in a patient with xeroderma pigmentosum. *Br J Radiol* 79(942): 510-7.

Armah, H. B., U. N. Rao & A. V. Parwani (2007). Primary angiosarcoma of the testis: report of a rare entity and review of the literature. *Diagn Pathol* 2: 23.

Arora, R., A. Sharma, R. Gupta & M. Vijayaraghavan (2008). Cutaneous angiosarcoma in a patient with xeroderma pigmentosum. *Indian J Pathol Microbiol* 51(4): 504-6.

Arvanitakis, L., E. Geras-Raaka, A. Varma, M. C. Gershengorn & E. Cesarman (1997). Human herpesvirus KSHV encodes a constitutively active G-protein-coupled receptor linked to cell proliferation. *Nature* 385(6614): 347-50.

Aust, M. R., K. D. Olsen, J. E. Lewis, A. G. Nascimento, N. B. Meland, R. L. Foote & V. J. Suman (1997). Angiosarcomas of the head and neck: clinical and pathologic characteristics. *Ann Otol Rhinol Laryngol* 106(11): 943-51.

Autenrieth, J. & S. Lange (1979). [Thorotrastoses--viewed in retrospect (author's transl)]. *Rontgenblatter* 32(2): 71-4.

Azuma, N., S. A. Duzgun, M. Ikeda, H. Kito, N. Akasaka, T. Sasajima & B. E. Sumpio (2000). Endothelial cell response to different mechanical forces. *J Vasc Surg* 32(4): 789-94.

Bais, C., B. Santomasso, O. Coso, L. Arvanitakis, E. G. Raaka, J. S. Gutkind, A. S. Asch, E. Cesarman, M. C. Gershengorn, E. A. Mesri & M. C. Gerhengorn (1998). G-protein-coupled receptor of Kaposi's sarcoma-associated herpesvirus is a viral oncogene and angiogenesis activator. *Nature* 391(6662): 86-9.

Bergman, P. (2010). Hemangiosarcoma. In: *Textbook of Veterinary Internal Medicine*. S. J. a. F. Ettinger, E.C. St. Louis, MO, Saunders. 2: 2175-2180.

Birchmeier, C., W. Birchmeier, E. Gherardi & G. F. Vande Woude (2003). Met, metastasis, motility and more. *Mol Biol Cell* 4: 915-925.

Bolt, H. M. (2005). Vinyl chloride-a classical industrial toxicant of new interest. *Crit Rev Toxicol* 35(4): 307-23.

Botros, M., J. F. Quevedo & R. C. Miler (2009). Angiosarcoma of the liver after multimodality therapy for gallbladder carcinoma. *Radiol Oncol* 43(2): 126-131.

Brash, D. & A. Bale (2001). Cancer of the Skin. In: *Cancer. Principles and practice of oncology*. V. DeVita Jr., S. Hellman&S. Rosenberg. Philadelpia, Lippincott Williams & Wilkins: 1971-2002.

Breiteneder-Geleff, S., A. Soleiman, H. Kowalski, R. Horvat, G. Amann, E. Kriehuber, K. Diem, W. Weninger, E. Tschachler, K. Alitalo & D. Kerjaschki (1999). Angiosarcomas express mixed endothelial phenotypes of blood and lymphatic capillaries: podoplanin as a specific marker for lymphatic endothelium. *Am J Pathol* 154(2): 385-94.

Brennan, M. F., K. M. Alektiar & R. G. Maki (2001). Sarcomas of the soft tissue and bone. In: *Cancer. Principles & Practice of Oncology*. V. DeVita Jr., S. Hellman&S. Rosenberg. Philadelphia, Lippincott Williams & Wilkins: 1841-1891.

Bulakowski, E. J., J. C. Philibert, S. Siegel, C. A. Clifford, R. Risbon, K. Zivin & K. L. Cronin (2008). Evaluation of outcome associated with subcutaneous and intramuscular hemangiosarcoma treated with adjuvant doxorubicin in dogs: 21 cases (2001-2006). *J Am Vet Med Assoc* 233(1): 122-8.

Burger, M., J. A. Burger, R. C. Hoch, Z. Oades, H. Takamori & I. U. Schraufstatter (1999). Point mutation causing constitutive signaling of CXCR2 leads to transforming activity similar to Kaposi's sarcoma herpesvirus-G protein-coupled receptor. *J Immunol* 163(4): 2017-22.

Cannon, M., N. J. Philpott & E. Cesarman (2003). The Kaposi's sarcoma-associated herpesvirus G protein-coupled receptor has broad signaling effects in primary effusion lymphoma cells. *J Virol* 77(1): 57-67.

Cannon, M. L. & E. Cesarman (2004). The KSHV G protein-coupled receptor signals via multiple pathways to induce transcription factor activation in primary effusion lymphoma cells. *Oncogene* 23(2): 514-23.

Casha, A. R., L. A. Davidson, P. Roberts & R. U. Nair (2002). Familial angiosarcoma of the heart. *J Thorac Cardiovasc Surg* 124(2): 392-4.

Cattel, L., M. Ceruti & F. Dosio (2003). From conventional to stealth liposomes: a new frontier in cancer chemotherapy. *Tumori* 89(3): 237-49.

Centeno, J. A., F. G. Mullick, L. Martinez, N. P. Page, H. Gibb, D. Longfellow, C. Thompson & E. R. Ladich (2002). Pathology related to chronic arsenic exposure. *Environ Health Perspect* 110 Suppl 5: 883-6.

Chandra, M. & C. H. Frith (1992). Spontaneous neoplasms in aged CD-1 mice. *Toxicol Lett* 61(1): 67-74.

Chandra, M. & C. H. Frith (1992). Spontaneous neoplasms in B6C3F1 mice. *Toxicol Lett* 60(1): 91-8.

Chang, Y., E. Cesarman, M. S. Pessin, F. Lee, J. Culpepper, D. M. Knowles & P. S. Moore (1994). Identification of herpesvirus-like DNA sequences in AIDS-associated Kaposi's sarcoma. *Science* 266(5192): 1865-9.

Chesterman, F. C., J. J. Harvey, R. R. Dourmashkin & M. H. Salaman (1966). The pathology of tumors and other lesions induced in rodents by virus derived from a rat with Moloney leukemia. *Cancer Res* 26(8): 1759-68.

Chlebowski, R. T. (1979). Adriamycin (doxorubicin) cardiotoxicity: a review. *West J Med* 131(5): 364-8.

Chun, R., H. B. Kellihan, R. A. Henik & R. L. Stepien (2010). Comparison of plasma cardiac troponin I concentrations among dogs with cardiac hemangiosarcoma, noncardiac hemangiosarcoma, other neoplasms, and pericardial effusion of nonhemangiosarcoma origin. *J Am Vet Med Assoc* 237(7): 806-11.

Cohen, S. M., R. D. Storer, K. A. Criswell, N. G. Doerrer, V. L. Dellarco, D. G. Pegg, Z. W. Wojcinski, D. E. Malarkey, A. C. Jacobs, J. E. Klaunig, J. A. Swenberg & J. C. Cook (2009). Hemangiosarcoma in rodents: mode-of-action evaluation and human relevance. *Toxicol Sci* 111(1): 4-18.

Corthals, S. M., L. M. Kamendulis & J. E. Klaunig (2006). Mechanisms of 2-butoxyethanol-induced hemangiosarcomas. *Toxicol Sci* 92(2): 378-86.

Creech, J. L., Jr. & M. N. Johnson (1974). Angiosarcoma of liver in the manufacture of polyvinyl chloride. *J Occup Med* 16(3): 150-1.

de Boer, J. & J. H. Hoeijmakers (2000). Nucleotide excision repair and human syndromes. *Carcinogenesis* 21(3): 453-60.

Depeille, P., J. J. Young, E. A. Boguslawski, B. D. Berghuis, E. J. Kort, J. H. Resau, A. E. Frankel & N. S. Duesbery (2007). Anthrax lethal toxin inhibits growth of and vascular endothelial growth factor release from endothelial cells expressing the human herpes virus 8 viral G protein coupled receptor. *Clin Cancer Res* 13(19): 5926-34.

Depeille, P. E., Y. Ding, J. L. Bromberg-White & N. S. Duesbery (2007). MKK signaling and vascularization. *Oncogene* 26(9): 1290-6.

Dickerson, E. B., R. Thomas, S. P. Fosmire, A. R. Lamerato-Kozicki, S. R. Bianco, J. W. Wojcieszyn, M. Breen, S. C. Helfand & J. F. Modiano (2005). Mutations of phosphatase and tensin homolog deleted from chromosome 10 in canine hemangiosarcoma. *Vet Pathol* 42(5): 618-32.

Dobson, J. M., S. Samuel, H. Milstein, K. Rogers & J. L. Wood (2002). Canine neoplasia in the UK: estimates of incidence rates from a population of insured dogs. *J Small Anim Pract* 43(6): 240-6.

Eaton, G. J., F. N. Johnson, R. P. Custer & A. R. Crane (1980). The Icr:Ha(ICR) mouse: a current account of breeding, mutations, diseases and mortality. *Lab Anim* 14(1): 17-24.

Eder, J. P., G. F. Vande Woude, S. A. Boerner & P. M. LoRusso (2009). Novel therapeutic inhibitors of the c-Met signaling pathway in cancer. *Clin Cancer Res* 15(7): 2207-14.

Falk, S., J. Krishnan & J. M. Meis (1993). Primary angiosarcoma of the spleen. A clinicopathologic study of 40 cases. *Am J Surg Pathol* 17(10): 959-70.

Farag, R., J. A. Schulak, F. W. Abdul-Karim & J. K. Wasman (2005). Angiosarcoma arising in an arteriovenous fistula site in a renal transplant patient: a case report and literature review. *Clin Nephrol* 63(5): 408-12.

Farhood, A. I., S. I. Hajdu, M. H. Shiu & E. W. Strong (1990). Soft tissue sarcomas of the head and neck in adults. *Am J Surg* 160(4): 365-9.

Fata, F., E. O'Reilly, D. Ilson, D. Pfister, D. Leffel, D. P. Kelsen, G. K. Schwartz & E. S. Casper (1999). Paclitaxel in the treatment of patients with angiosarcoma of the scalp or face. *Cancer* 86(10): 2034-7.

Fayette, J., E. Martin, S. Piperno-Neumann, A. Le Cesne, C. Robert, S. Bonvalot, D. Ranchere, P. Pouillart, J. M. Coindre & J. Y. Blay (2007). Angiosarcomas, a heterogeneous group of sarcomas with specific behavior depending on primary site: a retrospective study of 161 cases. *Ann Oncol* 18(12): 2030-6.

Fletcher, C. D., A. Beham, S. Bekir, A. M. Clarke & N. J. Marley (1991). Epithelioid angiosarcoma of deep soft tissue: a distinctive tumor readily mistaken for an epithelial neoplasm. *Am J Surg Pathol* 15(10): 915-24.

Flora, S. J. (2011). Arsenic-induced oxidative stress and its reversibility. *Free Radic Biol Med* 51(2): 257-81.

Fosmire, S. P., E. B. Dickerson, A. M. Scott, S. R. Bianco, M. J. Pettengill, H. Meylemans, M. Padilla, A. A. Frazer-Abel, N. Akhtar, D. M. Getzy, J. Wojcieszyn, M. Breen, S. C. Helfand & J. F. Modiano (2004). Canine malignant hemangiosarcoma as a model of primitive angiogenic endothelium. *Lab Invest* 84(5): 562-72.

Fury, M. G., C. R. Antonescu, K. J. Van Zee, M. F. Brennan & R. G. Maki (2005). A 14-year retrospective review of angiosarcoma: clinical characteristics, prognostic factors, and treatment outcomes with surgery and chemotherapy. *Cancer J* 11(3): 241-7.

Ge, Y., J. Y. Ro, D. Kim, C. H. Kim, M. J. Reardon, S. Blackmon, J. Zhai, D. Coffey, R. S. Benjamin & A. G. Ayala (2011). Clinicopathologic and immunohistochemical characteristics of adult primary cardiac angiosarcomas: analysis of 10 cases. *Ann Diagn Pathol*.

Gherghe, C. M., J. Duan, J. Gong, M. Rojas, N. Klauber-Demore, M. Majesky & A. Deb (2011). Wnt1 is a proangiogenic molecule, enhances human endothelial progenitor function, and increases blood flow to ischemic limbs in a HGF-dependent manner. *Faseb J* 25(6): 1836-43.

Gil-Benso, R., C. Lopez-Gines, P. Soriano, S. Almenar, C. Vazquez & A. Llombart-Bosch (1994). Cytogenetic study of angiosarcoma of the breast. *Genes Chromosomes Cancer* 10(3): 210-2.

Glazebrook, K. N., M. J. Magut & C. Reynolds (2008). Angiosarcoma of the breast. *AJR Am J Roentgenol* 190(2): 533-8.

Glickman, L. T., N. Glickman & R. Thorpe (1999). The Golden Retriever Club of America National Health Survey: 182.

Gong, Y., T. Hong, M. Chen & Y. Huo (2011). A right heart angiosarcoma with rapidly progressing hemorrhagic pericardial effusion. *Intern Med* 50(5): 455-8.

Gordon, I., M. Paoloni, C. Mazcko & C. Khanna (2009). The Comparative Oncology Trials Consortium: using spontaneously occurring cancers in dogs to inform the cancer drug development pathway. *PLoS Med* 6(10): e1000161.

Graveel, C., Y. Su, J. Koeman, L. M. Wang, L. Tessarollo, M. Fiscella, C. Birchmeier, P. Swiatek, R. Bronson & G. Vande Woude (2004). Activating Met mutations produce unique tumor profiles in mice with selective duplication of the mutant allele. *Proc Natl Acad Sci U S A* 101(49): 17198-203.

Guo, T., L. Zhang, N. E. Chang, S. Singer, R. G. Maki & C. R. Antonescu (2011). Consistent MYC and FLT4 gene amplification in radiation-induced angiosarcoma but not in other radiation-associated atypical vascular lesions. *Genes Chromosomes Cancer* 50(1): 25-33.

Hallel-Halevy, D., J. Yerushalmi, M. H. Grunwald, I. Avinoach & S. Halevy (1999). Stewart-Treves syndrome in a patient with elephantiasis. *J Am Acad Dermatol* 41(2 Pt 2): 349-50.

Hammond, T. N. & S. A. Pesillo-Crosby (2008). Prevalence of hemangiosarcoma in anemic dogs with a splenic mass and hemoperitoneum requiring a transfusion: 71 cases (2003-2005). *J Am Vet Med Assoc* 232(4): 553-8.

Hargis, A. M., P. J. Ihrke, W. L. Spangler & A. A. Stannard (1992). A retrospective clinicopathologic study of 212 dogs with cutaneous hemangiomas and hemangiosarcomas. *Vet Pathol* 29(4): 316-28.

Harvey, J. J. (1964). An Unidentified Virus Which Causes the Rapid Production of Tumours in Mice. *Nature* 204: 1104-5.

Haseman, J. K., J. R. Hailey & R. W. Morris (1998). Spontaneous neoplasm incidences in Fischer 344 rats and B6C3F1 mice in two-year carcinogenicity studies: a National Toxicology Program update. *Toxicol Pathol* 26(3): 428-41.

Holden, C. A., M. F. Spittle & E. W. Jones (1987). Angiosarcoma of the face and scalp, prognosis and treatment. *Cancer* 59(5): 1046-57.

Hollstein, M., M. J. Marion, T. Lehman, J. Welsh, C. C. Harris, G. Martel-Planche, I. Kusters & R. Montesano (1994). p53 mutations at A:T base pairs in angiosarcomas of vinyl chloride-exposed factory workers. *Carcinogenesis* 15(1): 1-3.

Huang, J. & W. J. Mackillop (2001). Increased risk of soft tissue sarcoma after radiotherapy in women with breast carcinoma. *Cancer* 92(1): 172-80.

Infante, P. F., S. E. Petty, D. H. Groth, G. Markowitz & D. Rosner (2009). Vinyl chloride propellant in hair spray and angiosarcoma of the liver among hairdressers and barbers: case reports. *Int J Occup Environ Health* 15(1): 36-42.

Jacks, T., L. Remington, B. O. Williams, E. M. Schmitt, S. Halachmi, R. T. Bronson & R. A. Weinberg (1994). Tumor spectrum analysis in p53-mutant mice. *Curr Biol* 4(1): 1-7.

Jakab, C., J. Halasz, A. Kiss, Z. Schaff, M. Rusvai, P. Galfi, T. Z. Abonyi & J. Kulka (2009). Claudin-5 protein is a new differential marker for histopathological differential diagnosis of canine hemangiosarcoma. *Histol Histopathol* 24(7): 801-13.

Ji, J. & K. Hemminki (2007). Familial blood vessel tumors and subsequent cancers. *Ann Oncol* 18(7): 1260-7.

Johnson, M. S., Martin, M., Binns, S., Day, M.J. (2004). A Retrospective Study of Clinical Findings, Treatment and Outcome in 143 Dogs with Pericardial Effusion. *Journal of Small Animal Practice* 45: 546-552.

Johnson, S. A., C. J. Bateman, M. E. Beard, J. M. Whitehouse & A. H. Waters (1977). Long-term haematological complications of thorotrast. *Q J Med* 46(182): 259-71.

Judson, I., J. A. Radford, M. Harris, J. Y. Blay, Q. van Hoesel, A. le Cesne, A. T. van Oosterom, M. J. Clemons, C. Kamby, C. Hermans, J. Whittaker, E. Donato di Paola, J. Verweij & S. Nielsen (2001). Randomised phase II trial of pegylated liposomal doxorubicin (DOXIL/CAELYX) versus doxorubicin in the treatment of advanced or metastatic soft tissue sarcoma: a study by the EORTC Soft Tissue and Bone Sarcoma Group. *Eur J Cancer* 37(7): 870-7.

Kaelin, W. G., Jr. (2007). The von hippel-lindau tumor suppressor protein: an update. *Methods Enzymol* 435: 371-83.

Kamendulis, L., S. Corthals & J. Klaunig (2010). Kupffer cells participate in 2-butoxyethanol-induced liver hemangiosarcomas. *Toxicology* 270(2-3): 131-136.

Karlsson, P., E. Holmberg, A. Samuelsson, K. A. Johansson & A. Wallgren (1998). Soft tissue sarcoma after treatment for breast cancer--a Swedish population-based study. *Eur J Cancer* 34(13): 2068-75.

Kato, Y., K. Asano, I. Mizutani, T. Konno, Y. Sasaki, K. Kutara, K. Teshima, K. Edamura, R. Kano, K. Suzuki, H. Shibuya, T. Sato, A. Hasegawa & S. Tanaka (2006). Gene expressions of canine angiopoietin-1 and -2 in normal tissues and spontaneous tumours. *Res Vet Sci* 81(2): 280-6.

Kemeny, L., M. Kiss, R. Gyulai, A. S. Kenderessy, E. Adam, F. Nagy & A. Dobozy (1996). Human herpesvirus 8 in classic Kaposi sarcoma. *Acta Microbiol Immunol Hung* 43(4): 391-5.

Kim, S. E., J. M. Liptak, T. T. Gall, G. J. Monteith & J. P. Woods (2007). Epirubicin in the adjuvant treatment of splenic hemangiosarcoma in dogs: 59 cases (1997-2004). *J Am Vet Med Assoc* 231(10): 1550-7.

Kindblom, L. G., G. Stenman & L. Angervall (1991). Morphological and cytogenetic studies of angiosarcoma in Stewart-Treves syndrome. *Virchows Arch A Pathol Anat Histopathol* 419(5): 439-45.

Kiyosawa, K., H. Imai, T. Sodeyama, S. T. Franca, M. Yousuf, S. Furuta, K. Fujisawa & C. Kido (1989). Comparison of anamnestic history, alcohol intake and smoking, nutritional status, and liver dysfunction between thorotrast patients who developed primary liver cancer and those who did not. *Environ Res* 49(2): 166-72.

Klaunig, J. E. & L. M. Kamendulis (2005). Mode of action of butoxyethanol-induced mouse liver hemangiosarcomas and hepatocellular carcinomas. *Toxicol Lett* 156(1): 107-15.

Kleinman, M. E., M. R. Greives, S. S. Churgin, K. M. Blechman, E. I. Chang, D. J. Ceradini, O. M. Tepper & G. C. Gurtner (2007). Hypoxia-induced mediators of stem/progenitor cell trafficking are increased in children with hemangioma. *Arterioscler Thromb Vasc Biol* 27(12): 2664-70.

Koch, M., G. P. Nielsen & S. S. Yoon (2008). Malignant tumors of blood vessels: angiosarcomas, hemangioendotheliomas, and hemangiopericytomas. *J Surg Oncol* 97(4): 321-9.

Kodama, A., H. Sakai, S. Matsuura, M. Murakami, A. Murai, T. Mori, K. Maruo, T. Kimura, T. Masegi & T. Yanai (2009). Establishment of canine hemangiosarcoma xenograft models expressing endothelial growth factors, their receptors, and angiogenesis-associated homeobox genes. *BMC Cancer* 9: 363.

Kraemer, K. H., M. M. Lee & J. Scotto (1987). Xeroderma pigmentosum. Cutaneous, ocular, and neurologic abnormalities in 830 published cases. *Arch Dermatol* 123(2): 241-50.

Lahat, G., A. R. Dhuka, S. Lahat, K. D. Smith, R. E. Pollock, K. K. Hunt, V. Ravi, A. J. Lazar & D. Lev (2009). Outcome of locally recurrent and metastatic angiosarcoma. *Ann Surg Oncol* 16(9): 2502-9.

Lamerato-Kozicki, A. R., K. M. Helm, C. M. Jubala, G. C. Cutter & J. F. Modiano (2006). Canine hemangiosarcoma originates from hematopoietic precursors with potential for endothelial differentiation. *Exp Hematol* 34(7): 870-8.

Lane, O. G. (1952). Cutaneous angiosarcoma with metastases. *Br J Cancer* 6(3): 230-5.

Lasota, J. & M. Miettinen (1999). Absence of Kaposi's sarcoma-associated virus (human herpesvirus-8) sequences in angiosarcoma. *Virchows Arch* 434(1): 51-6.

Lawley, L. P., F. Cerimele, S. W. Weiss, P. North, C. Cohen, H. P. Kozakewich, J. B. Mulliken & J. L. Arbiser (2005). Expression of Wilms tumor 1 gene distinguishes vascular malformations from proliferative endothelial lesions. *Arch Dermatol* 141(10): 1297-300.

Leaute-Labreze, C., E. Dumas de la Roque, T. Hubiche, F. Boralevi, J. B. Thambo & A. Taieb (2008). Propranolol for severe hemangiomas of infancy. *N Engl J Med* 358(24): 2649-51.

Lebel, M., R. D. Cardiff & P. Leder (2001). Tumorigenic effect of nonfunctional p53 or p21 in mice mutant in the Werner syndrome helicase. *Cancer Res* 61(5): 1816-9.

Lee, C.-S. & N. Duesbery (2010). Highly Selective MEK Inhibitors. *Current Enzyme Inhibition* 6(3): 146-157.

Lewis, T. S., P. S. Shapiro & N. G. Ahn (1998). Signal transduction through MAP kinase cascades. In: *Advances in Cancer Research*. G. F. V. Woude&G. Klein. San Diego, CA, Academic Press. 74: 49-139.

Lin, C. F., D. DeFrias & X. Lin (2010). Epithelioid angiosarcoma: a neoplasm with potential diagnostic challenges. *Diagn Cytopathol* 38(2): 154-8.

Looney, W. B. (1960). An investigation of the late clinical findings following thorotrast (thorium dioxide) administration. *Am J Roentgenol Radium Ther Nucl Med* 83: 163-85.

Lorusso, D., A. Di Stefano, V. Carone, A. Fagotti, S. Pisconti & G. Scambia (2007). Pegylated liposomal doxorubicin-related palmar-plantar erythrodysesthesia ('hand-foot' syndrome). *Ann Oncol* 18(7): 1159-64.

Ludolph-Hauser, D., E. Thoma-Greber, C. Sander, C. P. Sommerhoff & M. Rocken (2000). Mast cells in an angiosarcoma complicating xeroderma pigmentosum in a 13-year-old girl. *J Am Acad Dermatol* 43(5 Pt 2): 900-2.

Maeda, M., K. R. Johnson & M. J. Wheelock (2005). Cadherin switching: essential for behavioral but not morphological changes during an epithelium-to-mesenchyme transition. *J Cell Sci* 118(Pt 5): 873-87.

Mahony, B., R. B. Jeffrey & M. P. Federle (1982). Spontaneous rupture of hepatic and splenic angiosarcoma demonstrated by CT. *AJR Am J Roentgenol* 138(5): 965-6.

Marcon, I., P. Collini, M. Casanova, C. Meazza & A. Ferrari (2004). Cutaneous angiosarcoma in a patient with xeroderma pigmentosum. *Pediatr Hematol Oncol* 21(1): 23-6.

Marion, M. J., Froment, O., Trepo, C. (2005). Activation of Ki-ras gene by point mutation in human liver angiosarcoma associated with vinyl-chloride exposure. *Molecular Carcinogenesis* 4(6): 450-454.

Mark, R. J., J. C. Poen, L. M. Tran, Y. S. Fu & G. F. Juillard (1996). Angiosarcoma. A report of 67 patients and a review of the literature. *Cancer* 77(11): 2400-6.

Martin-Padura, I., C. De Castellarnau, S. Uccini, E. Pilozzi, P. G. Natali, M. R. Nicotra, F. Ughi, C. Azzolini, E. Dejana & L. Ruco (1995). Expression of VE (vascular endothelial)-cadherin and other endothelial-specific markers in haemangiomas. *J Pathol* 175(1): 51-7.

Matzke, L. A., M. A. Knowling, D. Grant, J. B. Cupples, J. Leipsic, A. Ignaszewski & M. F. Allard A rare cardiac neoplasm: case report of cardiac epithelioid angiosarcoma. *Cardiovasc Pathol.*

McDonagh, D. P., J. Liu, M. J. Gaffey, L. J. Layfield, N. Azumi & S. T. Traweek (1996). Detection of Kaposi's sarcoma-associated herpesvirus-like DNA sequence in angiosarcoma. *Am J Pathol* 149(4): 1363-8.

Mejia, A. F., L. Gierbolini, B. Jacob & S. V. Westmoreland (2009). Pediatric hepatic hemangiosarcoma in a rhesus macaque (Macaca mulatta). *J Med Primatol* 38(2): 121-4.

Mendenhall, W. M., C. M. Mendenhall, J. W. Werning, J. D. Reith & N. P. Mendenhall (2006). Cutaneous angiosarcoma. *Am J Clin Oncol* 29(5): 524-8.

Mesri, E. A., E. Cesarman & C. Boshoff (2010). Kaposi's sarcoma and its associated herpesvirus. *Nat Rev Cancer* 10(10): 707-19.

Miller, M. A., J. A. Ramos & J. M. Kreeger (1992). Cutaneous vascular neoplasia in 15 cats: clinical, morphologic, and immunohistochemical studies. *Vet Pathol* 29(4): 329-36.

Miura, K., Y. Kum, G. Han & Y. Tsutsui (2003). Radiation-induced laryngeal angiosarcoma after cervical tuberculosis and squamous cell carcinoma: case report and review of the literature. *Pathol Int* 53(10): 710-5.

Montaner, S., A. Sodhi, A. Molinolo, T. H. Bugge, E. T. Sawai, Y. He, Y. Li, P. E. Ray & J. S. Gutkind (2003). Endothelial infection with KSHV genes in vivo reveals that vGPCR initiates Kaposi's sarcomagenesis and can promote the tumorigenic potential of viral latent genes. *Cancer Cell* 3(1): 23-36.

Morgan, M. B., M. Swann, S. Somach, W. Eng & B. Smoller (2004). Cutaneous angiosarcoma: a case series with prognostic correlation. *J Am Acad Dermatol* 50(6): 867-74.

Muslin, A. J. (2008). MAPK signalling in cardiovascular health and disease: molecular mechanisms and therapeutic targets. *Clin Sci (Lond)* 115(7): 203-18.

Myers, D. D., Jr., R. C. Dysko, C. E. Chrisp & J. L. Decoster (2001). Subcutaneous hemangiosarcomas in a rhesus macaque (Macaca mulatta). *J Med Primatol* 30(2): 127-30.

Neuhauser, T. S., G. A. Derringer, L. D. Thompson, J. C. Fanburg-Smith, M. Miettinen, A. Saaristo & S. L. Abbondanzo (2000). Splenic angiosarcoma: a clinicopathologic and immunophenotypic study of 28 cases. *Mod Pathol* 13(9): 978-87.

Nickoloff, B. J. & C. E. Griffiths (1989). The spindle-shaped cells in cutaneous Kaposi's sarcoma. Histologic simulators include factor XIIIa dermal dendrocytes. *Am J Pathol* 135(5): 793-800.

Offori, T. W., C. C. Platt, M. Stephens & G. B. Hopkinson (1993). Angiosarcoma in congenital hereditary lymphoedema (Milroy's disease)--diagnostic beacons and a review of the literature. *Clin Exp Dermatol* 18(2): 174-7.

Ohsawa, M., N. Naka, Y. Tomita, D. Kawamori, H. Kanno & K. Aozasa (1995). Use of immunohistochemical procedures in diagnosing angiosarcoma. Evaluation of 98 cases. *Cancer* 75(12): 2867-74.

Paoloni, M. & C. Khanna (2008). Translation of new cancer treatments from pet dogs to humans. *Nat Rev Cancer* 8(2): 147-56.

Pawlik, T. M., A. F. Paulino, C. J. McGinn, L. H. Baker, D. S. Cohen, J. S. Morris, R. Rees & V. K. Sondak (2003). Cutaneous angiosarcoma of the scalp: a multidisciplinary approach. *Cancer* 98(8): 1716-26.

Penel, N., B. N. Bui, J. O. Bay, D. Cupissol, I. Ray-Coquard, S. Piperno-Neumann, P. Kerbrat, C. Fournier, S. Taieb, M. Jimenez, N. Isambert, F. Peyrade, C. Chevreau, E. Bompas, E. G. Brain & J. Y. Blay (2008). Phase II trial of weekly paclitaxel for unresectable angiosarcoma: the ANGIOTAX Study. *J Clin Oncol* 26(32): 5269-74.

Pitts, O. M., J. M. Powers & P. M. Hoffman (1983). Vascular neoplasms induced in rodent central nervous system by murine sarcoma viruses. *Lab Invest* 49(2): 171-82.

Pozo, A. L., E. M. Godfrey & K. M. Bowles (2009). Splenomegaly: investigation, diagnosis and management. *Blood Rev* 23(3): 105-11.

Prymak, C., L. J. McKee, M. H. Goldschmidt & L. T. Glickman (1988). Epidemiologic, clinical, pathologic, and prognostic characteristics of splenic hemangiosarcoma and splenic hematoma in dogs: 217 cases (1985). *J Am Vet Med Assoc* 193(6): 706-12.

Przygodzki, R. M., S. D. Finkelstein, P. Keohavong, D. Zhu, A. Bakker, P. A. Swalsky, Y. Soini, K. G. Ishak & W. P. Bennett (1997). Sporadic and Thorotrast-induced angiosarcomas of the liver manifest frequent and multiple point mutations in K-ras-2. *Lab Invest* 76(1): 153-9.

Quezado, M. M., L. P. Middleton, B. Bryant, K. Lane, S. W. Weiss & M. J. Merino (1998). Allelic loss on chromosome 22q in epithelioid sarcomas. *Hum Pathol* 29(6): 604-8.

Requena, L. & O. P. Sangueza (1998). Cutaneous vascular proliferations. Part III. Malignant neoplasms, other cutaneous neoplasms with significant vascular component, and disorders erroneously considered as vascular neoplasms. *J Am Acad Dermatol* 38(2 Pt 1): 143-75; quiz 176-8.

Sahmel, J., K. Unice, P. Scott, D. Cowan & D. Paustenbach (2009). The use of multizone models to estimate an airborne chemical contaminant generation and decay profile: occupational exposures of hairdressers to vinyl chloride in hairspray during the 1960s and 1970s. *Risk Anal* 29(12): 1699-725.

Sans, V., E. D. de la Roque, J. Berge, N. Grenier, F. Boralevi, J. Mazereeuw-Hautier, D. Lipsker, E. Dupuis, K. Ezzedine, P. Vergnes, A. Taieb & C. Leaute-Labreze (2009). Propranolol for severe infantile hemangiomas: follow-up report. *Pediatrics* 124(3): e423-31.

Schlemmer, M., P. Reichardt, J. Verweij, J. T. Hartmann, I. Judson, A. Thyss, P. C. Hogendoorn, S. Marreaud, M. Van Glabbeke & J. Y. Blay (2008). Paclitaxel in patients with advanced angiosarcomas of soft tissue: a retrospective study of the EORTC soft tissue and bone sarcoma group. *Eur J Cancer* 44(16): 2433-6.

Schmid, H. & C. Zietz (2005). Human herpesvirus 8 and angiosarcoma: analysis of 40 cases and review of the literature. *Pathology* 37(4): 284-7.

Schuborg, C., F. Mertens, A. Rydholm, O. Brosjo, M. Dictor, F. Mitelman & N. Mandahl (1998). Cytogenetic analysis of four angiosarcomas from deep and superficial soft tissue. *Cancer Genet Cytogenet* 100(1): 52-6.

Schultheiss, P. C. (2004). A retrospective study of visceral and nonvisceral hemangiosarcoma and hemangiomas in domestic animals. *J Vet Diagn Invest* 16(6): 522-6.

Shaw, S. P., E. A. Rozanski & J. E. Rush (2004). Cardiac troponins I and T in dogs with pericardial effusion. *J Vet Intern Med* 18(3): 322-4.

Sodhi, A., S. Montaner, V. Patel, M. Zohar, C. Bais, E. A. Mesri & J. S. Gutkind (2000). The Kaposi's sarcoma-associated herpes virus G protein-coupled receptor up-regulates vascular endothelial growth factor expression and secretion through mitogen-activated protein kinase and p38 pathways acting on hypoxia-inducible factor 1alpha. *Cancer Res* 60(17): 4873-80.

Soini, Y., J. A. Welsh, K. G. Ishak & W. P. Bennett (1995). p53 mutations in primary hepatic angiosarcomas not associated with vinyl chloride exposure. *Carcinogenesis* 16(11): 2879-81.

Sorenmo, K. U., J. L. Baez, C. A. Clifford, E. Mauldin, B. Overley, K. Skorupski, R. Bachman, M. Samluk & F. Shofer (2004). Efficacy and toxicity of a dose-intensified doxorubicin protocol in canine hemangiosarcoma. *J Vet Intern Med* 18(2): 209-13.

Spangler, W. L. & M. R. Culbertson (1992). Prevalence, type, and importance of splenic diseases in dogs: 1,480 cases (1985-1989). *J Am Vet Med Assoc* 200(6): 829-34.

Stewart, F. W. & N. Treves (1948). Lymphangiosarcoma in postmastectomy lymphedema; a report of six cases in elephantiasis chirurgica. *Cancer* 1(1): 64-81.

Stoica, G., J. Hoffman & P. H. Yuen (1990). Moloney murine sarcoma virus 349 induces Kaposi's sarcomalike lesions in Balb/c mice. *Am J Pathol* 136(4): 933-47.

Sutton, R. H. & M. W. McLennan (1982). Hemangiosarcoma in a cow. *Vet Pathol* 19(4): 456-8.

Suzuki, H., A. Komatsu, Y. Fujioka, K. Yamashiro, H. Takeda & T. Hamada (2010). Angiosarcoma-like metastatic carcinoma of the liver. *Pathol Res Pract* 206(7): 484-8.

Tamburini BA, P. T., Fosmire SP, Scott MC, Trapp SC, Duckett MM, Robinson SR, Slansky JE, Sharkey LC, Cutter GR, Wojcieszyn JW, Bellgrau D, Gemmill RM, Hunter LE, Modiano JF. (2010). Gene expression profiling identifies inflammation and angiogenesis as distinguishing features of canine hemangiosarcoma. *BMC Cancer* 10: 619.

Tanioka, M., A. Ikoma, K. Morita, H. Fujii, K. I. Toda, K. Takahashi, T. Tanaka, C. Nishigori, G. Jin, S. Higashi, S. Toyokuni & Y. Miyachi (2001). Angiosarcoma of the scalp: absence of vascular endothelial cadherin in primary and metastatic lesions. *Br J Dermatol* 144(2): 380-3.

Tate, G., T. Suzuki & T. Mitsuya (2007). Mutation of the PTEN gene in a human hepatic angiosarcoma. *Cancer Genet Cytogenet* 178(2): 160-2.

Thamm, D. H., E. B. Dickerson, N. Akhtar, R. Lewis, R. Auerbach, S. C. Helfand & E. G. MacEwen (2006). Biological and molecular characterization of a canine hemangiosarcoma-derived cell line. *Res Vet Sci* 81(1): 76-86.

Thompson, W. M., A. D. Levy, N. S. Aguilera, L. Gorospe & R. M. Abbott (2005). Angiosarcoma of the spleen: imaging characteristics in 12 patients. *Radiology* 235(1): 106-15.

Tuttle, A. D., Harms, C.A., Van Wettere, A., Grafinger, M.S., Lewbart, G.A. (2006). Splenic Hemangiosarcoma in a Corn Snake, *Elaphe guttata. Journal of Herpetological Medicine and Surgery* 16(4): 140-143.

Vakkalanka, B. & M. Milhem (2010). Paclitaxel as neoadjuvant therapy for high grade angiosarcoma of the spleen: a brief report and literature review. *Clin Med Insights Oncol* 4: 107-110.

Valenzuela, E. J., L. M. J. Lopez Poveda, P. F. J. Fuenzalida, G. C. Garre Sanchez, M. E. Barba & C. F. Alvarez (2009). Hepatic angiosarcoma. Presentation of two cases. *Rev Esp Enferm Dig* 101(6): 430-4, 434-7.

van Geel, A. N. & M. A. den Bakker (2009). Bilateral angiosarcoma of the breast in a fourteen-year-old child. *Rare Tumors* 1(2): e38.

Virtanen, A., E. Pukkala & A. Auvinen (2007). Angiosarcoma after radiotherapy: a cohort study of 332,163 Finnish cancer patients. *Br J Cancer* 97(1): 115-7.

Ward, H., L. E. Fox, M. B. Calderwood-Mays, A. S. Hammer & C. G. Couto (1994). Cutaneous hemangiosarcoma in 25 dogs: a retrospective study. *J Vet Intern Med* 8(5): 345-8.

Weihrauch, M., A. Markwarth, G. Lehnert, C. Wittekind, R. Wrbitzky & A. Tannapfel (2002). Abnormalities of the ARF-p53 pathway in primary angiosarcomas of the liver. *Hum Pathol* 33(9): 884-92.

Weiss, S. W. & F. M. Enzinger (1982). Epithelioid hemangioendothelioma: a vascular tumor often mistaken for a carcinoma. *Cancer* 50(5): 970-81.

Weisse, C., N. Soares, M. W. Beal, M. A. Steffey, K. J. Drobatz & C. J. Henry (2005). Survival times in dogs with right atrial hemangiosarcoma treated by means of surgical resection with or without adjuvant chemotherapy: 23 cases (1986-2000). *J Am Vet Med Assoc* 226(4): 575-9.

Withrow, S. & E. G. MacEwen (1996). *Small Animal Clinical Oncology*. Philadelphia, W.B. Saunders Co.

Wong, K. F., C. C. So, N. Wong, L. L. Siu, Y. L. Kwong & J. K. Chan (2001). Sinonasal angiosarcoma with marrow involvement at presentation mimicking malignant lymphoma: cytogenetic analysis using multiple techniques. *Cancer Genet Cytogenet* 129(1): 64-8.

Yang, X. J., J. W. Zheng, Q. Zhou, W. M. Ye, Y. A. Wang, H. G. Zhu, L. Z. Wang & Z. Y. Zhang (2010). Angiosarcomas of the head and neck: a clinico-immunohistochemical study of 8 consecutive patients. *Int J Oral Maxillofac Surg* 39(6): 568-72.

Yap, J., P. J. Chuba, R. Thomas, A. Aref, D. Lucas, R. K. Severson & M. Hamre (2002). Sarcoma as a second malignancy after treatment for breast cancer. *Int J Radiat Oncol Biol Phys* 52(5): 1231-7.

Yonemaru, K., H. Sakai, M. Murakami, A. Kodama, T. Mori, T. Yanai, K. Maruo & T. Masegi (2007). The significance of p53 and retinoblastoma pathways in canine hemangiosarcoma. *J Vet Med Sci* 69(3): 271-8.

Young, R. J., N. J. Brown, M. W. Reed, D. Hughes & P. J. Woll (2010). Angiosarcoma. *Lancet Oncol* 11(10): 983-91.

Yuen, P. H., C. M. Matherne & L. M. Molinari-Storey (1991). SV7, a molecular clone of Moloney murine sarcoma virus 349, transforms vascular endothelial cells. *Am J Pathol* 139(6): 1449-61.

Zanetta, L., M. Corada, M. Grazia Lampugnani, A. Zanetti, F. Breviario, L. Moons, P. Carmeliet, M. S. Pepper & E. Dejana (2005). Downregulation of vascular endothelial-cadherin expression is associated with an increase in vascular tumor growth and hemorrhagic complications. *Thromb Haemost* 93(6): 1041-6.

Zindy, F., L. M. Nilsson, L. Nguyen, C. Meunier, R. J. Smeyne, J. E. Rehg, C. Eberhart, C. J. Sherr & M. F. Roussel (2003). Hemangiosarcomas, medulloblastomas, and other tumors in Ink4c/p53-null mice. *Cancer Res* 63(17): 5420-7.

Zu, Y., M. A. Perle, Z. Yan, J. Liu, A. Kumar & J. Waisman (2001). Chromosomal abnormalities and p53 gene mutation in a cardiac angiosarcoma. *Appl Immunohistochem Mol Morphol* 9(1): 24-8.

10

Gastrointestinal Stromal Tumours: A Contemporary Review on Pathogenesis, Morphology and Prognosis

Muna Sabah
Connolly Hospital, Dublin,
Ireland

1. Introduction

Gastrointestinal stromal tumours (GISTs) comprise the largest subset of mesenchymal tumours of the digestive tract. Over the past 10 years, this group of tumours has emerged from a poorly understood neoplasm to a well defined tumour entity.

The first accurate description of mesenchymal neoplasms of the gastrointestinal tract was in 1941 (Golden T & Stout AP, 1941). Traditionally, these tumours were thought to be derived from smooth muscle cells, based on their resemblance to smooth muscle tumours. They were referred to as leiomyomas, bizarre leiomyomas (Stout AP, 1976), cellular leiomyomas (Appelman, 1977) and leiomyosarcomas. However, the advent of electron microscopy revealed that only a few of them have convincing ultrastructural evidence of smooth muscle differentiation. In addition, the application of immunohistochemistry clearly demonstrated that many of these tumours lack the features of smooth muscle differentiation. This led Mazur and Clark in 1983 to introduce the generic designation "stromal tumour" (Mazur & Clark, 1983).

A little later, in 1984, Herrera et al (Herrera et al., 1984) introduced the concept of "plexosarcoma" to acknowledge the existence of a small subset of stromal tumours with autonomic neuronal differentiation which became better known as gastrointestinal autonomic nerve tumours (GANTs) (Lauwers et al., 1993).

A considerable controversy arose as to the line of differentiation these tumours take. Some tumours exhibit a myogenic phenotype, while others may show a neural differentiation, mixed or no differentiation at all, the so called "null phenotype". Some enthusiasm was generated by the recognition that a significant proportion of stromal tumours express CD34 (Miettinen et al., 1995). However the diagnostic utility of this marker was hampered by its poor specificity. As a consequence of the lack of reproducible diagnostic criteria, GIST represented a generic term that indicates any mesenchymal tumour arising in the gastrointestinal tract.

The recognition of the central role of *c-kit* mutations in the pathogenesis of GISTs (Hirota et al., 1998; Rubin et al., 2000) and in most cases the associated expression of KIT protein in these tumours has provided a reproducible genotypic and phenotypic marker (Kindblom et al., 1998). Therefore KIT (CD117 in the standardised terminology of leucocyte antigens) expression has emerged as a marker for discriminating GISTs from other mesenchymal gastrointestinal neoplasms and some have equated immunoreactivity for KIT as definition of GISTs (Miettinen & Lasota, 2001).

Recently, it has become apparent that some GISTs that lacked *c-ki*t mutations were found to have activating mutations of *PDGFRA*. Therefore GISTs can be defined as specific CD117 positive and *c-kit* or *PDGFRA* mutation-driven mesenchymal tumours of the gastrointestinal tract.

2. Histogenesis

GISTs are either derived from or differentiate towards the interstitial cell of Cajal (ICC), or their stem cell precursors which have the capacity to differentiate towards both the ICC and smooth muscle phenotype (Kindblom et al., 1998; Rubin et al., 2000). The ICCs are intercalated between the autonomic nerves and smooth muscle cells. Their principle function is to generate autonomous rhythmic contractions, involved in digestion and peristalsis. Therefore these cells are known as the "pacemaker" cells of the gastrointestinal tract.

Morphologically, these cells are slender with ovoid nuclei and scanty cytoplasm. They have incomplete features of both neural and myoid differentiation.

Immunohistochemical studies revealed that GISTs have similar features to ICC, being positive with CD34 and CD117 and negative or variably positive for other neural and smooth muscle markers (Kindblom et al., 1998).

3. Molecular biology (*c-kit* and *PDGFRA*)

The *c-kit* proto-oncogene is a cellular homolog of the *v-kit* oncogene present in the genome of Hardy-Zuckerman-feline sarcoma virus (Besmer et al., 1986). It encodes a transmembrane tyrosine kinase receptor (Vliagoftis et al., 1997). The ligand for KIT is a growth factor called the stem cell factor.

Extracellular binding of stem cell factor results in dimerisation of the receptor, triggering phosphorylation of the kinase domain. This induces a signalling cascade that propagates through the cytoplasm into the nucleus. This signalling cascade affects many aspects of cellular behaviour including proliferation, differentiation, adhesion and apoptosis (Vliagoftis et al., 1997).

KIT expression is extremely important in the development of several cell types including the haematopoietic stem cells, mast cells, germ cells, melanocytes, some epithelial cells and the ICC (Vliagoftis et al., 1997).

The majority of GISTs have gain of function mutations of *c-kit* (Corless et al., 2004). These mutations have been observed in sporadic GISTs and less commonly as germline mutations in familial GISTs (Hirota et al., 1998; Isozaki et al., 2000), suggesting that constitutive expression of KIT plays a significant role in the tumourigenesis of GISTs. However, around 10-15% of GISTs lack *c-kit* mutations (Debiec-Rychter et al., 2004b). Within this group a large subset would have gain of function mutations of *PDGFRA* (Heinrich et al., 2003a; Heinrich et al., 2003b; Hirota et al., 2003).

3.1 *c-kit* mutations

Approximately 85%-90%of sporadic GISTs harbour a mutation of *c-kit* (Corless et al., 2002; Heinrich et al., 2002; Heinrich et al., 2003a; Hirota et al., 1998; Rubin et al., 2001). *c-kit* contains a total of 21 exons. However, mutations cluster within only four exons. They are in decreasing order of frequency, exon 11 encoding the intracellular juxtamembrane domain, exon 9 encoding the extracellular domain , exon 13 encoding the first portion of the kinase domain and exon 17 encoding the kinase activation loop (Giuly et al., 2003; Heinrich et al., 2002) (Figure 1A).

Mutations affecting exon 11 have been reported in 60-70% of GISTs (Corless et al., 2002; Corless et al., 2004; Heinrich et al., 2003a; Hirota et al., 1998; Rubin et al., 2001). The juxtamembrane region exerts a negative regulatory effect on KIT receptor (Longley et al., 2001) and therefore mutations in this region lead to loss of its inhibitory function. Mutations in exon 11 are fairly heterogenous and different types of mutations cluster within different regions. These mutations correlate with the best response to imatinib.

Approximately 60-70% of exon 11 mutations are in-frame deletions of 1 to several codons and the majority occur at the 5' and cluster between codons Gln^{550} and Glu^{561} (Corless et al., 2004; Hirota et al., 1998).

Missense point mutations in exon 11 occur in 20-30% of GISTs. They affect codons Trp^{557}, Val^{559} and Val^{560} and Leu^{576}. Internal tandem duplications are found at the 3′ end of the exon (codon 576-580) (Lasota et al., 2003a; Lasota & Miettinen, 2006; Rubin, 2006) and are typically seen in gastric GISTs (Lasota & Miettinen, 2006).

Exon 9 mutations are found in approximately 10% of cases (Antonescu et al., 2003; Hirota et al., 2001; Lasota et al., 2000b; Lux et al., 2000; Sakurai et al., 2001). Nearly all mutations affecting exon 9 are insertion of six nucleotides that result in Ala^{502}-Tyr^{503} duplication at the protein level (Heinrich et al., 2003a; Hostein et al., 2006; Lasota et al., 2000b; Lasota et al., 2003a; Lux et al., 2000; Willmore et al., 2004). This type of mutation is associated with small intestinal localisation and aggressive behaviour (Antonescu et al., 2003; Antonescu, 2006; Corless et al., 2004; Lasota et al., 2003a). Patients with this type of mutation respond less well to imatinib. More recently, another duplication leading to Phe^{506}-Phe^{508} duplication was reported (Heinrich et al., 2003a).

Mutations affecting exon 13 occur in approximately 1% of GISTs (Heinrich et al., 2003a; Kinoshita et al., 2003; Lasota et al., 2000b; Lux et al., 2000). All exon 13 mutations identified to date are missense mutations resulting in substitution of Glu for Lys^{642} (Lasota et al., 2000b; Lux et al., 2000) and are associated with resistance to imatinib treatment (Chen et al., 2004; Willmore et al., 2004).

Mutations affecting exon 17 are very rare and are found in less than 1% of all GISTs (Heinrich et al., 2003a; Rubin et al., 2001) and are typically missense substitution at codons 820 and 822 (Tornillo & Terracciano, 2006), whereas mutations at codon 817 are usually observed in non GISTs, including seminomas and mastocytomas (Corless et al., 2004).

3.2 *PDGFRA* mutations

Approximately 5%-10% of GISTs have mutations within *PDGFRA* (Corless et al., 2005; Heinrich et al., 2003b; Hirota et al., 2003). These mutations are functionally similar to *c-kit* mutations and are usually seen in epithelioid, gastric GISTs which show weak or no immunoreactivity for KIT (Corless, 2004; Corless et al., 2004; Corless et al., 2005; Heinrich et al., 2003a; Hornick & Fletcher, 2007; Lasota et al., 2004; Medeiros et al., 2004). Three different regions of *PDGFRA* have been reported to be mutated in GISTs (Figure 1B). These mutations, in decreasing order of frequency affect exon 18, exon 12 and exon 14 (Corless et al., 2005; Heinrich et al., 2003b).

Exon 18 encodes the kinase activation loop (TK2). The majority of exon 18 mutations are missense mutations leading to substitution of Val for Asp[842]. These mutations are usually seen in gastric tumours and are associated with resistance to imatinib (Heinrich et al., 2003a; Heinrich et al., 2003b; Hirota et al., 2003; Hornick & Fletcher, 2007; Ohashi et al., 2004).
Exon 12 encodes the juxtamembrane. Mutations affecting exon 12 are rare and lead to Asp for Val[561] substitution. In-frame deletions and insertions have also been reported around codon Val[561] (Corless et al., 2005; Miettinen & Lasota, 2006b).
Exon 14 encodes the kinase I domain (TK1). A single missense mutation leading to substitution of Lys for Asn[659] has been described (Corless et al., 2005).
Approximately 5-10% of GISTs are negative for both *c-kit* and *PDGFRA* mutations. This subset of GISTs may have an activating mutation either in a tyrosine kinase receptor similar to KIT and PDGFRA or in downstream signalling molecule of KIT or PDGFRA signalling cascade (Hornick & Fletcher, 2007; Rubin, 2006).

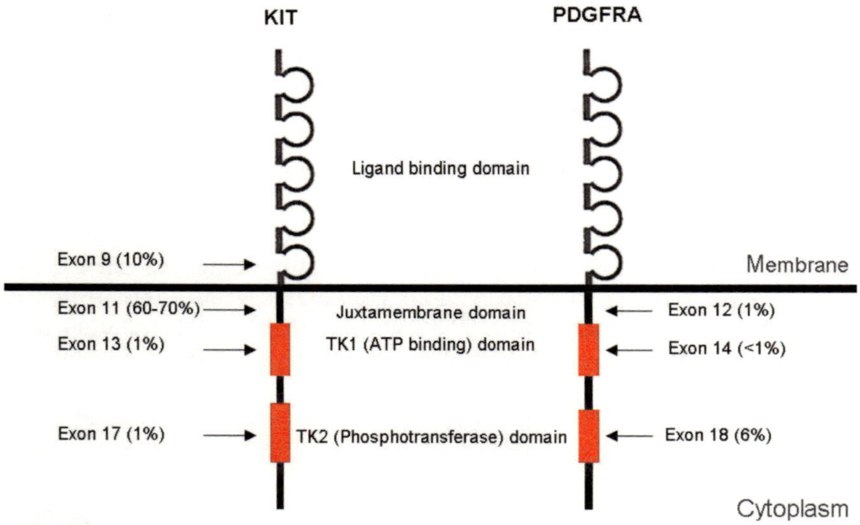

Fig. 1. Mutations of *c-kit* and *PDGFRA*.

3.3 *DOG1* gene

DOG1 "discovered on GIST" is a new gene, which encodes a protein of unknown function. It is expressed in GISTs independent of mutation type and is absent in non GISTs (West et al., 2004).

4. Epidemiology and risk factors

The lack of accepted diagnostic criteria for GISTs has led to variations in the current estimate of disease incidence. GIST is a relatively rare neoplasm representing less than 1% of all primary tumours of the gastrointestinal tract with an incidence of approximately 0.68-1.45/100,000 (Miettinen & Lasota, 2001; Nilsson et al., 2005; Tran et al., 2005). These figures do not account for benign GISTs, which are usually not included in cancer registries and are usually lost to clinical follow-up. Disease incidence seems to be uniform across all geographic and ethnic populations. More than 90% of GISTs occur in adults, mostly in middle-aged or

older individuals (Nilsson et al., 2005; Tran et al., 2005). There is no gender preference except in the setting of Carney's triad (Carney, 1999). Although there are no known predisposing risk factors, there are reports of familial GISTs (Isozaki et al., 2000) and GISTs in association with Von Recklinghausen's disease (Giuly et al., 2003), pointing to a genetic role.
Although GISTs may arise anywhere in the gastrointestinal tract, they are most common in the stomach (60%), followed by the jejenum and ileum (30%), duodenum (5%) and colorectum (<5%) (Miettinen & Lasota, 2006a; Miettinen & Lasota, 2006b). Very few cases have been described in the oesophagus (Miettinen et al., 2000a) or appendix (Miettinen & Sobin, 2001). A small proportion of GISTs arise in extra-gastrointestinal tract sites including the omentum, mesentery and retroperitoneum (Miettinen et al., 1999) with a few case reports of primary GISTs occurring in the gallbladder, pancreas, liver and urinary bladder (Bussolati, 2005; Hu et al., 2003; Lasota et al., 2000a; Mendoza-Marin et al., 2002). It is important to make sure that these do not represent spread from a primary lesion in the gastrointestinal tract.

5. GISTs syndromes

Although the vast majority of GISTs are sporadic, approximately 5% are associated with tumour syndromes. These include:

5.1 Familial GIST syndrome

This syndrome is inherited as an autosomal dominant disease. Patients with familial GISTs have germline activating mutations involving *c-kit* (Hirota et al., 2000; Isozaki et al., 2000; Li et al., 2005; Maeyama et al., 2001; Nishida et al., 1998; O'Brien et al., 1999) or *PDGFRA* (Chompret et al., 2004). These patients develop multiple GISTs, some of which in association with hyperplasia of the ICC (Chen et al., 2002). Other patients may also have the clinical manifestations of *c-kit* activation such as mastocytosis and hyperpigmentation (Kang et al., 2007).

5.2 Carney's triad and Carney Stratakis syndrome

Carney's triad consists of multicentric functioning extra-adrenal paraganglioma, pulmonary chondroma and multifocal epithelioid GIST of the stomach (Carney, 1999). There is a striking female predominance with approximately 85% of cases occurring in females. Most patients are less than 30 years of age at the time of diagnosis. Only subsets of patients have all of the three tumour types. Extra-adrenal parganglíomas and pulmonary chondromas may develop many years after the occurrence of GIST.
Carney Stratakis syndrome is a recently recognised autosomal dominant syndrome which represents a separate condition that affects both males and females and lacks the association with pulmonary chondromas. Mutations of the genes coding for succinate dehydrogenase subunits, typically associated with familial paragangliomas, are most likely implicated in the pathogenesis of Carney Stratakis syndrome (Pasini et al., 2008).
Mutations of *c-kit* or *PDGFRA* have not been identified in patients with Carney's triad or Carney Stratakis syndrome (Corless et al., 2004; Matyakhina et al., 2007; Prakash et al., 2005).

5.3 Neurofibromatosis type 1 (von Recklinghausen's disease)

Some patients with classic neurofibromatosis type 1 develop GISTs (Giuly et al., 2003; Takazawa et al., 2005). The tumours are usually in the small bowel and often multifocal.

They tend to be small, mitotically inactive and have a bland morphology. They are often accompanied by ICC hyperplasia. Most GISTs arising in the setting of NF1 do not have *c-kit* or *PDGFRA* mutations (Takazawa et al., 2005; Yantiss et al., 2005).

6. Clinical presentations

The clinical picture of GISTs depends on site, size and aggressiveness of these tumours which can vary from the benign to frank sarcoma. The symptoms can also vary, depending on the size and location of the lesion. Small tumours may be asymptomatic and may be found incidentally at laparotomy, endoscopy or during radiological studies for other conditions. Symptomatic tumours often present with abdominal pain or discomfort. They may ulcerate and cause gastrointestinal bleeding. This may be acute or insidious leading to anaemia or fatigue. Lesions in the oesophagus may present with dysphagia, while those of the intestine may present with an abdominal mass, obstruction or perforation. Occasionally, duodenal GISTs cause obstructive jaundice.

Patients with GISTs may also present with metastases, particularly to the liver. Malignancies reported in association with GISTs include carcinomas of the gastrointestinal tract as well as those of the breast, kidney, lung, uterus and prostate (Agaimy et al., 2006; Dematteo et al., 2000).

7. Morphology

7.1 Gross features

GISTs develop in any part of the gastrointestinal tract and tend to be primarily intramural tumours, usually involving the submucosa and muscularis propria.

GISTs vary in size from being several millimetres in diameter to over 30cms. Most lesions are well circumscribed, but are unencapsulated. Some are multinodular. They may have either a whorled fibroid-like cut surface or may be fleshy in appearance. They may protrude inward, leading to ulceration of the mucosa, or outward resulting in serosal based lesion. Large tumours may protrude into the lumen and from the serosa, resulting in a dumbbell appearance.

Areas of haemorrhage, cystic degeneration and central necrosis may be seen. The overlying mucosa may be intact or ulcerated, a feature that can be seen in either benign or malignant tumours.

7.2 Microscopic features

GISTs show a wide range of histologic features. Morphologically the cells of GISTs are spindle, epithelioid, mixed pattern and occasionally pleomorphic.

Spindle cell type is the predominant pattern, seen in 70% of GIST cases (Figure 2A). The tumour cells are arranged in short fascicles, whorls or a storiform growth pattern. The neoplastic cells have light fibrillary eosinophilic cytoplasm with indistinct cell borders. Perinuclear vacuoles are present and indent the nucleus at one pole (Figure 2B). These vacuoles are an artefact of fixation since they are not present in frozen sections (Appelman, 1977). The Nuclei tend to have relatively pointed ends as compared with blunt-ended nuclei in smooth muscle tumours, often with vesicular chromatin. Nuclear palisading reminiscent of that seen in schwannoma may be seen.

GISTs with epithelioid morphology account for 20% of cases (Figure 2C). The tumour cells are arranged in sheets or they may have a nested organoid growth pattern, reminiscent of paraganglioma or carcinoid. The tumour cells exhibit eosinophilic or clear cytoplasm (Figure 2D). The cytoplasm may be retracted simulating inclusions. The nuclei tend to be round to ovoid and may be pushed to an eccentric location.

GISTs with a mixed pattern (Figure 2E) are more common in the stomach. It may feature an abrupt transition between spindle and epithelioid areas or may show intermediate ovoid cytologic appearance.

A small minority of GISTs (<5%) have extensive nuclear pleomorphism (Figure 2F).

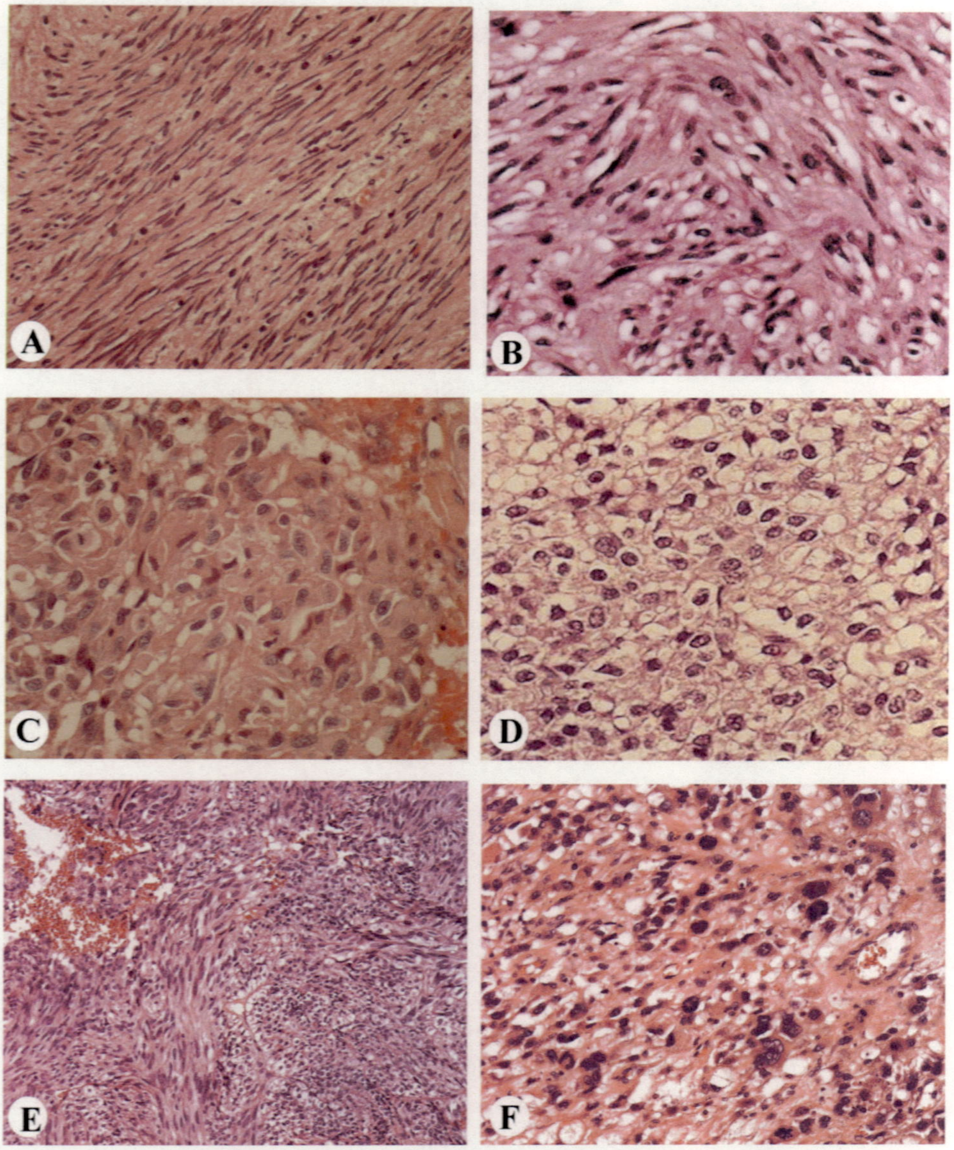

Fig. 2. Haematoxylin and Eosin sections of GISTs with a spindle cell morphology (A, B), GISTs with an epithelioid morphology (C, D), mixed cell pattern (E) and pleomorphic GIST (F).

The stroma in GISTs may be myxoid or it may be hyalinised (Figure 3A) or calcified. Delicate thin walled blood vessels may be prominent and may be associated with stromal haemorrhage (Figure 3B). Necrosis may be present. Lymphocytes can be seen.

Gastric GISTs have spindle cell morphology in 50% of cases, while 30% are epithelioid and 20% are mixed (Miettinen et al., 2005).

Small intestinal GISTs are more often spindled and may show extracellular bright eosinophilic collagen globules termed "skenoid fibres" (Figure 3C). These structures are periodic acid-Schiff (PAS) positive (Figure 3D). Small bowel tumours with an epithelioid morphology are usually associated with an aggressive behaviour.

Studies on oesophageal, colonic, ano-rectal and extra-gastrointestinal GISTs are sparse. Oesophageal GISTs involve the lower third of the oesophagus or gastro-oesophageal junction. They typically resemble gastric GISTs and usually show spindle cell morphology (Greenson, 2003). The majority of oesophageal GISTs are malignant.

Colonic GISTs and ano-rectal GISTs appear to be morphologically more similar to intestinal than gastric GISTs (Greenson, 2003). The majority are malignant with pleomorphic or overtly malignant spindle cell morphology.

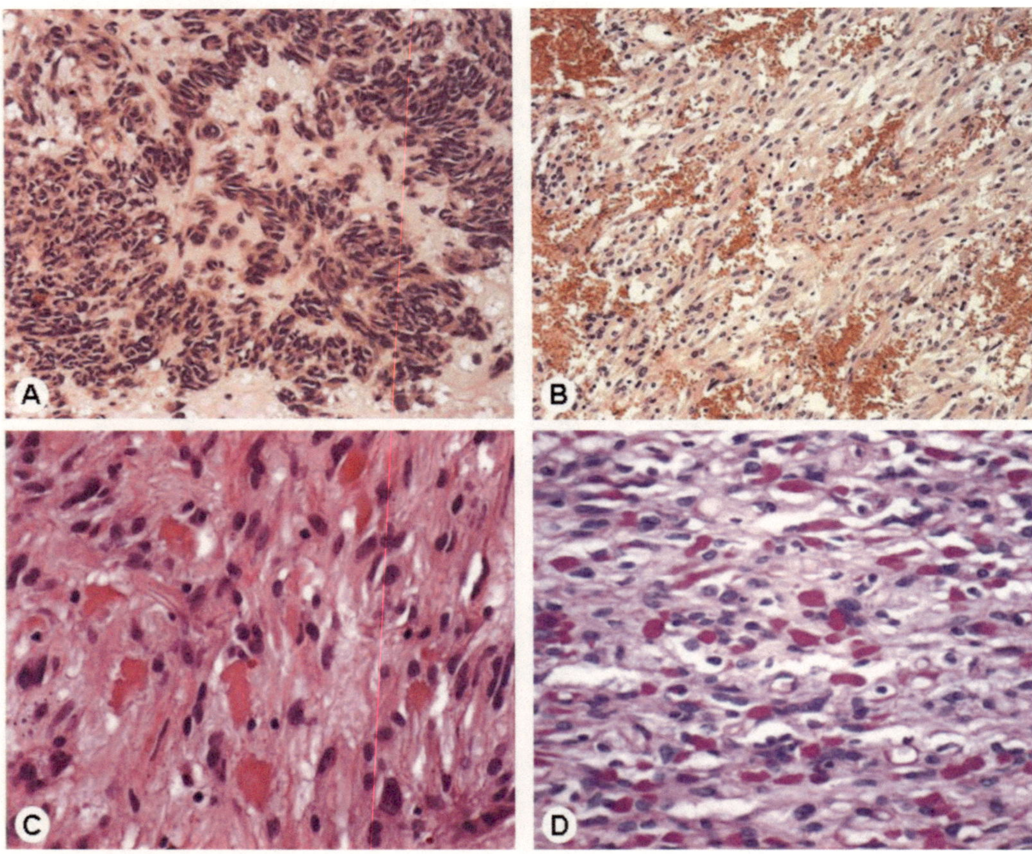

Fig. 3. GIST with a myxoid stroma (A), stromal haemorrhage (B), Skenoid fibres (C) and PAS positive skenoid fibres (D).

8. Gastrointestinal autonomic nerve tumours

GANTs were originally designated "plexoma" and "plexosarcoma" based on ultrastructural resemblance to cells of autonomic nervous system. GANTs are uncommon tumours which can occasionally develop in the context of von Recklinghausen's disease (Lespi & Drut, 1997) and Carney's triad (Segal et al., 1994). Familial multiple GANTs have been described in an association with intestinal neuronal dysplasia (O'Brien et al., 1999).

The characteristic ultrastructural features include complex interdigitating cell processes with bulbulous synaptic structures, dense core neurosecretory granules, rudimentary cell junctions and intermediate filaments.

Although originally believed to be a distinct tumour, recent evidence supports the concept that GANTs represent a phenotyptic variant of GISTs (Segal et al., 1994). These tumours tend to be KIT positive and a most have gain of function mutation in the juxtamembrane domain of *c-kit* (Lee et al., 2001).

9. Immunohistochemical features

The overwhelming majority of GISTs express KIT protein (detected as CD117). The results of KIT immunostaining depend on several technical factors including fixation, tissue preparation, variations in antibody clones in terms of specificity and sensitivity, antibody dilutions and staining techniques. This may account in part for the reported immunophenotypic heterogeneity in GISTs. It has been emphasised that CD117 should be performed without epitope retrieval (Fletcher & Fletcher, 2002).

The monoclonal antibodies currently available react inconsistently in formalin fixed paraffin embedded tissue and identify only a minority of GISTs (Miettinen et al., 2002b).

Given the potential clinical importance of CD117 immunostaining, optimisation of the staining techniques and reproducibility are critical.

The pattern of staining is variable (Figure 4). Diffuse strong pancytoplasmic staining is the predominant pattern. Membranous staining and dot-like "golgi zone pattern" staining can be identified. It has been suggested that different staining patterns correlate with different types of *c-kit* mutations (Fletcher et al., 2002a). Stromal mast cells and ICC are useful internal positive controls to supplement the normal positive and negative controls.

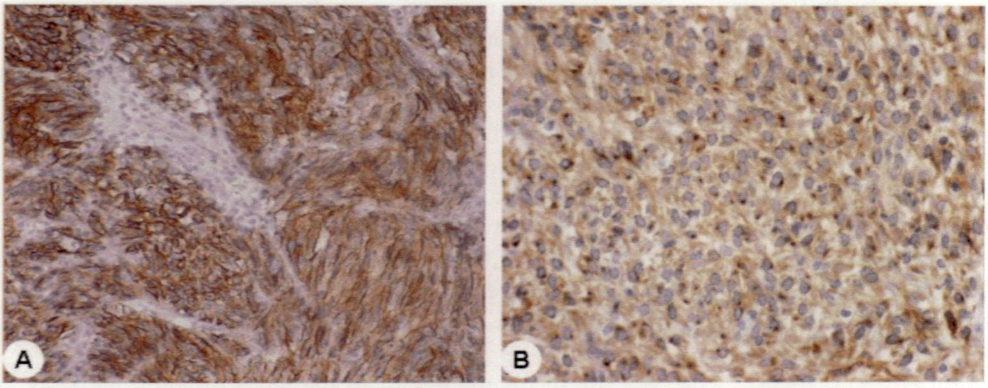

Fig. 4. Pattern of CD117 immunostaining. GIST showing membranous and cytoplasmic staining (A) and golgi zone-like staining (B).

Immunoreactivity may also be patchy, and thus false negative staining can be encountered in small biopsy specimens.

Immunohistochemical detection of KIT does not necessarily imply *c-kit* activation. Indeed CD117 is expressed by other tumour types such as melanoma and soft tissue sarcomas including dermatofibrosarcoma protuberans, synovial sarcoma and angiosarcoma (Sabah et al., 2003). The CD117 immunoreactivity should therefore, be interpreted in the context of morphology and clinical setting.

Approximately 5% of GISTs are KIT negative (Debiec-Rychter et al., 2004b; Medeiros et al., 2004). In these exceptional circumstances, KIT-negative mesenchymal lesions in the gastrointestinal tract with typical morphological features of GISTs may be referred to as "A stromal neoplasm most consistent with GIST". Such rare scenarios include GISTs that are either immunohistochemically inert for technical reasons, the subject of sampling error (biopsy of tumour with only focal KIT staining), the product of clonal evolution with emergence of KIT negative clone following imatinib therapy, or a rare example of a true GIST lacking KIT expression (Fletcher et al., 2002a; Parfitt et al., 2006). In such cases, pathologists should consider consultation with those experienced in dealing with large numbers of GISTs, as well as mutational analysis to look for mutations in *c-kit* and, if negative, *PDGFRA* (Corless et al., 2004; Medeiros et al., 2004).

DOG1 expression is found to be specific and sensitive for GISTs including KIT negative tumours (Espinosa et al., 2008; West et al., 2004). It has been reported in over 95% of cases.

CD34 is a transmembrane glycoprotein present on human haematopoietic progenitor cells and vascular endothelium. CD34 is detectable in approximately 60-70%. The oesophageal and rectal GISTs have the highest frequency of CD34 positivity, whereas small intestinal tumours have the lowest percentage of CD34 positivity (Miettinen et al., 2000b).

Muscle markers such as actin, calponin and h-caldesmon are positive in approximately 30% of cases (Miettinen et al., 2000b). α-smooth muscle actin (SMA) expression is often reciprocal with CD34 expression: the SMA positive tumours are often CD34 negative and vice versa. Some tumours may show mosaic pastern with actin positive and CD34 negative areas and vice versa (Miettinen et al., 2000b). Desmin positive immunostaining is uncommon (2%) (Fletcher et al., 2002a) and is often limited to scattered tumour cells. Prominent staining is more common in epithelioid tumours.

Positive staining for S100 protein occurs in 5-10% of GISTs, especially in small bowel tumours (Fletcher et al., 2002a). These tumours are usually negative for other neural markers including neurofilament and glial fibrillary protein.

Focal positive staining for cytokeratin markers can be seen especially in malignant epithelioid GISTs.

Data on immunohistochemical staining for PDGFRA protein are scant. Rossi et al (Rossi et al., 2005) evaluated the role of PDGFR immunohistochemistry in the differential diagnosis of KIT-negative GISTs. They reported positive expression of PDGFR, in KIT-negative GISTs, while KIT-positive GISTs, smooth muscle tumours, schwannomas and solitary fibrous tumours did not; however, 27% of desmoid tumours were also positive for PDGFRA. PDGFRA immunohistochemistry has not been standardised to be of practical diagnostic value in GISTs and many available antibodies do not appear reliable on paraffin-embedded material.

Protein kinase C theta (PKCθ) is a downstream effector in the KIT signalling pathway and has been suggested as an immunohistochemical marker for GISTs with a high specificity and sensitivity (Blay et al., 2004; Duensing et al., 2004). The expression of PKCθ has been reported in 98% of GISTs, including several CD117- negative tumours (Motegi et al., 2005). However, experience with this marker is limited.

10. Differential diagnosis

The differential diagnosis of GISTs is wide and includes the following:

10.1 Smooth muscle tumours

Intramural leiomyomas are most common in the oesophagus, and in fact, leiomyomas in this location outnumber GISTs by 3:1 (Dow et al., 2006). Oesophageal leiomyomas arise typically in young men, usually in the lower third of the oesophagus. Intramural leiomyomas are rare in the stomach and small intestine, but are common in the colon (Miettinen et al., 2001). Muscularis mucosae leiomyomas are usually small polypoid lesions found incidentally at colonoscopy and are most often found in the colon and rectum (Miettinen et al., 2001).

Morphologically, leiomyomas are generally less cellular than GISTs and are composed of bland spindle cells with eosinophilic cytoplasm and cigar shaped nuclei. Rare cases may show nuclear atypia without mitotic activity. Calcifications may be seen. The cells are positive for desmin and actin and negative for CD117. Approximately 10-15% of smooth muscle tumours are positive for CD34 (Fletcher et al., 2002a).

Pelvic uterine leiomyomas may become attached to the colon and therefore may mimic GISTs. These tumours resemble uteric leiomyomas morphologically and are positive for actin and desmin. The tumours are also oestrogen and progesterone receptors positive, whereas GISTs are negative for hormonal receptors.

Leiomyomatosis peritonealis disseminate represents numerous small (2-3mm), smooth muscle nodules on the peritoneum (Tavassoli & Norris, 1982). The nodules are composed of smooth muscle cells with no atypia and low mitotic activity, usually less than 2/10 high power fields (HPFs) (Dow et al., 2006). The cells have similar immunohistochemical features to uterine leiomyoma (Dow et al., 2006).

Leiomyosarcomas of the gastrointestinal tract are rare. They usually occur in older adults with a female predilection and are most common in the colon (Dow et al., 2006). The tumour cells show nuclear pleomorphism, mitotic activity and necrosis. They are actin and desmin positive and CD117 negative.

10.2 Schwannoma

This is a rare mesenchymal tumours of the gastrointestinal tract. It occurs most frequently in the stomach with a peak incidence in 6th and 7th decades. The tumour typically involves the submucosa and the muscularis propria. Histologically, it appears as a sharply demarcated but unencapsulated lesion often surrounded by a lymphoid cuff. The tumour is usually small in size (< 5cm) and is composed of spindle cells with wavy nuclei and occasional intranuclear inclusions. Mitoses are rare (< 5/50 HPFs). The cells are positive for S100 protein. Antoni B areas may express CD34 (Fletcher et al., 2002a), however the cells are negative for CD117.

Gastrointestinal schwannoma lack *NF2* gene alterations found in many soft tissue schwannomas. In addition, they frequently exhibit glial fibrillary acidic protein (GFAP) which is not a feature in soft tissue sarcomas. On this basis, it has been suggested that gastrointestinal schwannomas may represent a distinctive group of peripheral nerve sheath tumours (Lasota et al., 2003b).

10.3 Intra-abdominal fibromatosis

These are locally aggressive lesions but they usually do not metastasise. They occur either sporadically or in association with Gardner's syndrome, typically in young and middle-ages adults. Intra-abdominal fibromatoses are the most common primary tumours of the mesentery. The most common site is the mesentery of the small bowel, but some originate from the ileocolic mesentery, gastrocolic ligament or omentum. They may also occur in the reteroperitoneum and may involve the bowel wall. Most patients present with an asymptomatic mass, but some present with gastrointestinal bleeding or an acute abdomen secondary to bowel perforation.

These lesions are usually large in size, more than 10cm in diameter. Although grossly well circumscribed, they tend to infiltrate the surrounding tissue. Histologically, they are composed of spindle cell proliferation arranged in parallel with evenly spaced blood vessels. The stroma is typically collagenous with keloid-like fibres and thin-walled blood vessels. Mitotic figures can be identified.

CD117 has been reported to be positive depending on the antibody used (Miettinen, 2001; Yantiss et al., 2000). However, studies have suggested that under optimum technical conditions, intra-abdominal fibromatosis are CD117- negative tumours (Lucas et al., 2003). Nuclear immunoreactivity for β-catenin in these tumours has been reported to be useful in distinguishing these tumours from GISTs (Montgomery et al., 2002). CD34 is negative.

10.4 Inflammatory myofibroblastic tumour

Inflammatory myofibroblastic tumour known as "inflammatory psuedo tumour". The lesion often occurs in children but may be present in adults. It is commonly located on the peritoneal surface, but may involve the omentum, mesentery, stomach or intestinal wall. Patients with inflammatory myofibroblastic tumours present with abdominal pain and abdominal mass which may be associated with obstruction. Some patients present with fever, night sweats, malaise and weight loss. Whilst some of these lesions are felt to be benign reactions to infectious processes, others have been shown to be clonal in origin (Cook et al., 2001). Inflammatory myofibroblastic tumours are lobular or multinodular.

Histologically, they are characterised by spindled or stellate shaped cellular proliferation admixed with lymphocytes and plasma cells with streaks of fibrosis. The cells are positive for desmin and actin and negative for CD117 and CD34. A high proportion of these lesions are also positive for anaplastic lymphoma kinase (ALK1) (Cook et al., 2001).

10.5 Inflammatory fibroid polyp

This is a tumour-like lesion that occurs in adults and most often encountered in the small intestine, especially ileum and the stomach. The peak incidence is in the 6th to 7th decade of life. The lesion arises in the submucosa and is usually well circumscribed. It is composed of spindle cell proliferation admixed with granulation tissue-like blood vessels in a loose oedematous stroma. The cells may show concentric arrangement around the blood vessels, the so called "onion-skin pattern". Mixed inflammatory cells are present, comprising plasma cells, lymphocytes and mast cells. Eosinophils are usually prominent. The majority of these lesions are positive for CD34 but are negative for CD1117.

10.6 Solitary fibrous tumour

Solitary fibrous tumour may involve the peritoneal cavity and adhere to the bowel. It is characterised by a spindle cell proliferation admixed with collagen and "staghorn" blood vessels. The tumour cells are positive for CD34 but negative for CD117.

Predicting the clinical behaviour of solitary fibrous tumour is notoriously difficult, but large size, infiltrative margins, high cellularity, nuclear pleomorphism, tumour necrosis and high mitotic count (> 4/10 HPFs) are all associated with an increased risk of malignant behaviour (Gengler & Guillou, 2006).

10.7 Sclerosing mesenteritis

This tumour-like lesion affects the small bowel mesentery. It consists of fibrous bands infiltrating and encasing fat lobules with fat necrosis. Chronic inflammatory cells including lymphocytes, plasma cells and eosinophils are usually present. The cells are negative for CD34 and CD117.

10.8 Glomus tumours

These tumours rarely occur in the gastrointestinal tract. They are found almost exclusively in the stomach and mainly in women (Dow et al., 2006). They are usually benign and similar to peripheral glomus tumours. They are made up of round uniform cells arranged around prominent dilated haemangiopericytoma-like vessels. The cells are positive for smooth muscle actin and negative for desmin, S100 protein and CD117. CD34 positive staining is seen in 30% of cases (Miettinen et al., 2002c).

10.9 Miscellaneous lesions

GISTs with epithelioid morphology may be mistaken for paraganglioma, metastatic carcinoma, melanoma and clear cell sarcoma.

Paragangliomas arise outside the adrenal gland in approximately 10% of the cases. They occur anywhere along the midline of the retroperitoneum.

Metastatic carcinoma is the most common type of solid tumour of the mesentry and in most cases the primary site is an intra-abdominal neoplasm.

Malignant melanoma has a tendency to metastasise to the gastrointestinal tract. They are CD117 positive but can be distinguished from GISTs by the expression of S100 protein, HMB45 and Melan-A.

Clear cell sarcoma may rarely involve the gastrointestinal tract. The tumour cells are diffusely positive for S100 protein, but unlike peripheral clear cell sarcoma, they are negative for HMB45 and Melan-A. They are characterised by the presence of t(12;22) translocation with EWS-ATF1 gene fusions.

Mesothelioma with a sarcomatoid morphology may also mimic GIST if it involves the bowel. Mesothelioma cells are positive for calretinin and negative for CD34 and CD117.

Follicular dendritic cells sarcoma affects the spleen, but may extend into the adjacent structures. The tumour is composed of sheets and whorls of cells with ovoid nuclei. The cells are intimately associated with small lymphocytes and are positive for CD21 and CD35 and negative for CD117 and CD34.

Dedifferentiated retroperitoneal liposarcoma may be attached to the bowel wall and sometimes simulate GISTs. Thorough sampling usually reveals a lipomatous component.

Angiosarcoma can simulate GIST and can be positive for CD117, but the specific histologic and immunohistochemical features allow for the differential diagnosis from GIST.
Synovial sarcoma may rarely occur in the gastrointestinal tract, abdominal wall and retropeitoneum. Some immunohistochemical studies have shown KIT expression in synovial sarcomas (Sabah et al., 2003; Tamborini et al., 2001). However, synovial sarcoma exhibits (X;18) (p11.2;q11.2) translocation.

11. Prognostic factors

Several clinicopathological and cytogenetic features have prognostic relevance:

11.1 Clinicopathologic factors

11.1.1 Tumour stage at presentation

The presence of peritoneal or liver metastases at presentation is an adverse prognostic factor and is associated with a shorter survival (Dematteo et al., 2000). Invasion of adjacent organs also correlates with a poor outcome.

11.1.2 Tumour size, site and mitotic activity

The subset of GISTs that has a high likelihood of malignant behaviour is generally identified by increased tumour size and mitotic activity in the context of tumour location (Miettinen et al., 2002a; Miettinen et al., 2005; Miettinen et al., 2006; Miettinen & Lasota, 2006b). The size of the tumour should be measured along the greatest axis of the tumour. The mitotic count is most accurately expressed as the number of mitoses per 50 HPFs and should be performed on areas with highest mitotic activity. This requires adequate sampling of the tumour.
Based on the size of the tumour and mitotic count, GISTs can be classified into very low risk, low risk, intermediate risk and high risk (Fletcher et al., 2002a; Fletcher et al., 2002b) (Table 1).

GIST categories	Tumour size (cm)	Mitotic count (per 50 HPFs)
Very low risk	< 2	<5
Low risk	2-5	<5
Intermediate risk	<5 5-10	6-10 <5
High risk	> 5 > 10 Any size	> 5 Any mitotic rate > 10

Table 1. Tumour size and mitotic rate as guides to the evaluation of GIST malignancy (Fletcher et al., 2002b).

In recent years, it has become clear that GISTs require site evaluation because of differing behaviour (Emory et al., 1999; Miettinen et al., 2002a). It has been suggested that the site of the tumour is a prognostic factor independent of the tumour size and mitotic count (Emory et al., 1999) with small bowel tumours having the worst prognosis. This provided a rationale for the proposed site specific evaluation of GIST. In this classification, GIST is classified according to the site, size and mitotic count into three categories: benign, malignant and uncertain or low malignant potential (Miettinen et al., 2002a) (Table 2).

GIST categories	Criteria for diagnosis
Probably benign	**Intestinal tumours**: Maximum diameter ≤ 2 cm *and* no more than 5/50 HPFs **Gastric tumours**: Maximum diameter ≤ 5 cm *and* no more than 5/50 HPFs
Probably malignant	**Intestinal tumours**: Maximum diameter > 5 cm *or* more than 5/50 HPFs **Gastric tumours**: Maximum diameter > 10 cm *or* more than 5/50 HPFs
Uncertain (low malignant potential)	**Intestinal tumours**: Maximum diameter >2 cm but ≤ 5 cm *and* no more than 5/50 HPFs **Gastric tumours**: Maximum diameter > 5 cm and ≤ 10 cm *and* no more than 5/50 HPFs

Table 2. Tumour size, mitotic rate and tumour site as guides to the evaluation of GIST malignancy (Miettinen et al., 2002a).

Recent large series have evaluated the behaviour of large number of gastric and small intestinal GISTs. Because the data antedates imatinib application, it gives an insight into the natural history of GISTs. Based on the tumour size, mitotic count and the anatomic location of the tumour, GISTs are classified into different groups (Miettinen et al., 2005; Miettinen et al., 2006; Miettinen & Lasota, 2006b) (Table 3).

GIST groups	Tumour size (cm)	Mitotic count (per 50 HPFs)	Risk of progressive disease and malignant potential
1	≤ 2	≤5	Gastric: very low if any (0%) Small intestinal: very low if any (0%)
2	>2 ≤5	≤5	Gastric: low (1.9%) Small intestinal: low (4.3%)
3a	>5 ≤10	≤5	Gastric: low (3.6%) Small intestinal: intermediate (24%)
3b	> 10	≤5	Gastric: intermediate (12%) Small intestinal: high (52%)
4	≤ 2	> 5	Gastric: low (0% but too few cases to predict) Small intestinal: high (50% but too few cases to predict)
5	>2 ≤5	> 5	Gastric: intermediate (16%) Small intestinal: high (73%)
6a	>5 ≤10	> 5	Gastric: high (55%) Small intestinal: high (85%)
6b	> 10	> 5	Gastric: high (86%) Small intestinal: high (90%)

Table 3. Risk assessment of GISTs based on tumour size, mitotic count and tumour site (Miettinen & Lasota, 2006b).

A scheme proposed under the aegis of the National Institutes of Health (NIH) defined the risk of aggressive behaviour using the twin criteria of tumour size and mitotic activity count irrespective of tumour location. A significant body of opinion holds that the NIH scheme underestimates the risk of small bowel tumours and overestimates those of gastric origin. It is now widely held that this scheme should be replaced by one derived from the data collected by Lasota and Miettinen (Miettinen & Lasota, 2006a) (Table 4).
This scheme requires validation on independent data. Based on tumour size (maximum dimension in cm) and mitotic activity (number of mitoses per 50 HPFs), the categories of prognosis are defined as follows:

Tumour Parameters		Risk of progressive disease (metastasis or tumour-related death)			
Mitotic index ≤5/50HPFs	Size	Gastric	Duodenum	Jejenum/Ileum	Rectum
	≤ 2cm	None (0%)	None (0%)	None (0%)	None (0%)
	>2 - ≤5	Very low (1.9%)	Low (8.3%)	Low (4.3%)	Low (8.5%)
	>5 - ≤10	Low (3.6%)	Insufficient data	Moderate (24%)	Insufficient data
	>10 cm	Moderate (10%)	High (34%)	High (52%)	High (57%)
Mitotic index >5/50 HPFs	≤ 2cm	Insufficient data	Insufficient data	High (limited data)	High (54%)
	>2 - ≤5	Moderate (16%)	High (50%)	High (73%)	High (52%)
	>5 - ≤10	High (55%)	Insufficient data	High (85%)	Insufficient data
	>10 cm	High (86%)	High (86%)	High (90%)	High (71%)

Table 4. Risk stratification of GIST by mitotic count, tumour size and anatomic site (Miettinen & Lasota, 2006a).

11.1.3 Resection margins

The principal treatment for GISTs is surgery with wide local resection including a margin of 10–20mm for most tumours. Radical resection such as total gastrectomy with lymphadenectomy is not required. Involvement of the circumferential and surgical margins indicates a higher likelihood of local recurrence and therefore poorer outcome regardless of all other factors.

11.1.4 Epithelioid morphology

This cellular pattern is present in one third of gastric tumours, but is usually associated with more aggressive behaviour when found in the small intestine.

11.1.5 Mucosal invasion

Mucosal invasion is rarely seen in GISTs but is an adverse prognostic sign (Goldblum & Appelman, 1995) as it is confined to malignant GISTs (Miettinen et al., 2002a). Mucosal invasion should be distinguished from mucosal ulceration by its diffuse "lymphoma-like" pattern of growth between the glandular elements (Miettinen et al., 2002a). The presence of mucosal ulceration has no prognostic significance as it is found in benign and malignant GISTs

11.1.6 Cellularity

Low cellularity has emerged as a favourable prognostic feature according to some studies (Goldblum & Appelman, 1995).

11.1.7 Nuclear pleomorphism

Marked nuclear pleomorphism in a spindle cell tumour suggests a malignant behavior, on the other hand, scattered bizarre multinucleated cells are characteristic of benign lesions.

11.1.8 Immunohistochemical markers

Proliferation markers (Ki-67, MIB-1 and proliferating cell nuclear antigen (PCNA)) may aid in tumour evaluation. It has been reported that tumours with more than 10% of nuclei for Ki-67 analogue are associated with metastases and poor survival rate (Amin et al., 1993; Panizo-Santos et al., 2000; Reith et al., 2000; Rudolph et al., 1998; Wang et al., 2002). One study has reported that MIB-1 index was not superior to mitotic count as a prognostic factor (Wong et al., 2003).

Alterations affecting certain cell cycle regulators have been implicated in the pathogenesis and tumour progression of many tumours.

The tumour suppressor gene *p16*^{INK4} encodes a nuclear protein that belongs to the INK4A family of cyclin dependent kinase inhibitors and blocks cell cycle progression at the G1-S transition (Serrano et al., 1993). It has been reported that loss of p16 immunostaining is associated with high risk GISTs (Haller et al., 2005; Liang et al., 2007; Ricci et al., 2004; Sabah et al., 2004b; Sabah et al., 2006; Schneider-Stock et al., 2003; Schneider-Stock et al., 2005; Steigen et al., 2008).

Another gene, *p27*^{KIP1} is also a cyclin dependent kinase inhibitor that belongs to the CIP/KIP family. An inverse correlation between p27^{KIP1} protein expression and the degree of malignancy has been observed. Low p27^{KIP1} expression seems to be associated with aggressive clinical behaviour in GISTs (Gelen et al., 2003; Nemoto et al., 2006; Pruneri et al., 2003; Sabah et al., 2006).

E2F1 is a transcription factor. Phosphorylation of the Rb protein results in the release of E2F proteins, that are necessary for progression into S phase. Expression of E2F1 has been reported to be an adverse prognostic factor (Haller et al., 2005; Sabah et al., 2006).

Finally, the expression of p53, a transcription factor and a cell cycle regulator, has been extensively investigated in human malignancies including GISTs. Most studies have suggested that p53 expression correlates with histologically malignant GISTs (Al Bozom, 2001; Cunningham et al., 2001; Feakins, 2005; Gumurdulu et al., 2007; Haller et al., 2005; Hata et al., 2006; Hillemanns et al., 1998; Ryu et al., 2007; Sabah et al., 2006; Wang & Kou, 2007; Wang et al., 2002; Wong et al., 2003; Yalcinkaya et al., 2007).

11.2 Cytogenetic markers as prognostic factors

Prediction of clinical outcome on the basis of morphology alone is not always reliable. Other new and promising parameters that may aid prognostic evaluation may emerge from genetic studies.

11.2.1 Mutations of *c-kit* and *PDGFRA*

Both are known to be critical steps in initiating primary oncogenic events. The prognostic value and the therapeutic significance of *c-kit* mutations remain under investigation.

The presence of deletion/insertion mutations involving exon 11 has been identified as an independent negative predictor of disease-free survival (Lasota et al., 1999; Martin et al., 2005; Singer et al., 2002). In addition the type of *c-kit* mutation was found to be of prognostic relevance. For instance deletions; particularly deletions affecting codon 557 to 558 indicate a poor prognosis (Antonescu, 2006; Martin et al., 2005). In contrast, GIST patients harbouring point mutations or internal tandem duplications, follow a more indolent clinical course (Antonescu, 2006; Corless, 2004; Corless et al., 2004; Martin et al., 2005; Miettinen et al., 2005; Wardelmann et al., 2003).

Moreover an association between KIT exon 9 mutations and aggressive behaviour and non gastric site was reported (Antonescu et al., 2003; Corless et al., 2004).

It has been shown that the type of kinase receptor mutation influences response to imatinib treatment. Patients with GISTs expressing mutant exon 11 isoforms have a better response to STI-571 compared with patients harbouring mutations in exon 9 or without detectable *c-kit* or *PDGFRA* mutations (Heinrich et al., 2003a). In contrast, tumours with exon 17 or exon 13 mutations are primarily resistant to STI-571 (Chen et al., 2004; Debiec-Rychter et al., 2004a; Heinrich et al., 2003a; Tornillo & Terracciano, 2006). Similarly, mutations in exon 12 of *PDGFRA* have shown in vivo sensitivity to STI-571 compared with *PDGFRA* exon 18 (Debiec-Rychter et al., 2004a) which are resistant to both imatinib and sunitinib.

11.2.2 Chromosomal losses and gains

Certain cytogenetic aberrations have been identified in benign, malignant and metastatic GISTs, irrespective of their sites or degree of differentiation (Breiner et al., 2000; El Rifai et al., 1996; El Rifai et al., 2000; Gunawan et al., 2002; Kim et al., 2000; Lasota et al., 2005; Sandberg & Bridge, 2002; Sarlomo-Rikala et al., 1998; Wozniak et al., 2007), suggesting that these changes are early events in GIST tumourigenesis. These include losses at chromosome arms 14q and 22q.

Cytogenetic studies have reported correlations between the acquisition of additional chromosomal changes and aggressive behaviour such as gains at 5p and 20q and losses at chromosomes 1p, 9q and 9p. Gains at 8q and 17q have been detected in metastatic GISTs far more frequently than in primary tumours (Breiner et al., 2000; Debiec-Rychter et al., 2001; Derre et al., 2001; Gunawan et al., 2004; Kim et al., 2000; Miettinen et al., 2002a; O'Leary et al., 1999). Therefore, these chromosomal aberrations appear to be secondary events and may play an important role in tumour progression (Heinrich et al., 2003a) (Figure 5).

The loss of heterozygosity of the 9p region in malignant and low malignant potential GISTs has been investigated. It has been shown that loss of heterozygosity at the 9p region was absent in low malignant potential GISTs but was a common finding in high risk tumours (malignant and recurrent group). Recurrent GISTs showed more frequent deletions than their primary tumours (Sabah et al., 2004b). These findings support the theory that loss of 9p may contribute to the progression and/or malignant transformation of GISTs.

11.2.3 Telomerase activity

Telomerase is an enzyme that extends telomeric repeats on the ends of eukaryotic chromosomes, protecting them from loss, fusion and degradation. Most normal somatic cells do not express telomerase. Telomerase activity has been detected exclusively in malignant GISTs (Gunther et al., 2000; Sakurai et al., 1998; Wang & Kou, 2007). The expression of human telomerase reverse transcriptase (hTERT) by immunohistochemistry was investigated and was found that hTERT expression occurs preferentially in malignant GISTs and that the signal intensity correlated with the mitotic count of the tumour (Sabah et al., 2004a).

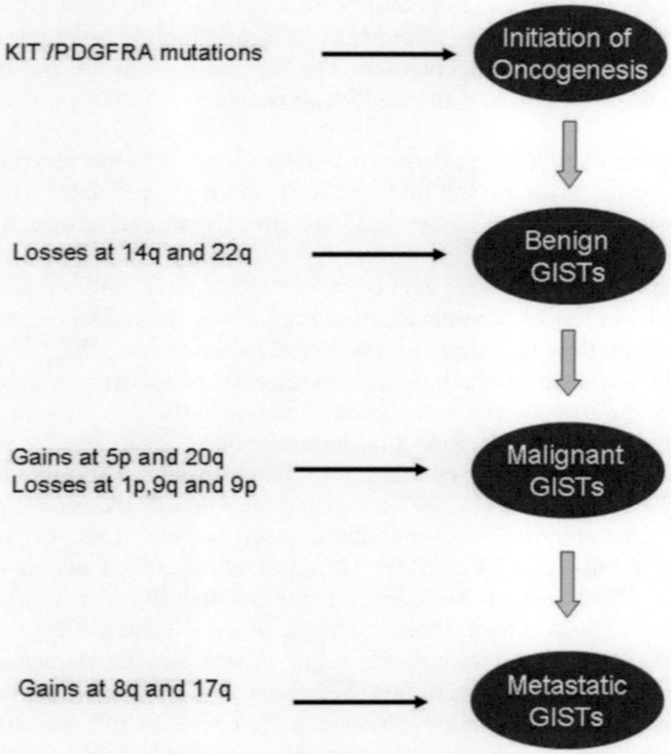

Fig. 5. Molecular events involved in the tumourigenesis of GISTs and chromosomal losses and gains involved in the progression of GISTs.

12. Imaging

Several radiological techniques are used to image GISTs. These include double contrast gastrointestinal X-ray series with barium, endoscopic ultrasound, computed tomography scanning and magnetic resonance. These modalities allow preoperative assessment of the size and involvement of other structures. They are also useful in identifying metastatic lesions.

Recently positron emission tomography (PET) scanning has been shown to be a useful and non-invasive mean of monitoring effectiveness of treatment of GISTs. Moreover, GIST response assessed by PET scan eight days after the start of imatinib mesylate treatment correlates with prognosis and survival at one year in patients with non-resectable GIST (Stroobants et al., 2003).

13. Treatment options

Until recently surgery was the only effective treatment for GISTs and complete surgical resection is still the only treatment that can cure the disease. However even for patients whose tumour was completely removed with clear margins there is still high probability of local recurrence.

Treatment options for recurrent or metastatic GISTs are even more limited. Radiation therapy is rarely used to treat GISTs because of the radio-sensitivity of adjacent organs and the high radio-resistance of these tumours. GISTs are highly resistant to conventional chemotherapy, regardless of the agent used. The reasons for this are not fully understood but may relate to the expression of the multidrug resistance protein products of the *MDR1* gene.

This bleak prognostic picture for patients with metastatic GISTs has recently changed with the advent of the tyrosine kinase inhibitor (STI-571, Imatinib mesylate). This drug binds to the ATP binding site of the target kinase and interrupts the signal transduction (Dematteo et al., 2002; Heinrich et al., 2002).

Imatinib is currently the first line agent for metastatic and unresectable GISTs and is currently under trial to test its possible effect of minimising the risk of recurrence in patients with high risk GISTs following complete resection (Dematteo et al., 2002). However, there is an ongoing debate on the duration, dose and the selection of patients for adjuvant therapy.

The effects of imatinib on GISTs morphology include reduction in tumour size, loss of cellularity, decreased mitoses or Ki67 proliferation index, degenerative changes such as myxoid stroma, cyst formation, necrosis and haemorrhage (Abdulkader et al., 2005; Loughrey et al., 2005; Pauwels et al., 2005). Additional potential diagnostic pitfalls include a possible shift from spindled to epithelioid morphology, loss of KIT and CD34 immunoreactivity (Abdulkader et al., 2005; Loughrey et al., 2005; Pauwels et al., 2005; Sciot & Debiec-Rychter, 2006) and positive desmin immunostaining in a tumours which were previously completely negative for desmin (Sciot & Debiec-Rychter, 2006).

Some 90% of patients obtain symptomatic relief. About two thirds achieve an objective response, as defined by a reduction of 50% or greater in tumour volume (van Oosterom et al., 2001). Another 20% of patients remain stable. However, in 10% the disease progresses despite of imatinib therapy due the occurrence of secondary mutations or clonal selection which cause drug resistance.

In such cases other tyrosine kinase inhibitors or downstream targets such as protein kinase theta can be tried (Sakamoto, 2004). Sunitinib malate (SU11248) has shown promising activity in imatinib resistant GISTs. In addition to KIT and PDGFRA, this drug also targets FLT3 and VEGF receptors (Demetri et al., 2003; Sakamoto, 2004).

Other drugs that are being evaluated in imatinib-refractory patients include Nilotinib (Montemurro et al., 2009) (inhibitor of KIT and PDGFRA); Sorafenib (a multi kinase inhibitor of raf kinase, VEGFR, PDGFR and KIT)(Demetri, 2011); RAD001 (a rapamycin analogue inhibitor of the protein kinase mammalian target of rapamycin); Oblimersen (an antisense oligonucleotide to bcl-2 mRNA); heat shock protein 90 inhibitor (17-allyylamino-18-demethoxy-geldanamycin, 17-AAG) (Bauer et al., 2006); Bevacizumab (a neutralising antibody to vascular endothelial growth factor); CCI 779 (a rapamycin analogue inhibitor of the protein kinase mammalian target of rapamycin); PKC 412 (an inhibitor of protein kinase C) and neutralising antibodies against vascular endothelial growth factor and several multi kinase inhibitors (De Giorgi & Verweij, 2005; Rubin, 2006).

14. Conclusion

GISTs constitute the largest group of mesenchymal tumours of the gastrointestinal tract. These tumours originate from the ICC or their precursors. Most GISTs express KIT and have gain of function mutations of *c-kit* or *PDGFRA*. Therefore, KIT expression has emerged as an important defining feature for these tumours. However, KIT expression is not specific for GISTs and should be interpreted in the context of clinical setting and appropriate morphology. A minority of GISTs are negative for KIT. In such cases, analysis of *c-kit* or *PDGFRA* genes is necessary for accurate diagnosis. Clinically and pathologically, GISTs represent a spectrum of tumours that include benign, malignant and borderline variants.

Prognostic features indicative of malignancy or high risk for aggressive clinical behaviour are generally identified by increased tumour size and mitotic activity in the context of tumour location. Cytogenetic parameters aid prognostic evaluation and may play a role in the prognostication of GISTS in the future.

Imatinib has revolutionised the management of advanced and metastatic GISTs. Alternative therapeutic strategies are currently being evaluated. These may benefit patients who are refractory to imatinib or may be useful as adjuvant/neoadjuvant therapy to improve the outlook for GIST patients.

15. References

Abdulkader, I., Cameselle-Teijeiro, J., & Forteza, J. (2005). Pathological changes related to Imatinib treatment in a patient with a metastatic gastrointestinal stromal tumour. *Histopathology, 46,* 470-472.

Agaimy, A., Wunsch, P. H., Sobin, L. H., Lasota, J., & Miettinen, M. (2006). Occurrence of other malignancies in patients with gastrointestinal stromal tumors. *Semin.Diagn.Pathol., 23,* 120-129.

Al Bozom, I. A. (2001). p53 expression in gastrointestinal stromal tumors. *Pathol.Int., 51,* 519-523.

Amin, M. B., Ma, C. K., Linden, M. D., Kubus, J. J., & Zarbo, R. J. (1993). Prognostic value of proliferating cell nuclear antigen index in gastric stromal tumors. Correlation with mitotic count and clinical outcome. *Am.J.Clin.Pathol, 100,* 428-432.

Antonescu, C. R. (2006). Gastrointestinal stromal tumor (GIST) pathogenesis, familial GIST, and animal models. *Semin.Diagn.Pathol., 23,* 63-69.

Antonescu, C. R., Sommer, G., Sarran, L., Tschernyavsky, S. J., Riedel, E., Woodruff, J. M. et al. (2003). Association of KIT exon 9 mutations with nongastric primary site and aggressive behavior: KIT mutation analysis and clinical correlates of 120 gastrointestinal stromal tumors. *Clin.Cancer Res., 9,* 3329-3337.

Appelman, H. D. (1977). Cellular leiomyomas of the stomach in 49 patients. *Arch.Pathol Lab Med., 101,* 373-377.

Bauer, S., Yu, L. K., Demetri, G. D., & Fletcher, J. A. (2006). Heat shock protein 90 inhibition in imatinib-resistant gastrointestinal stromal tumor. *Cancer Res., 66,* 9153-9161.

Besmer, P., Lader, E., George, P. C., Bergold, P. J., Qiu, F. H., Zuckerman, E. E. et al. (1986). A new acute transforming feline retrovirus with fms homology specifies a C-terminally truncated version of the c-fms protein that is different from SM-feline sarcoma virus v-fms protein. *J.Virol., 60,* 194-203.

Blay, P., Astudillo, A., Buesa, J. M., Campo, E., Abad, M., Garcia-Garcia, J. et al. (2004). Protein kinase C theta is highly expressed in gastrointestinal stromal tumors but not in other mesenchymal neoplasias. *Clin.Cancer Res., 10,* 4089-4095.

Breiner, J. A., Meis-Kindblom, J., Kindblom, L. G., McComb, E., Liu, J., Nelson, M. et al. (2000). Loss of 14q and 22q in gastrointestinal stromal tumors (pacemaker cell tumors). *Cancer Genet.Cytogenet., 120,* 111-116.

Bussolati, G. (2005). Of GISTs and EGISTs, ICCs and ICs. *Virchows Arch., 447,* 907-908.

Carney, J. A. (1999). Gastric stromal sarcoma, pulmonary chondroma, and extra-adrenal paraganglioma (Carney Triad): natural history, adrenocortical component, and possible familial occurrence. *Mayo Clin.Proc., 74,* 543-552.

Chen, H., Hirota, S., Isozaki, K., Sun, H., Ohashi, A., Kinoshita, K. et al. (2002). Polyclonal nature of diffuse proliferation of interstitial cells of Cajal in patients with familial and multiple gastrointestinal stromal tumours. *Gut, 51,* 793-796.

Chen, L. L., Trent, J. C., Wu, E. F., Fuller, G. N., Ramdas, L., Zhang, W. et al. (2004). A missense mutation in KIT kinase domain 1 correlates with imatinib resistance in gastrointestinal stromal tumors. *Cancer Res., 64,* 5913-5919.

Chompret, A., Kannengiesser, C., Barrois, M., Terrier, P., Dahan, P., Tursz, T. et al. (2004). PDGFRA germline mutation in a family with multiple cases of gastrointestinal stromal tumor. *Gastroenterology, 126,* 318-321.

Cook, J. R., Dehner, L. P., Collins, M. H., Ma, Z., Morris, S. W., Coffin, C. M. et al. (2001). Anaplastic lymphoma kinase (ALK) expression in the inflammatory myofibroblastic tumor: a comparative immunohistochemical study. *Am.J.Surg Pathol, 25,* 1364-1371.

Corless, C. L. (2004). Assessing the prognosis of gastrointestinal stromal tumors: a growing role for molecular testing. *Am.J.Clin.Pathol., 122,* 11-13.

Corless, C. L., Fletcher, J. A., & Heinrich, M. C. (2004). Biology of gastrointestinal stromal tumors. *J.Clin.Oncol., 22,* 3813-3825.

Corless, C. L., McGreevey, L., Haley, A., Town, A., & Heinrich, M. C. (2002). KIT mutations are common in incidental gastrointestinal stromal tumors one centimeter or less in size. *Am.J.Pathol., 160,* 1567-1572.

Corless, C. L., Schroeder, A., Griffith, D., Town, A., McGreevey, L., Harrell, P. et al. (2005). PDGFRA mutations in gastrointestinal stromal tumors: frequency, spectrum and in vitro sensitivity to imatinib. *J.Clin.Oncol., 23,* 5357-5364.

Cunningham, R. E., Abbondanzo, S. L., Chu, W. S., Emory, T. S., Sobin, L. H., & O'Leary, T. J. (2001). Apoptosis, bcl-2 expression, and p53 expression in gastrointestinal stromal/smooth muscle tumors. *Appl.Immunohistochem.Mol.Morphol., 9,* 19-23.

De Giorgi, U. & Verweij, J. (2005). Imatinib and gastrointestinal stromal tumors: Where do we go from here? *Mol.Cancer Ther., 4,* 495-501.

Debiec-Rychter, M., Dumez, H., Judson, I., Wasag, B., Verweij, J., Brown, M. et al. (2004a). Use of c-KIT/PDGFRA mutational analysis to predict the clinical response to imatinib in patients with advanced gastrointestinal stromal tumours entered on phase I and II studies of the EORTC Soft Tissue and Bone Sarcoma Group. *Eur.J.Cancer, 40,* 689-695.

Debiec-Rychter, M., Lasota, J., Sarlomo-Rikala, M., Kordek, R., & Miettinen, M. (2001). Chromosomal aberrations in malignant gastrointestinal stromal tumors: correlation with c-KIT gene mutation. *Cancer Genet.Cytogenet., 128,* 24-30.

Debiec-Rychter, M., Wasag, B., Stul, M., De Wever, I., van Oosterom, A., Hagemeijer, A. et al. (2004b). Gastrointestinal stromal tumours (GISTs) negative for KIT (CD117 antigen) immunoreactivity. *J.Pathol, 202,* 430-438.

Dematteo, R. P., Heinrich, M. C., El Rifai, W. M., & Demetri, G. (2002). Clinical management of gastrointestinal stromal tumors: before and after STI-571. *Hum.Pathol., 33,* 466-477.

Dematteo, R. P., Lewis, J. J., Leung, D., Mudan, S. S., Woodruff, J. M., & Brennan, M. F. (2000). Two hundred gastrointestinal stromal tumors: recurrence patterns and prognostic factors for survival. *Ann.Surg, 231,* 51-58.

Demetri, G. D., George, S., Heinrich, M. C., & et al. (2003). Clinical activity and tolerability of the multi-targated tyrosine kinase inhibitor SU11248 in patients with metastatic gastrointestinal stromal tumour refractory to imatinib mesylate. Proc.Am.Soc.Clin.Oncol 22[814], abstract (3273).

Demetri, G. D. (2011). Differential properties of current tyrosine kinase inhibitors in gastrointestinal stromal tumors. *Semin.Oncol., 38 Suppl 1,* S10-S19.

Derre, J., Lagace, R., Terrier, P., Sastre, X., & Aurias, A. (2001). Consistent DNA losses on the short arm of chromosome 1 in a series of malignant gastrointestinal stromal tumors. *Cancer Genet.Cytogenet., 127,* 30-33.

Dow, N., Giblen, G., Sobin, L. H., & Miettinen, M. (2006). Gastrointestinal stromal tumors: differential diagnosis. *Semin.Diagn.Pathol., 23,* 111-119.

Duensing, A., Joseph, N. E., Medeiros, F., Smith, F., Hornick, J. L., Heinrich, M. C. et al. (2004). Protein Kinase C theta (PKCtheta) expression and constitutive activation in gastrointestinal stromal tumors (GISTs). *Cancer Res., 64,* 5127-5131.

El Rifai, W., Sarlomo-Rikala, M., Andersson, L. C., Knuutila, S., & Miettinen, M. (2000). DNA sequence copy number changes in gastrointestinal stromal tumors: tumor progression and prognostic significance. *Cancer Res., 60,* 3899-3903.

El Rifai, W., Sarlomo-Rikala, M., Miettinen, M., Knuutila, S., & Andersson, L. C. (1996). DNA copy number losses in chromosome 14: an early change in gastrointestinal stromal tumors. *Cancer Res., 56,* 3230-3233.

Emory, T. S., Sobin, L. H., Lukes, L., Lee, D. H., & O'Leary, T. J. (1999). Prognosis of gastrointestinal smooth-muscle (stromal) tumors: dependence on anatomic site. *Am.J.Surg.Pathol., 23,* 82-87.

Espinosa, I., Lee, C. H., Kim, M. K., Rouse, B. T., Subramanian, S., Montgomery, K. et al. (2008). A novel monoclonal antibody against DOG1 is a sensitive and specific marker for gastrointestinal stromal tumors. *Am.J.Surg.Pathol., 32,* 210-218.

Feakins, R. M. (2005). The expression of p53 and bcl-2 in gastrointestinal stromal tumours is associated with anatomical site, and p53 expression is associated with grade and clinical outcome. *Histopathology, 46,* 270-279.

Fletcher, C. D., Berman, J. J., Corless, C., Gorstein, F., Lasota, J., Longley, B. J. et al. (2002a). Diagnosis of gastrointestinal stromal tumors: A consensus approach. *Hum.Pathol., 33,* 459-465.

Fletcher, C. D., Berman, J. J., Corless, C., Gorstein, F., Lasota, J., Longley, B. J. et al. (2002b). Diagnosis of gastrointestinal stromal tumors: a consensus approach. *Int.J.Surg.Pathol., 10,* 81-89.

Fletcher, C. D. & Fletcher, J. A. (2002). Testing for KIT (CD117) in gastrointestinal stromal tumors: another HercepTest? *Am.J.Clin.Pathol, 118,* 163-164.

Gelen, M. T., Elpek, G. O., Aksoy, N. H., Ogus, M., Suleymanlar, I., & Isitan, F. (2003). p27 expression and proliferation in gastrointestinal stromal tumors. *Turk.J.Gastroenterol., 14,* 132-137.

Gengler, C. & Guillou, L. (2006). Solitary fibrous tumour and haemangiopericytoma: evolution of a concept. *Histopathology, 48,* 63-74.

Giuly, J. A., Picand, R., Giuly, D., Monges, B., & Nguyen-Cat, R. (2003a). Von Recklinghausen disease and gastrointestinal stromal tumors. *Am.J.Surg, 185,* 86-87.

Goldblum, J. R. & Appelman, H. D. (1995). Stromal tumors of the duodenum. A histologic and immunohistochemical study of 20 cases. *Am.J.Surg.Pathol., 19,* 71-80.

Golden T & Stout AP (1941). Smooth muscle tumours of the gastrointestinal tract and retroperitoneal tissues. *Surg Gynecol Obstet, 73,* 784-810.

Greenson, J. K. (2003). Gastrointestinal stromal tumors and other mesenchymal lesions of the gut. *Mod.Pathol., 16,* 366-375.

Gumurdulu, D., Erdogan, S., Kayaselcuk, F., Seydaoglu, G., Parsak, C. K., Demircan, O. et al. (2007). Expression of COX-2, PCNA, Ki-67 and p53 in gastrointestinal stromal tumors and its relationship with histopathological parameters. *World J.Gastroenterol., 13,* 426-431.

Gunawan, B., Bergmann, F., Hoer, J., Langer, C., Schumpelick, V., Becker, H. et al. (2002). Biological and clinical significance of cytogenetic abnormalities in low-risk and high-risk gastrointestinal stromal tumors. *Hum.Pathol., 33,* 316-321.

Gunawan, B., Schulten, H. J., von Heydebreck, A., Schmidt, B., Enders, C., Hoer, J. et al. (2004). Site-independent prognostic value of chromosome 9q loss in primary gastrointestinal stromal tumours. *J.Pathol., 202,* 421-429.

Gunther, T., Schneider-Stock, R., Hackel, C., Pross, M., Schulz, H. U., Lippert, H. et al. (2000). Telomerase activity and expression of hTRT and hTR in gastrointestinal stromal tumors in comparison with extragastrointestinal sarcomas. *Clin.Cancer Res., 6,* 1811-1818.

Haller, F., Gunawan, B., von Heydebreck, A., Schwager, S., Schulten, H. J., Wolf-Salgo, J. et al. (2005). Prognostic role of E2F1 and members of the CDKN2A network in gastrointestinal stromal tumors. *Clin.Cancer Res., 11,* 6589-6597.

Hata, Y., Ishigami, S., Natsugoe, S., Nakajo, A., Okumura, H., Miyazono, F. et al. (2006). P53 and MIB-1 expression in gastrointestinal stromal tumor (GIST) of the stomach. *Hepatogastroenterology, 53,* 613-615.

Heinrich, M. C., Corless, C. L., Demetri, G. D., Blanke, C. D., von Mehren, M., Joensuu, H. et al. (2003a). Kinase mutations and imatinib response in patients with metastatic gastrointestinal stromal tumor. *J.Clin.Oncol., 21,* 4342-4349.

Heinrich, M. C., Corless, C. L., Duensing, A., McGreevey, L., Chen, C. J., Joseph, N. et al. (2003b). PDGFRA activating mutations in gastrointestinal stromal tumors. *Science, 299,* 708-710.

Heinrich, M. C., Rubin, B. P., Longley, B. J., & Fletcher, J. A. (2002). Biology and genetic aspects of gastrointestinal stromal tumors: KIT activation and cytogenetic alterations. *Hum.Pathol., 33,* 484-495.

Herrera, G. A., Pinto de Moraes H., Grizzle, W. E., & Han, S. G. (1984). Malignant small bowel neoplasm of enteric plexus derivation (plexosarcoma). Light and electron microscopic study confirming the origin of the neoplasm. *Dig.Dis.Sci., 29,* 275-284.

Hillemanns, M., Pasold, S., Bottcher, K., & Hofler, H. (1998). [Prognostic factors of gastrointestinal stromal tumors of the stomach]. *Verh.Dtsch.Ges.Pathol., 82,* 261-266.

Hirota, S., Isozaki, K., Moriyama, Y., Hashimoto, K., Nishida, T., Ishiguro, S. et al. (1998). Gain-of-function mutations of c-kit in human gastrointestinal stromal tumors. *Science, 279,* 577-580.

Hirota, S., Nishida, T., Isozaki, K., Taniguchi, M., Nakamura, J., Okazaki, T. et al. (2001). Gain-of-function mutation at the extracellular domain of KIT in gastrointestinal stromal tumours. *J.Pathol., 193,* 505-510.

Hirota, S., Ohashi, A., Nishida, T., Isozaki, K., Kinoshita, K., Shinomura, Y. et al. (2003). Gain-of-function mutations of platelet-derived growth factor receptor alpha gene in gastrointestinal stromal tumors. *Gastroenterology, 125,* 660-667.

Hirota, S., Okazaki, T., Kitamura, Y., O'Brien, P., Kapusta, L., & Dardick, I. (2000). Cause of familial and multiple gastrointestinal autonomic nerve tumors with hyperplasia of interstitial cells of Cajal is germline mutation of the c-kit gene. *Am.J.Surg.Pathol., 24,* 326-327.

Hornick, J. L. & Fletcher, C. D. (2007). The role of KIT in the management of patients with gastrointestinal stromal tumors. *Hum.Pathol., 38,* 679-687.

Hostein, I., Longy, M., Gastaldello, B., Geneste, G., & Coindre, J. M. (2006). Detection of a new mutation in KIT exon 9 in a gastrointestinal stromal tumor. *Int.J.Cancer, 118,* 2089-2091.

Hu, X., Forster, J., & Damjanov, I. (2003). Primary malignant gastrointestinal stromal tumor of the liver. *Arch.Pathol.Lab Med., 127,* 1606-1608.

Isozaki, K., Terris, B., Belghiti, J., Schiffmann, S., Hirota, S., & Vanderwinden, J. M. (2000). Germline-activating mutation in the kinase domain of KIT gene in familial gastrointestinal stromal tumors. *Am.J.Pathol., 157,* 1581-1585.

Kang, D. Y., Park, C. K., Choi, J. S., Jin, S. Y., Kim, H. J., Joo, M. et al. (2007). Multiple gastrointestinal stromal tumors: Clinicopathologic and genetic analysis of 12 patients. *Am.J.Surg.Pathol., 31,* 224-232.

Kim, N. G., Kim, J. J., Ahn, J. Y., Seong, C. M., Noh, S. H., Kim, C. B. et al. (2000). Putative chromosomal deletions on 9P, 9Q and 22Q occur preferentially in malignant gastrointestinal stromal tumors. *Int.J.Cancer, 85,* 633-638.

Kindblom, L. G., Remotti, H. E., Aldenborg, F., & Meis-Kindblom, J. M. (1998). Gastrointestinal pacemaker cell tumor (GIPACT): gastrointestinal stromal tumors show phenotypic characteristics of the interstitial cells of Cajal. *Am.J.Pathol., 152,* 1259-1269.

Kinoshita, K., Isozaki, K., Hirota, S., Nishida, T., Chen, H., Nakahara, M. et al. (2003). c-kit gene mutation at exon 17 or 13 is very rare in sporadic gastrointestinal stromal tumors. *J.Gastroenterol.Hepatol., 18,* 147-151.

Lasota, J., Carlson, J. A., & Miettinen, M. (2000a). Spindle cell tumor of urinary bladder serosa with phenotypic and genotypic features of gastrointestinal stromal tumor. *Arch.Pathol.Lab Med., 124,* 894-897.

Lasota, J., Jasinski, M., Sarlomo-Rikala, M., & Miettinen, M. (1999). Mutations in exon 11 of c-Kit occur preferentially in malignant versus benign gastrointestinal stromal tumors and do not occur in leiomyomas or leiomyosarcomas. *Am.J.Pathol., 154,* 53-60.

Lasota, J., Kopczynski, J., Sarlomo-Rikala, M., Schneider-Stock, R., Stachura, T., Kordek, R. et al. (2003a). KIT 1530ins6 mutation defines a subset of predominantly malignant gastrointestinal stromal tumors of intestinal origin. *Hum.Pathol., 34,* 1306-1312.

Lasota, J. & Miettinen, M. (2006). KIT and PDGFRA mutations in gastrointestinal stromal tumors (GISTs). *Semin.Diagn.Pathol., 23,* 91-102.

Lasota, J., Dansonka-Mieszkowska, A., Sobin, L. H., & Miettinen, M. (2004). A great majority of GISTs with PDGFRA mutations represent gastric tumors of low or no malignant potential. *Lab Invest, 84,* 874-883.

Lasota, J., Wasag, B., Dansonka-Mieszkowska, A., Karcz, D., Millward, C. L., Rys, J. et al. (2003b). Evaluation of NF2 and NF1 tumor suppressor genes in distinctive gastrointestinal nerve sheath tumors traditionally diagnosed as benign schwannomas: s study of 20 cases. *Lab Invest, 83,* 1361-1371.

Lasota, J., Wozniak, A., Kopczynski, J., Dansonka-Mieszkowska, A., Wasag, B., Mitsuhashi, T. et al. (2005). Loss of heterozygosity on chromosome 22q in gastrointestinal stromal tumors (GISTs): a study on 50 cases. *Lab Invest, 85,* 237-247.

Lasota, J., Wozniak, A., Sarlomo-Rikala, M., Rys, J., Kordek, R., Nassar, A. et al. (2000b). Mutations in exons 9 and 13 of KIT gene are rare events in gastrointestinal stromal tumors. A study of 200 cases. *Am.J.Pathol., 157,* 1091-1095.

Lauwers, G. Y., Erlandson, R. A., Casper, E. S., Brennan, M. F., & Woodruff, J. M. (1993). Gastrointestinal autonomic nerve tumors. A clinicopathological, immunohistochemical, and ultrastructural study of 12 cases. *Am.J.Surg Pathol, 17,* 887-897.

Lee, J. R., Joshi, V., Griffin, J. W., Jr., Lasota, J., & Miettinen, M. (2001). Gastrointestinal autonomic nerve tumor: immunohistochemical and molecular identity with gastrointestinal stromal tumor. *Am.J.Surg.Pathol., 25,* 979-987.

Lespi, J. & Drut, R. (1997). [Gastrointestinal autonomic tumor associated with von Recklinghausen's disease]. *Acta Gastroenterol.Latinoam., 27,* 271-274.

Li, F. P., Fletcher, J. A., Heinrich, M. C., Garber, J. E., Sallan, S. E., Curiel-Lewandrowski, C. et al. (2005). Familial gastrointestinal stromal tumor syndrome: phenotypic and molecular features in a kindred. *J.Clin.Oncol., 23,* 2735-2743.

Liang, J. F., Zheng, H. X., Li, N., Cheng, C. X., Xiao, H., & Wang, H. K. (2007). [Prognostic value of P16 gene methylation and P16 protein expression in gastrointestinal stromal tumor]. *Zhonghua Wei Chang Wai Ke.Za Zhi., 10,* 372-375.

Longley, B. J., Reguera, M. J., & Ma, Y. (2001). Classes of c-KIT activating mutations: proposed mechanisms of action and implications for disease classification and therapy. *Leuk.Res., 25,* 571-576.

Loughrey, M. B., Mitchell, C., Mann, G. B., Michael, M., & Waring, P. M. (2005). Gastrointestinal stromal tumour treated with neoadjuvant imatinib. *J.Clin.Pathol., 58,* 779-781.

Lucas, D. R., al-Abbadi, M., Tabaczka, P., Hamre, M. R., Weaver, D. W., & Mott, M. J. (2003). c-Kit expression in desmoid fibromatosis. Comparative immunohistochemical evaluation of two commercial antibodies. *Am.J.Clin.Pathol., 119,* 339-345.

Lux, M. L., Rubin, B. P., Biase, T. L., Chen, C. J., Maclure, T., Demetri, G. et al. (2000). KIT extracellular and kinase domain mutations in gastrointestinal stromal tumors. *Am.J.Pathol., 156,* 791-795.

Maeyama, H., Hidaka, E., Ota, H., Minami, S., Kajiyama, M., Kuraishi, A. et al. (2001). Familial gastrointestinal stromal tumor with hyperpigmentation: association with a germline mutation of the c-kit gene. *Gastroenterology, 120,* 210-215.

Martin, J., Poveda, A., Llombart-Bosch, A., Ramos, R., Lopez-Guerrero, J. A., Garcia del, M. J. et al. (2005). Deletions affecting codons 557-558 of the c-KIT gene indicate a poor prognosis in patients with completely resected gastrointestinal stromal tumors: a study by the Spanish Group for Sarcoma Research (GEIS). *J.Clin.Oncol., 23,* 6190-6198.

Matyakhina, L., Bei, T. A., McWhinney, S. R., Pasini, B., Cameron, S., Gunawan, B. et al. (2007). Genetics of carney triad: recurrent losses at chromosome 1 but lack of germline mutations in genes associated with paragangliomas and gastrointestinal stromal tumors. *J.Clin.Endocrinol.Metab, 92,* 2938-2943.

Mazur, M. T. & Clark, H. B. (1983). Gastric stromal tumors. Reappraisal of histogenesis. *Am.J.Surg.Pathol., 7,* 507-519.

Medeiros, F., Corless, C. L., Duensing, A., Hornick, J. L., Oliveira, A. M., Heinrich, M. C. et al. (2004). KIT-negative gastrointestinal stromal tumors: proof of concept and therapeutic implications. *Am.J.Surg.Pathol., 28,* 889-894.

Mendoza-Marin, M., Hoang, M. P., & Albores-Saavedra J. (2002). Malignant stromal tumor of the gallbladder with interstitial cells of Cajal phenotype. *Arch.Pathol.Lab Med., 126,* 481-483.

Miettinen, M. (2001). Are desmoid tumors kit positive? *Am.J.Surg.Pathol., 25,* 549-550.

Miettinen, M., El Rifai, W., Sobin, H. L., & Lasota, J. (2002a). Evaluation of malignancy and prognosis of gastrointestinal stromal tumors: a review. *Hum.Pathol., 33,* 478-483.

Miettinen, M. & Lasota, J. (2001). Gastrointestinal stromal tumors--definition, clinical, histological, immunohistochemical, and molecular genetic features and differential diagnosis. *Virchows Arch., 438,* 1-12.

Miettinen, M. & Lasota, J. (2006a). Gastrointestinal stromal tumors: pathology and prognosis at different sites. *Semin.Diagn.Pathol., 23,* 70-83.

Miettinen, M. & Lasota, J. (2006b). Gastrointestinal stromal tumors: review on morphology, molecular pathology, prognosis, and differential diagnosis. *Arch.Pathol.Lab Med., 130,* 1466-1478.

Miettinen, M., Majidi, M., & Lasota, J. (2002b). Pathology and diagnostic criteria of gastrointestinal stromal tumors (GISTs): a review. *Eur.J.Cancer, 38 Suppl 5,* S39-S51.

Miettinen, M., Makhlouf, H., Sobin, L. H., & Lasota, J. (2006). Gastrointestinal stromal tumors of the jejunum and ileum: a clinicopathologic, immunohistochemical, and molecular genetic study of 906 cases before imatinib with long-term follow-up. *Am.J.Surg.Pathol., 30,* 477-489.

Miettinen, M., Monihan, J. M., Sarlomo-Rikala, M., Kovatich, A. J., Carr, N. J., Emory, T. S. et al. (1999). Gastrointestinal stromal tumors/smooth muscle tumors (GISTs) primary in the omentum and mesentery: clinicopathologic and immunohistochemical study of 26 cases. *Am.J.Surg.Pathol., 23,* 1109-1118.

Miettinen, M., Paal, E., Lasota, J., & Sobin, L. H. (2002c). Gastrointestinal glomus tumors: a clinicopathologic, immunohistochemical, and molecular genetic study of 32 cases. *Am.J.Surg.Pathol., 26,* 301-311.

Miettinen, M., Sarlomo-Rikala, M., & Sobin, L. H. (2001). Mesenchymal tumors of muscularis mucosae of colon and rectum are benign leiomyomas that should be separated from gastrointestinal stromal tumors-a clinicopathologic and immunohistochemical study of eighty-eight cases. *Mod.Pathol., 14,* 950-956.

Miettinen, M., Sarlomo-Rikala, M., Sobin, L. H., & Lasota, J. (2000a). Esophageal stromal tumors: a clinicopathologic, immunohistochemical, and molecular genetic study of 17 cases and comparison with esophageal leiomyomas and leiomyosarcomas. *Am.J.Surg.Pathol., 24,* 211-222.

Miettinen, M. & Sobin, L. H. (2001). Gastrointestinal stromal tumors in the appendix: a clinicopathologic and immunohistochemical study of four cases. *Am.J.Surg.Pathol., 25,* 1433-1437.

Miettinen, M., Sobin, L. H., & Lasota, J. (2005). Gastrointestinal stromal tumors of the stomach: a clinicopathologic, immunohistochemical, and molecular genetic study of 1765 cases with long-term follow-up. *Am.J.Surg.Pathol., 29,* 52-68.

Miettinen, M., Sobin, L. H., & Sarlomo-Rikala, M. (2000b). Immunohistochemical spectrum of GISTs at different sites and their differential diagnosis with a reference to CD117 (KIT). *Mod.Pathol., 13,* 1134-1142.

Miettinen, M., Virolainen, M., & Maarit, S. R. (1995). Gastrointestinal stromal tumors--value of CD34 antigen in their identification and separation from true leiomyomas and schwannomas. *Am.J.Surg Pathol, 19,* 207-216.

Montemurro, M., Schoffski, P., Reichardt, P., Gelderblom, H., Schutte, J., Hartmann, J. T. et al. (2009). Nilotinib in the treatment of advanced gastrointestinal stromal tumours resistant to both imatinib and sunitinib. *Eur.J.Cancer, 45,* 2293-2297.

Montgomery, E., Torbenson, M. S., Kaushal, M., Fisher, C., & Abraham, S. C. (2002). Beta-catenin immunohistochemistry separates mesenteric fibromatosis from gastrointestinal stromal tumor and sclerosing mesenteritis. *Am.J.Surg.Pathol., 26,* 1296-1301.

Motegi, A., Sakurai, S., Nakayama, H., Sano, T., Oyama, T., & Nakajima, T. (2005). PKC theta, a novel immunohistochemical marker for gastrointestinal stromal tumors (GIST), especially useful for identifying KIT-negative tumors. *Pathol.Int., 55,* 106-112.

Nemoto, Y., Mikami, T., Hana, K., Kikuchi, S., Kobayashi, N., Watanabe, M. et al. (2006). Correlation of enhanced cell turnover with prognosis of gastrointestinal stromal tumors of the stomach: relevance of cellularity and p27kip1. *Pathol.Int., 56,* 724-731.

Nilsson, B., Bumming, P., Meis-Kindblom, J. M., Oden, A., Dortok, A., Gustavsson, B. et al. (2005). Gastrointestinal stromal tumors: the incidence, prevalence, clinical course, and prognostication in the preimatinib mesylate era--a population-based study in western Sweden. *Cancer, 103,* 821-829.

Nishida, T., Hirota, S., Taniguchi, M., Hashimoto, K., Isozaki, K., Nakamura, H. et al. (1998). Familial gastrointestinal stromal tumours with germline mutation of the KIT gene. *Nat.Genet., 19,* 323-324.

O'Brien, P., Kapusta, L., Dardick, I., Axler, J., & Gnidec, A. (1999). Multiple familial gastrointestinal autonomic nerve tumors and small intestinal neuronal dysplasia. *Am.J.Surg Pathol, 23,* 198-204.

O'Leary, T., Ernst, S., Przygodzki, R., Emory, T., & Sobin, L. (1999). Loss of heterozygosity at 1p36 predicts poor prognosis in gastrointestinal stromal/smooth muscle tumors. *Lab Invest, 79,* 1461-1467.

Ohashi, A., Kinoshita, K., Isozaki, K., Nishida, T., Shinomura, Y., Kitamura, Y. et al. (2004). Different inhibitory effect of imatinib on phosphorylation of mitogen-activated protein kinase and Akt and on proliferation in cells expressing different types of mutant platelet-derived growth factor receptor-alpha. *Int.J.Cancer, 111,* 317-321.

Panizo-Santos, A., Sola, I., Vega, F., de Alava, E., Lozano, M. D., Idoate, M. A. et al. (2000). Predicting Metastatic Risk of Gastrointestinal Stromal Tumors: Role of Cell Proliferation and Cell Cycle Regulatory Proteins. *Int.J.Surg.Pathol., 8,* 133-144.

Parfitt, J. R., Streutker, C. J., Riddell, R. H., & Driman, D. K. (2006). Gastrointestinal stromal tumors: a contemporary review. *Pathol.Res.Pract., 202,* 837-847.

Pasini, B., McWhinney, S. R., Bei, T., Matyakhina, L., Stergiopoulos, S., Muchow, M. et al. (2008). Clinical and molecular genetics of patients with the Carney-Stratakis syndrome and germline mutations of the genes coding for the succinate dehydrogenase subunits SDHB, SDHC, and SDHD. *Eur.J.Hum.Genet., 16,* 79-88.

Pauwels, P., Debiec-Rychter, M., Stul, M., De Wever, I., van Oosterom, A. T., & Sciot, R. (2005). Changing phenotype of gastrointestinal stromal tumours under imatinib mesylate treatment: a potential diagnostic pitfall. *Histopathology, 47,* 41-47.

Prakash, S., Sarran, L., Socci, N., Dematteo, R. P., Eisenstat, J., Greco, A. M. et al. (2005). Gastrointestinal stromal tumors in children and young adults: a clinicopathologic, molecular, and genomic study of 15 cases and review of the literature. *J.Pediatr.Hematol.Oncol., 27,* 179-187.

Pruneri, G., Mazzarol, G., Fabris, S., Del Curto, B., Bertolini, F., Neri, A. et al. (2003). Cyclin D3 immunoreactivity in gastrointestinal stromal tumors is independent of cyclin D3 gene amplification and is associated with nuclear p27 accumulation. *Mod.Pathol., 16,* 886-892.

Reith, J. D., Goldblum, J. R., Lyles, R. H., & Weiss, S. W. (2000). Extragastrointestinal (soft tissue) stromal tumors: an analysis of 48 cases with emphasis on histologic predictors of outcome. *Mod.Pathol., 13,* 577-585.

Ricci, R., Arena, V., Castri, F., Martini, M., Maggiano, N., Murazio, M. et al. (2004). Role of p16/INK4a in gastrointestinal stromal tumor progression. *Am.J.Clin.Pathol., 122,* 35-43.

Rossi, G., Valli, R., Bertolini, F., Marchioni, A., Cavazza, A., Mucciarini, C. et al. (2005). PDGFR expression in differential diagnosis between KIT-negative gastrointestinal stromal tumours and other primary soft-tissue tumours of the gastrointestinal tract. *Histopathology, 46,* 522-531.

Rubin, B. P. (2006). Gastrointestinal stromal tumours: an update. *Histopathology, 48,* 83-96.

Rubin, B. P., Fletcher, J. A., & Fletcher, C. D. (2000). Molecular Insights into the Histogenesis and Pathogenesis of Gastrointestinal Stromal Tumors. *Int.J.Surg.Pathol., 8,* 5-10.

Rubin, B. P., Singer, S., Tsao, C., Duensing, A., Lux, M. L., Ruiz, R. et al. (2001). KIT activation is a ubiquitous feature of gastrointestinal stromal tumors. *Cancer Res., 61,* 8118-8121.

Rudolph, P., Gloeckner, K., Parwaresch, R., Harms, D., & Schmidt, D. (1998). Immunophenotype, proliferation, DNA ploidy, and biological behavior of gastrointestinal stromal tumors: a multivariate clinicopathologic study. *Hum.Pathol., 29,* 791-800.

Ryu, M. H., Kang, Y. K., Jang, S. J., Kim, T. W., Lee, H., Kim, J. S. et al. (2007). Prognostic significance of p53 gene mutations and protein overexpression in localized gastrointestinal stromal tumours. *Histopathology, 51,* 379-389.

Sabah, M., Cummins, R., Leader, M., & Kay, E. (2004a). Expression of human telomerase reverse transcriptase in gastrointestinal stromal tumors occurs preferentially in malignant neoplasms. *Hum.Pathol., 35,* 1231-1235.

Sabah, M., Cummins, R., Leader, M., & Kay, E. (2004b). Loss of heterozygosity of chromosome 9p and loss of p16(INK4A) expression are associated with malignant gastrointestinal stromal tumors. *Mod.Pathol.*.

Sabah, M., Cummins, R., Leader, M., & Kay, E. (2006). Altered expression of cell cycle regulatory proteins in gastrointestinal stromal tumors: markers with potential prognostic implications. *Hum.Pathol., 37,* 648-655.

Sabah, M., Leader, M., & Kay, E. (2003). The problem with KIT: clinical implications and practical difficulties with CD117 immunostaining. *Appl.Immunohistochem.Mol.Morphol., 11,* 56-61.

Sakamoto, K. M. (2004). Su-11248 Sugen. *Curr.Opin.Investig.Drugs, 5,* 1329-1339.

Sakurai, S., Fukayama, M., Kaizaki, Y., Saito, K., Kanazawa, K., Kitamura, M. et al. (1998). Telomerase activity in gastrointestinal stromal tumors. *Cancer, 83,* 2060-2066.

Sakurai, S., Oguni, S., Hironaka, M., Fukayama, M., Morinaga, S., & Saito, K. (2001). Mutations in c-kit gene exons 9 and 13 in gastrointestinal stromal tumors among Japanese. *Jpn.J.Cancer Res., 92,* 494-498.

Sandberg, A. A. & Bridge, J. A. (2002). Updates on the cytogenetics and molecular genetics of bone and soft tissue tumors. Gastrointestinal stromal tumors. *Cancer Genet.Cytogenet., 135,* 1-22.

Sarlomo-Rikala, M., El Rifai, W., Lahtinen, T., Andersson, L. C., Miettinen, M., & Knuutila, S. (1998). Different patterns of DNA copy number changes in gastrointestinal stromal tumors, leiomyomas, and schwannomas. *Hum.Pathol, 29,* 476-481.

Schneider-Stock, R., Boltze, C., Lasota, J., Miettinen, M., Peters, B., Pross, M. et al. (2003). High prognostic value of p16INK4 alterations in gastrointestinal stromal tumors. *J.Clin.Oncol., 21,* 1688-1697.

Schneider-Stock, R., Boltze, C., Lasota, J., Peters, B., Corless, C. L., Ruemmele, P. et al. (2005). Loss of p16 protein defines high-risk patients with gastrointestinal stromal tumors: a tissue microarray study. *Clin.Cancer Res., 11,* 638-645.

Sciot, R. & Debiec-Rychter, M. (2006). GIST under imatinib therapy. *Semin.Diagn.Pathol., 23,* 84-90.

Segal, A., Carello, S., Caterina, P., Papadimitriou, J. M., & Spagnolo, D. V. (1994). Gastrointestinal autonomic nerve tumors: a clinicopathological, immunohistochemical and ultrastructural study of 10 cases. *Pathology, 26,* 439-447.

Serrano, M., Hannon, G. J., & Beach, D. (1993). A new regulatory motif in cell-cycle control causing specific inhibition of cyclin D/CDK4. *Nature, 366,* 704-707.

Singer, S., Rubin, B. P., Lux, M. L., Chen, C. J., Demetri, G. D., Fletcher, C. D. et al. (2002). Prognostic value of KIT mutation type, mitotic activity, and histologic subtype in gastrointestinal stromal tumors. *J.Clin.Oncol., 20,* 3898-3905.

Steigen, S. E., Bjerkehagen, B., Haugland, H. K., Nordrum, I. S., Loberg, E. M., Isaksen, V. et al. (2008). Diagnostic and prognostic markers for gastrointestinal stromal tumors in Norway. *Mod.Pathol., 21,* 46-53.

Stout AP (1976). Bizarre smooth muscle tumours of the stomach. *Cancer, 15,* 400-409.

Stroobants, S., Goeminne, J., Seegers, M., Dimitrijevic, S., Dupont, P., Nuyts, J. et al. (2003). 18FDG-Positron emission tomography for the early prediction of response in advanced soft tissue sarcoma treated with imatinib mesylate (Glivec). *Eur.J.Cancer, 39,* 2012-2020.

Takazawa, Y., Sakurai, S., Sakuma, Y., Ikeda, T., Yamaguchi, J., Hashizume, Y. et al. (2005). Gastrointestinal stromal tumors of neurofibromatosis type I (von Recklinghausen's disease). *Am.J.Surg.Pathol., 29,* 755-763.

Tamborini, E., Papini, D., Mezzelani, A., Riva, C., Azzarelli, A., Sozzi, G. et al. (2001). c-KIT and c-KIT ligand (SCF) in synovial sarcoma (SS): an mRNA expression analysis in 23 cases. *Br.J.Cancer, 85,* 405-411.

Tavassoli, F. A. & Norris, H. J. (1982). Peritoneal leiomyomatosis (leiomyomatosis peritonealis disseminata): a clinicopathologic study of 20 cases with ultrastructural observations. *Int.J.Gynecol.Pathol., 1,* 59-74.

Tornillo, L. & Terracciano, L. M. (2006). An update on molecular genetics of gastrointestinal stromal tumours. *J.Clin.Pathol., 59,* 557-563.

Tran, T., Davila, J. A., & El-Serag, H. B. (2005). The epidemiology of malignant gastrointestinal stromal tumors: an analysis of 1,458 cases from 1992 to 2000. *Am.J.Gastroenterol., 100,* 162-168.

van Oosterom, A. T., Judson, I., Verweij, J., Stroobants, S., Donato di Paola, E., Dimitrijevic, S. et al. (2001). Safety and efficacy of imatinib (STI571) in metastatic gastrointestinal stromal tumours: a phase I study. *Lancet, 358,* 1421-1423.

Vliagoftis, H., Worobec, A. S., & Metcalfe, D. D. (1997). The protooncogene c-kit and c-kit ligand in human disease. *J.Allergy Clin.Immunol., 100,* 435-440.

Wang, Q. & Kou, Y. W. (2007). Study of the expressions of p53 and bcl-2 genes, the telomerase activity and apoptosis in GIST patients. *World J.Gastroenterol., 13,* 2626-2628.

Wang, X., Mori, I., Tang, W., Utsunomiya, H., Nakamura, M., Nakamura, Y. et al. (2002). Helpful parameter for malignant potential of gastrointestinal stromal tumors (GIST). *Jpn.J.Clin.Oncol., 32,* 347-351.

Wardelmann, E., Losen, I., Hans, V., Neidt, I., Speidel, N., Bierhoff, E. et al. (2003). Deletion of Trp-557 and Lys-558 in the juxtamembrane domain of the c-kit protooncogene is associated with metastatic behavior of gastrointestinal stromal tumors. *Int.J.Cancer, 106,* 887-895.

West, R. B., Corless, C. L., Chen, X., Rubin, B. P., Subramanian, S., Montgomery, K. et al. (2004). The novel marker, DOG1, is expressed ubiquitously in gastrointestinal stromal tumors irrespective of KIT or PDGFRA mutation status. *Am.J.Pathol., 165,* 107-113.

Willmore, C., Holden, J. A., Zhou, L., Tripp, S., Wittwer, C. T., & Layfield, L. J. (2004). Detection of c-kit-activating mutations in gastrointestinal stromal tumors by high-resolution amplicon melting analysis. *Am.J.Clin.Pathol., 122,* 206-216.

Wong, N. A., Young, R., Malcomson, R. D., Nayar, A. G., Jamieson, L. A., Save, V. E. et al. (2003). Prognostic indicators for gastrointestinal stromal tumours: a clinicopathological and immunohistochemical study of 108 resected cases of the stomach. *Histopathology, 43,* 118-126.

Wozniak, A., Sciot, R., Guillou, L., Pauwels, P., Wasag, B., Stul, M. et al. (2007). Array CGH analysis in primary gastrointestinal stromal tumors: cytogenetic profile correlates with anatomic site and tumor aggressiveness, irrespective of mutational status. *Genes Chromosomes.Cancer, 46,* 261-276.

Yalcinkaya, U., Yerci, O., & Koc, E. U. (2007). Significance of p53 expression in gastrointestinal stromal tumors. *Hepatogastroenterology, 54,* 140-143.

Yantiss, R. K., Rosenberg, A. E., Sarran, L., Besmer, P., & Antonescu, C. R. (2005). Multiple gastrointestinal stromal tumors in type I neurofibromatosis: a pathologic and molecular study. *Mod.Pathol., 18,* 475-484.

Yantiss, R. K., Spiro, I. J., Compton, C. C., & Rosenberg, A. E. (2000). Gastrointestinal stromal tumor versus intra-abdominal fibromatosis of the bowel wall: a clinically important differential diagnosis. *Am.J.Surg.Pathol., 24,* 947-957.

Part 4

Treatment of Soft Tissue Tumors

11

Treatment of Synovial Sarcoma in Children

Shvarova Anna Viktorovna[1], Rykov Maxim Yurjevich[1],
Karseladze Appolon Irodionovich[2] and Ivanova Nadezhda Mikhailovna[1]
[1]*Institute of Paediatric Oncology and Hematology,
N. N. Blokhin Cancer Research Center, Department of Surgery №3
(The Musculo-Sceletal Tumors Department), Moscow,*
[2]*Institute of Clinical Oncology N. N. Blokhin Cancer Research Centre,
Department of Human Tumor Pathologic Anatomy, Moscow
Russia*

1. Introduction

A synovial sarcoma (SS) is a rare soft tissue sarcoma; in children and adolescents it accounts for 4 % of all non-rhabdomyosarcoma soft tissue sarcomas. The most common site of primary disease is the lower limbs. Although relatively rare, SS is the third most common extremity STS. In both children and adults three histopathologic subtypes of SS are described (monophasic, biphasic and poorly differentiated); it is associated with a characteristic translocation t(x;18) [23;17]. Despite considerable progress and achievements in child oncology, treating children with synovial sarcoma still remains a pressing problem. Numerous treatment options available today to children with SS and dispute among researchers show high importance of the issue and necessity of its complex study.

2. Materials and methods

Herein, we analyze the outcomes in 48 patients with various localizations of synovial sarcoma who were treated in N. N. Blokhin Cancer Research Centre between 1990 and 2007. The results were evaluated on 31 December 2010. The analyzed group was divided into two subgroups – the control group (historical control group) and the study group (experimental group) – matched for sex, age, localization of cancer, extent of tumor spread and recurrence. The mean age in the historical control group (1990-1999) was 10.41±4.03 years (range, 1.0 to 15.0 years). The group included 29 pediatric patients – 13 males (44.8 %), 16 females (55.2%). 20 (69.9%) test subjects were diagnosed with biphasic synovial sarcoma, 8 (27.6%) – with monophasic subtype and 1 (3.4%) – with poorly differentiated subtype. In all cases the diagnosis was based upon morphological study. Immunohistochemistry was used in 14 (48.2%) cases to verify the diagnosis. The most likely localization of lesions was the lower extremity – 14 (48.3%) cases. 10 (34.5%) patients had lesions in upper extremities and 4 (13.8%) in the trunk. One patient was diagnosed with retroperitoneal synovial sarcoma. Mean tumor volume in the control group was 49.1 cm^3. 22 patients (75.9 %) had tumor size above 5 cm.

At the beginning of therapy 11 pediatric patients (37.9 %) had metastatic disease. Lung and lymph node (regional and distant) metastases were present in 8 (27.6%) and 2 (6.9%) patients respectively. One (3.4%) test subject had both lung and lymph node metastases. 15 (51.7%) patients had recurrent disease. Control group therapy strategy included induction polychemotherapy (in the study we refer to induction PCT as chemotherapy courses given before local control which consisted of radiation therapy (RT) ± surgical treatment). Induction CT included IVA chemotherapy: Vincristine 1.5 mg/m^2 o.d. IV push, Actinomycin 1500 mkg/m^2 o.d. IV drip, Ifosfomide 3 g/m^2 b.i.d. IV drip. Chemotherapeutic regimens used in the control group were rather inefficient - induction efficacy (Complete response + Partial response) was 28.6 %.

Having analyzed the causes of low treatment efficacy in the control group, The Muscular - Skeletal Department and The Intensive Care, Reanimation and Bone Marrow Transplantation Department of N. N. Blokhin Cancer Research Centre developed an intensive CT protocol which included reinfusion of autologous haematopoetic stem cells derived from peripheral blood. The protocol was used in patients who developed soft tissue sarcomas with poor prognosis including synovial sarcoma. The article describes complex treatment of high-risk soft tissue sarcomas in pediatric patients with intensive consolidation CT (Cyclophosphamid - Etoposid - Carboplatin) and peripheral haematopoetic stem cell infusion. General therapy strategy included 4 induction CT courses, harvesting and cryoconservation of peripheral stem cells following hematopoetic stimulation by G-CSF, local control of primary tumor and consolidation CT. Local control consisted of surgical removal of primary tumor provided the technical resources were present and irradiation of primary tumor and metastases surviving induction CT. Consolidation CT included 4 courses (additional to 4 main courses) analogous to induction CT. Intensive CT consisted of treatment with Etoposid 100 mg/m^2 on day 1 - 5, Cyclophosphamid 400 mg/m^2 on day 1 - 5, Carboplatin 500 mg/m^2 on day 4.

Between 1999 and 2007 19 pediatric patients with synovial sarcoma were included in the treatment protocol: 9 (47.9 %) male, 10 female (52.6 %) with mean age 10.84±3.28 (range, 2.0 to 15.0 years). Synovial sarcoma was diagnosed by light microscopy: 5 (26.3%) patients had a biphasic subtype, 12 (63.2 %) - a monophasic subtype and 2 (10.5%) - a poorly differentiated subtype. Verification of histological origin was performed with immunohistochemistry in 17 (89.4%) cases. In 13 (68.4 %) experimental group patients the diagnosis was verified through FISH (fluorescence in situ hybridization) with detection of a characteristic translocation t(X;18) and SYT - SSX (1 or 2) fusion genes. From 2004 till 2007 year was performed 34 cytogenesis analysis by fluorescence in situ hybridization from 22 biopsy for the histologic subtyping of soft tissue sarcomas, from 20 patients, none of whom had a previously established sarcoma diagnosis, and from 2 patients with recurrence of the disease. Cytogenetic analysis confirmed the t(X;18)(p11;q11) in 13 cases, the t(11;22)(q24;q12) in 9 cases and t(2;13)(q35;q14) in 1 case, t(1;13)(p36;q14) in 2 cases. The samples were presented in impression smear -10 cases, fine-needle aspiration biopsy specimens - in 12 cases. We successfully verified the diagnosis of synovial sarcoma in 13 cases, included relapses in 2 cases, extraosseous localization of Ewing's sarcoma in 6 cases and alveolar rhabdomyosarcoma in 3 cases. FISH allowed for establishing the diagnosis before obtaining microscopy results due to the study taking only 1 - 2 days and requiring an impression smear made right after biopsy.

The experimental group included 14 (73.7%) patients with primary tumor and 5 (26.3%) patients with recurrent disease. Primary tumor was classified according to the TNM staging system. In the study the patients were staged as follows: 7 (36.8%) patients had T2bN0M0, 2 (10.5%) - T2bN1M0, 3 (15.8%) - T2bN0M1, 1 (5.3%) - TxN1M1 and 1 (5.3%) - TxN1M0. The most likely localization of lesions was the lower extremity - 10 (52.6%) cases. 3 (15.8%) patients had lesions in upper extremities and 5 (26.3%) in the trunk. One patient was diagnosed with synovial sarcoma of the lesser pelvis. Mean tumor volume in the experimental group was 59.8 cm^3; 13 patients (68.4 %) had tumor size above 5 cm^3 (12 - primary, 1 - recurring). In 2 (10.5%) patients with metastatic disease no primary tumor was found. Evident metastases were present at diagnosis in 8 (42.1%) experimental group patients. 1 (5.3%) patient had multiple metastases to the lungs, 1 (5.3%) - multiple metastases to bones and lungs, 1 (5.3%) - to regional lymph nodes and lungs, 1 (5.3%) - multiple metastases to lungs and soft tissues. Metastases to regional and distant lymph nodes were found in 4 (21.1%) cases. The above mentioned (tumor size, recurring and metastatic disease) made it possible to classify the experimental group as high-risk patients.

Harvesting of peripheral stem cells was done after 2 induction CT courses provided bone marrow was intact on light microscopy. Leucopheresis was performed by continuous flow cell separators Baxter CS-3000 plus or CobeSpectra. Separation results (quantity of $CD34^+$-cells) were evaluated by a Becton Dickenson flow cytometer (USA) with the use of anti-HPCA-2 monoclonal antibodies to CD34 in a Radioimmunology Laboratory of N. N. Blokhin Cancer Research Centre. Harvested peripheral stem cells underwent liquid nitrogen freezing with dimetylsulphoxide as a cryopreservation agent and were stored in the N. N. Blokhin Cancer Research Centre marrow bank.

A total of 76 courses of induction CT were given. The mean interval between the courses was 23.33±0.49 days (range, 18 to 27 days). Evaluation of the induction CT toxicity showed that severe leucopenia (IV) developed during 61.0% of CT courses. The decline in leukocyte count to the absolute leukocyte count (ALC) of less than 1000 cells/µL was observed on the 9.23±0.45 day since the beginning of CT. The maximum and minimum decline was up to 100 cells/µL and 1600 cells/µL respectively. The peak of the decline was observed on the 11.72±0.38 day. The mean duration of leucopenia (ALC < 1000 cells/µL) was 7.32±0.42 days (range, 1 to 13 days). The rise of leukocyte count to ALC > 1000 cells/µL was seen on the 16.47±0.43 day. 44.1% of CT courses were associated with severe thrombocytopenia (IV). The decline in thrombocyte count to the absolute thrombocyte count (ATC) of less than 75000 cells/µL was observed on the 11.92±0.37 day since the beginning of CT. The minimum and maximum decline was up to 20500 cells/µL and 1000 cells/µL respectively. The peak of the decline was observed on the 15.07±0.41 day. The mean duration of thrombocytopenia (ATC < 75000 cells/µL) was 10.66±1.25 days (range, 4 to 46 days). The rise of thrombocyte count to ATC > 75000 cells/µL was seen on the 21.72±0.56 day. 23.7% of the CT courses were associated with severe anemia (IV).

The decline in hemoglobin to 79 g/L was observed on the 10.43±0.65 day since the beginning of CT. The peak of the decline was observed on the 14.14±0.61 day. The mean duration of anemia (Hb < 79 g/L) was 8.00±0.8 days (range, 1 to 20 days). The rise of hemoglobin above 79 g/L was seen on the 18.69±0.94 day.

Local control included 18 surgeries: 14 (73.7%) radical excisions, 2 (10.5%) non-radical excisions (with tumor cells at resection margins), 2 (10.5%) amputations and exarticulations. In 1 (5.3%) case no surgical local treatment was performed due to impossibility of radical surgery. Therapeutic pathomorphosis in the remaining tumor was observed in 13 cases: 1 st. - 4 (30.7%), 2 st. - 7 (53.8%), 4 st. - 2 (15.5%). 17 (89.5%) patients underwent irradiation of primary tumor with total dose ranging from 45.6 to 32.2 Gy (1 patient received RT without surgical treatment, 16 patients had the site of an excised tumor irradiated). 2 (10.5%) patients did not receive RT due to amputation and exarticulation. 4 (21.0%) patients with multiple metastases to the lungs received large-field regional RT (total dose 12 Gy). Consolidation CT included 4 additional PCT courses analogous to induction CT with autologous peripheral stem cell infusion. A total of 76 courses of consolidation CT with hematopoetic support via peripheral blood stem cells without G-CSF stimulation were given. Median interval between courses was 26.00±0.54 days (range, 21 to 27 days). In order to provide hematopoietic support on the 7th day each PCT course was followed by reinfusion of low doses ($CD34^+$ = 0.9-1.5±0,1x10^6/kg) of peripheral stem cells. Evaluation of the consolidation CT toxicity showed that severe leucopenia (IV) developed during 74.6% of CT courses. The decline in leukocyte count to the absolute leukocyte count (ALC) of less than 1000 cells/µL was observed on the 8.35±0.36 day since the beginning of CT. The maximum and minimum decline was up to 100 cells/µL and 1800 cells/µL respectively. The peak of the decline was observed on the 11.35±0.34 day. The mean duration of leucopenia (ALC < 1000 cells/µL) was 7.47±0.49 days (range, 1 to 21 days). The rise of leukocyte count to ALC > 1000 cells/µL was seen on the 16.00±0.45 day. 53.7% of CT courses were associated with severe thrombocytopenia (IV). The decline in thrombocyte count to the absolute thrombocyte count (ATC) of less than 75000 cells/µL was observed on the 9.64±0.5 day since the beginning of CT. The maximum and minimum decline was up to 142000 cells/µL and 4000 cells/µL respectively. The peak of the decline occurred on the 13.26±0.4 day. The mean duration of thrombocytopenia (ATC < 75000 cells/µL) was 11.45±0.73 days (range, 5 to 23 days). The rise of thrombocyte count to ATC > 75000 cells/µL was seen on the 21.58±0.74 day. 29.9% of the CT courses were associated with severe anemia (IV). The decline in hemoglobin to 79 g/L was observed on the 8.39±0.56 day since the beginning of CT. The peak of the decline occurred on the 12.79±0.62 day. The mean duration of anemia (Hb < 79 g/L) was 8.70±0.71 days (range, 1 to 20 days). The rise of hemoglobin above 79 g/L was seen on the 16.72±0.68 day.

3. Results

Induction efficacy (Complete response + Partial response) was high (80% according to WHO criteria). Long-term outcome analysis has shown that of 18 patients in the control group 8 (44.4%) patients are currently alive and 10 (55.6%) died due to disease progression after cessation of treatment. Disease recurrence was observed in 1.88±3.0 months (range, 0 to 9 months). Of 11 patients in the experimental group only 2 (18.2%) died; metastatic disease developed on the 79th and 25th month. Of 11 control group patients with metastatic dissemination only 1 (9.0%) is alive - a female with synovial sarcoma of the right hip and metastases to regional lymph nodes. It should be noted that despite inductive PCT inefficiency, she underwent conservative surgery, namely tumor, soft tissue and regional inguinofemoral lymph node excision; no cancerous cells were found at resection margins. The patient received RT (total dose 45 Gy) to the site of an excised tumor and has been alive for 158 months. Other 10 (91.0%) patients died of underlying disease; recurrence developed within 5.3±10.8 months (range, 0 - 34 months). Of 8 experimental group patients with metastases 4 (50.0%) died: 1 - with metastases to the lymph nodes, 1 - with multiple metastases to the lungs, 2 – with metastases to multiple sites (lungs + lymph nodes, lungs + bones). Death occurred on the 14th, 15th, 24th and 9th month; 3 patients died of recurring disease and metastatic dissemination to the lungs, 1 patient died of metastatic disease progression in the lungs and local recurrence. 4 (50.0%) test subjects are currently alive. 1 patient is inoperable, having had metastases to the lungs, soft tissues and retroperitoneal lymph nodes upon first presentation; underwent PCT and RT, is currently alive. 1 patient had right calf tumor, metastases to popliteal and inguinofemoral lymph nodes; underwent complex treatment, was stabilized after PCT, is currently alive for 109 months with recurring metastases to the lungs. 2 patients with primary lesions in inguinofemoral lymph nodes and soft tissues of the thigh and calf are alive for 116 and 47 months with no signs of disease.

The experimental and control group were compared on the basis of therapy results. The study analyzes relapse-free and overall survival in patients with synovial sarcoma. Worthy of note was the statistically significant (more than twofold) increase in relapse-free survival upon use of intensive CT regimen (Etoposid, Cyclophosphamid, Carboplatin) and hematopoetic support with autologous haematopoetic stem cells instead of standard therapy regimens. Thus, 2-year relapse-free survival of patients was 31.0±8.5% in the control group (who received standard treatment) and 66.1±11.3% in the experimental group. The difference was statistically significant (p=0.0097). Overall survival was also significantly higher: 3-year overall survival was 31.0±8.5% in the control group (who received standard treatment) and 75.6±10.6% in the experimental group (p=0,003).

Characteristic	Control group	Experimental group
Number of patients	18	11
Alive	8(44,4%)	9 (81,8%)
Died	10 (55,6%)	2 (18,2%)
2-year relapse-free survival	31,0±8.5%	66.1±11.3%
2-year overall survival	31.0±8.5%	75.6±10.6%
Patients with metastases	11 (61,1%)	8 (72,7%)
Died patients with metastases	10 (91%)	4 (50,0%)

Table 1. Patient Characteristics

4. Discussion

Synovial sarcoma is characterized by infrequent occurrence and demand of histologic verification [12]. The use of fine-needle aspiration of the tumor and molecular genetic study as standard diagnostic methods allows for prompt establishment of diagnosis and therapy start [14]. Multiple research groups have proven the prognostic value of primary tumor size [7;10;11;4;9]. The majority of patients (75.9% in the control group and 68.4% in the experimental group) had tumor size more than 5 cm (in the study the largest diameter was taken to represent tumor size); median tumor volume in the control and experimental group was 49.1 cm^3 and 59.8 cm^3 respectively. At the beginning of therapy metastases were present in 37.9% and 42.1% of cases which led to attributing poor prognosis to these patients. It should be noted that no primary tumor was visualized in 2 pediatric patients with metastatic disease which shows high tumor aggressiveness and proneness to metastatic dissemination even with small tumor size. The study has proven high efficacy (80%) of induction PCT in the experimental group which enabled conservative surgery to be performed due to tumor size regression. Adequate tumor excision (radical resection or broad surgical resection with "clean" cancer cell-free margins) is the cornerstone of therapy [19;21]; it was achieved in 89.5% of experimental group patients what correlates with data provided by foreign researchers [20].

The advisability of postoperative RT in patients with synovial sarcoma remains a highly controversial issue. According to data [19;21;5;20] provided by the multi-factor analysis, the best relapse-free survival was shown in patients who underwent postoperative RT, especially with large primary tumor. Taking account of our experience and that of our foreign colleagues, we provided adjuvant RT to 84.2% of the experimental group; only 10.5% of the patients did not receive RT due to operative mutilation. Adjuvant PCT was essential in patients with poor prognosis [6]: age - 10 years, lesion localization - trunk and extremities, primary tumor size above 5 cm (T2b), recurrent disease and regional/distant metastases upon diagnosis. Having analyzed the experience of 2 decades, European oncology pediatrics physicians came to the conclusion that PCT in children with SS is an essential asset of treatment (contrary to adult patients who do not respond to PCT). Thus pediatric patients with SS were included in rhabdomyosarcoma treatment protocol and received adjuvant PCT regardless of the risk [15;8;19]. J.J. Lewis et. al, 2000 [16] studied 112 cases of adult and adolescent SS; they observed 11 cases of local recurrence following only surgical treatment and 34 cases of metastatic dissemination to distant sites. Despite adequate operative treatment, almost 40% of patients developed distant metastases within 5 years after treatment cessation, which undoubtedly calls for the development of a new effective systemic treatment. With 33-year experience M.F. Okcu et al, 2001 [18] believe complex therapy to provide better outcome. In 50% of inoperable pediatric patients with cancer preoperative CT yielded good results which enabled broad surgical resection to be performed. In high-risk pediatric patients (with primary tumor size above 5 cm and tumor extending outside the organ (T2b)) with localized synovial sarcoma who received complex treatment, 5-year relapse-free survival is 44 - 68% [10;11;4]. Worthy of note is the fact that the main factor limiting therapy intensification is hematological toxicity which increases with higher doses of anti-cancer drugs. Subtransplantation doses of peripheral blood stem cells as substitution treatment during hematopoetic suppression should be considered effective hematopoetic support. D.S. Hawkins et al., 2002 [13] used a combination of multi-cycle high-dose chemotherapy and hematopoetic support with peripheral blood stem cells to show that this method could be used in patients with stage IV rhabdomyosarcoma, desmoplastic small round cell tumor and malignant schwannoma. I. S. Dolgopolov et al., 1999 [1;2] gathered data indicating the possibility of giving multiple intensive CT courses with hematopoetic support via peripheral blood stem cells. Mobilizing peripheral blood stem cells with colony-stimulating factors after 1 - 2 PCT courses following their reinfusion in subtransplantation doses after 3 subsequent courses of PCT may facilitate the decrease of neutropenic fever. This, in turn, allows physicians to shorten intervals between PCT courses which may improve outcomes in high-risk pediatric patients with soft tissue sarcomas [3]. 2-year overall and relapse-free survival in young high-risk patients with synovial sarcoma in the experimental group was 75.6±10.6% and 66.1±11.3% which corresponds to international data on analogous patient groups [22;6;20].

5. Conclusions

Intensive induction CT (Cyclophosphamid - Etopsid - Carboplatin) in high-risk patients with soft tissue sarcomas proved rather efficient (Complete response + Partial response = 80.0%) compared to standard treatment strategies (28.6%) as well as tolerable provided there was adequate additional therapy.

Collection of peripheral stem cells can be carried out after 1 - 2 induction CT courses (Cyclophosphamid - Etopsid - Carboplatin) and G-CSF administration in all patients. Reinfusion of low doses of peripheral blood stem cells ($CD34^+ = 0.9\text{-}1.5 \pm 0.1 \times 10^6$/kg) during adjuvant CT decreases hematological toxicity which allows consolidation CT to be done earlier when induction CT is already possible.

Intensive CT regimen (Cyclophosphamid - Etopsid - Carboplatin) with hematopoetic support via infusion of autologous haematopoetic stem cells derived from peripheral blood significantly improves 2-year relapse-free survival compared to standard therapy strategies from 31.0±8.5% (control group) to 66.1±11.3% (experimental group).

6. References

[1] Dolgopolov I. S., Yankelevich M. J. et al. Poluchenije i ispolzovanije periphericheskih stvolovih kletok v pediatrii - novie puti intensifikatsii lechenija oncologicheskih bolnih. Pediatria (Rossija). (Collection and use of peripheral stem cells in pediatrics - new means of treatment intensification in oncology. Pediatrics (Russia)), №3, 1999 p.126-131.

[2] Dolgopolov I. S., Yankelevich M. J., Andreeva L. U. et al. Mobilizatsija i separatsija stvolovih kletok iz periphericheskoj krovi v detskoj oncologii: rezultati tshetirehletnego poiska effektivnoj i bezopasnoj metodiki. Pediatrija (Peripheral blood stem cell mobilization and separation in pediatric oncology: the results of a 4-year-long search for an effective and safe method. Pediatrics) 1999; 3:58-65.

[3] Mentkevich G. L. Perspektyvy primenenija visokodoznoj himioterapii s autotransplantatsiej stvolovih kletok v detskoj onkologii. Vserossijskaja nauchno-prakticheskaya konferentsiya s mezhdunarodnim uchastiem. Problemy transplantatsii kostnogo mozga I stvolovih kletok periphericheskoj krovi. (Perspectives of high dose chemotherapy in combination with stem cell autotransplantation in pediatric oncology. Russian Scientific Practical Conference with International Participation Challenges of bone marrow and peripheral blood stem cell transplantation). 19th Jan 1999, Moscow, p. 124 - 125.

[4] Brecht IB, Ferrari A, et al. Grossly-resected synovial sarcoma treated by the German and Italian Pediatric Soft Tissue Sarcoma Cooperative Groups: discussion on the role of adjuvant therapies. Pediatr Blood Cancer. 2006 Jan; 46(1):11-7.

[5] Casali PG, Jost L, Sleijfer S, et al. ESMO Guidelines Working Group. Soft tissue sarcomas: ESMO clinical recommendations. *Ann Oncol.* 2008; 19(suppl 2): ii89-ii93.

[6] Casanova M, Meazza C, et al. Soft-tissue sarcomas of the extremities in patients of pediatric age. J Child Orthop. 2007 Sep;1(3):195-203.

[7] Eilber FC, Brennan MF, Eilber FR, et al. Chemotherapy is associated with improved survival in adult patients with primary extremity synovial sarcoma. *Ann Surg.* 2007; 246: 105-113.

[8] Ferrari A, Casanova M., et al. Synovial sarcoma: Report of a series of 25 consecutive children from a single institution. Med. and Pediat. Oncol. 32 (1), 1999, 32-37.

[9] Ferrari A, Gronchi A, Casanova M, et al. Synovial sarcoma: a retrospective analysis of 271 patients of all ages treated at a single institution. *Cancer.* 2004; 101: 627-634.

[10] Gofman A, Issakov J et al. Synovial sarcoma of the extremities and trunk: a long-lasting disease. Oncol Rep. 2007 Dec; 18(6):1577-81

[11] Guadagnolo BA, Zagars GK, et al. Long-term outcomes for synovial sarcoma treated with conservation surgery and radiotherapy. Int J Radiat Oncol Biol Phys. 2007 Nov 15;69(4):1173-80. Epub 2007 Aug 6.

[12] Hasegawa T, Yamamoto S, Yokoyama R, et al. Prognostic significance of grading and staging systems using MIB-1 score in adult patients with soft tissue sarcoma of the extremities and trunk. *Cancer.* 2002; 95: 843-851.

[13] Hawkins D., Felgenhauer J. et al. Peripheral blood stem cell support reduces the toxicity of intensive chemotherapy for children and adolescents with metastatic sarcomas. Cancer, 2002, 95(6): 1356-1365.

[14] Kilpatrick S. E., Bergman S., et al. The usefulness of cytogenetic analysis in fine needle aspirates for the histologic subtyping of sarcomas. *Modern Pathology* (2006) 19, 815–819.

[15] Ladenstein R., Treuner J. et al. Synovial sarcoma of childhood and adolescence. Report of the German CWS-81 study. Cancer, 1993; 71: 3647-3655.

[16] Lewis JJ, Antonescu CR, et al. Synovial Sarcoma: A Multevariate Analysis of Prognostic Factors in 112 Patients with Primary Localized Tumors of the Extremity. J Clin Oncol , 2000, 18 (10): 2087- 2094.

[17] Miser JS, Pappo AS, Triche TJ,et al. Other soft tissue sarcomas of childhood. In: Pizzo PA, PoplackDG, editors. Principles and practice of pediatric oncology. Philadelphia, PA: Lippincott Williams&Wilkins; 2002. pp 1017 - 1050.

[18] Okcu MF, Despa S, et al. Synovial sarcoma in children and adolescents: thirty three years of experience with multimodal therapy. Med Pediatr Oncol. 2001 Aug;37(2):90-96.

[19] Okcu MF, Munsell M et al. Synovial sarcoma of childhood and adolescence: a multicenter, multivariate analysis of outcome. J Clin Oncol. 2003 Apr 15;21(8):1602-1611.

[20] Palmerini E., Staals E.L., et al. Synovial sarcoma: retrospective analysis of 250 patients treated at a single institution. Cancer. 2009 Jul 1;115(13):2988-98.

[21] Pisters PW, O'Sullivan B, Maki RG. Evidence-based recommendations for local therapy for soft tissue sarcomas. *J Clin Oncol.* 2007; 25: 1003-1008.

[22] Ulmer C, Kettelhack C, et al. Synovial sarcoma of the extremities. Results of surgical and multimodal therapy. Chirurg. 2003 Apr;74(4):370-4.

[23] Weiss S.W., Goldblum J. Malignant soft tissue tumors of uncertain type. In: Weiss SW, Goldblum JR, editors. Enzingerand Weiss soft tissue tumors. St.Louis, Missouri:CV Mosby; 2001. pp1483-1571.

12

Novel Therapeutic Targets in Soft Tissue Sarcomas

Quincy S.C. Chu and Karen E. Mulder
[1]Department of Medical Oncology, Cross Cancer Institute, Edmonton, Alberta
[2]Department of Oncology, Faculty of Medicine, University of Alberta, Edmonton, Alberta
Canada

1. Introduction

Approximately 1% of all malignancies or 10,000 cases diagnosed in North American are sarcomas. Amongst which, soft tissue sarcoma comprises of the majority. Local disease is managed with the use of pre-operative or post-operative radiation and surgery, yielding over 90% local control rate.[1] In the meta-analysis reported by Figueredo et al.,[2] adjuvant chemotherapy yielded an absolute overall survival benefit of 4% and the benefit was mainly observed in tumours in the extremity, at a deep location, larger than 5 cm or high histological grade. Unfortunately, a recently reported adjuvant trial comparing doxorubicin/ifosfamide combination with observation enrolling patients with such features failed to demonstrate any overall survival benefit.[3]

Upon follow-up, 50% of localized soft tissue sarcomas will recur either locally, or systemically or both. The benefit of systemic therapy in the recurrent and/or metastatic setting, including doxorubicin, ifsofamide and DTIC, has been shown to be modest with an overall response rate of 10-15%, as single agent, and of 30% in combination at the expense of toxicity without any improvement to the median overall survival rate of 12 months.[4]

In the past 10 years, the most significant advancement has been observed in gastrointestinal stromal sarcoma (GIST), a rare form of gastrointestinal (GI) tract sarcoma. GIST originates from the interstitial cell of Cajal, a pacemaker cell in the muscularis mucosa of the GI tract.[5,6] It is characterized by the expression of CD117 or c-KIT. Eighty-five to 90% of GIST harbour activating mutation in c-KIT, predominantly at exon 11 (70-75%), followed by exon 9 (10%) and rarely exons 13 and 17 (1-2%). About 5-10% of GISTs have platelet derived growth factor receptor-α mutation, predominantly in exons 12 and 18.[7-11] The rest harbour mutation in neither tyrosine kinase receptors are considered as wild type.[7,11,12] Imatinib, a tyrosine kinase inhibitor targeting both wild type and mutated c-KIT and PDGFR, as well as ABL kinase and BCR-ABL, was the first therapy licensed in metastatic GIST with or without mutations in C-KIT and PDGFR with an impressive improvement in response (80% response rate as compared to no response for conventional chemotherapy) and a median progression-free survival (PFS) of 2-2.5 years and overall survival (OS) of almost 5 years.[13-16] More recently, imatinib has been licensed as adjuvant therapy for resected GIST more than 3 cm for 1 year with an improvement in progression-free survival.[17] In the annual meeting of the American Society of Clinical Oncology Meeting in 2011, GISTs with c-KIT expression and either over 10 cm in diameter or >10 mitotic figures per 50 high power fields were randomized to 1 versus 3 years of adjuvant imatinib treatment. There was not only an improvement in 5-year recurrence-free survival (47.9% versus 65.6%, HR=0.46 and p<0.001) but OS (81.7% versus 92%, HR=0.45, p=0.019).[18] Upon failure of imatinib, sunitinib has been shown in a randomized controlled trial to improve the median PFS as compared to placebo (24.1 weeks versis 6 weeks, HR=0.33).[19] Unfortunately, recent trials with a more potent c-KIT and PDGFR-α inhibitor, nilotinib, as compared to imatinib in the first-line and as compared to best supportive care in the previously pretreated population failed to provide any PFS or OS benefit.

One of the most important barriers for the management of soft tissue sarcomas is that there are more than 50 histological subtypes with diverse clinical, biological and molecular characteristics. At the molecular level, soft tissue sarcomas can be divided into 2 categories: those with a characteristic chromosomal translocation as in Table 1[20-22] and those with complex karyotypes, including liposarcomas, except for mxyoid/round cell liposarcoma, leiomyosarcoma, malignant nerve sheath tumours, etc. Over the years, significant gain in the knowledge through translational research in soft tissues sarcoma help identifying novel targets for all subtypes or specific subtypes, which has been reflected in design of recent trials in this population.[23] One would hope therapeutic strategies based on molecular or biological characteristic will yield an improvement in the overall survival of patients with metastatic soft tissue sarcomas and possibly in the curative setting.

Despite the impressive improvement in the management and outcome of GIST, resistance to imatinib and sunitinib occurs. Through ongoing translational research, secondary resistance mechanisms, including secondary mutations in c-KIT or PDGFR-α or activation of downstream pathways, have been partially elucidated, which will help developing novel agents alone or in combination with imatinib and/or sunitinib.[24]

In this chapter, we will focus on the biology of selected targets in soft tissue sarcomas, and their current development in all or certain subtypes of soft tissue sarcomas.

2. Growth signalling pathway

Insulin Growth Factor Receptor (IGF-R)/PI3 Kinase (PI3K)/mTOR pathway

Insulin Growth Factor Receptor and Insulin Receptor

The insulin growth factor pathway consists of 3 ligands, IGF-1, IGF-2 and insulin, IGF binding proteins, and 4 receptors, IGF-1R, IGF-2R, insulin receptor (IR) and hybrid IGF-1R/IR.[25-27]

IGF-1R is a transmembrane receptor tyrosine kinase that comprised of 2 α and 2 β subunits. Upon binding of ligands, with the highest affinity for IGF-1, followed by IGF-2 and the least for insulin, the tyrosine residues in the intracellular domain will be autophosphorylated leading to activation of downstream signalling Raf/MAPK/ERK and c-Raf proliferation pathways and the PI3K/Akt/mTOR survival pathway.[26-28] Structurally, IGF-1R and IR share 84% homology in the intracellular domain and 100% in the ATP-binding domain, which permits heterodimeration of IGF-1R and IR. [26-28] Complicating by the fact that IR exists in 2 isoforms, IR-A or fetal IR which is overexpressed in cancer, and IR-B which is present in normal tissues. The 2 isoforms differ by 12 amino acids in exon 11.[29] The IR-A isoform has high affinity for IGF-2 and insulin but less so for IGF-1.[30-32] In the contrary, IGF-2R is a mannose-6-phophate receptor devoid of any ATP-binding domain, making it a dead receptor which can modulate the growth stimulation activity of IGF-1R and IR through binding and internalization of IGF-2.[32]

At least six different IGFBPs have been identified, which modulate the plasma concentrations of IGF-1 and IGF-2, thus the activation of the receptors in this pathway.[25-27]

Various mechanisms of aberrancy of this pathway have been identified and summarized in Table 2. In short, the fusion protein from the translocation-associated sarcomas binds to either the IGF-2[33-36] or IGF-1R promoter,[37-40] leading to pathway activation. Whereas, for those soft tissue sarcomas that harbour complex karyotypes, the pathway is activated through overexpression of ligands, IGF-2,[36,41,42] IGF-1,[42] overexpression of IGF-1R and IR,[36] activation of downstream PI3K/AKT/mTOR pathway.[43,44]

Pediatric GISTs are less common to have mutation in c-KIT and PDGFR-α. Agaram et al.[45] and others reported that as compared to wild-type (WT) GISTs in adult, the transcriptome of WT pediatric GISTs have an increased expression in IGF-1R without amplification.[46,47] However Tarn et al. reported either overexpression or amplification of IGF-1R in adult WT GISTs.[48] IGF1-R expression was found to be increased in all 188 patient derived samples with at least moderate expression of IGF1/2 in 115 samples. Elevated IGF-1 or IGF-2 expression is associated with increased mitotic rate and high risk for relapsed in resected samples and elevated IGF-1 level is also found to be related to increased risk for metastatic disease and relapsed disease in the metastatic setting.[49] Inhibition of IGF1-R by a tyrosine kinase inhibitor leads to apoptosis via the inhibition of the AKT and MAPK.[48] Synergistic anti-tumor activity is observed when an IGF-1R tyrosine kinase inhibitor is combined with imatinib. Therefore, targeting IGF-1R with or without imatinib is of interest in metastatic WT GISTs.

Currently, there are three different strategies targeting this pathway.

1. Antibody to IGF-1R was the first therapeutic strategy that entered the clinical and current clinical development in sarcoma was summarized in Table 3. These antibodies block the binding of IGF-1 and possibly IGF-2 to IGF-1R. The antibody/IGF-1R complexes will be internalized and then degraded by the proteosome pathway, leading to downregulation of IGF-1R. It has been reported that the activity of these antibody depends on the level of membrane IGF-1R expression.[50] A number of phase 2 studies in soft tissue sarcomas have been reported and stable disease as best response was the most common.[51,52] Toxicities include hyperglycemia, headache, skin rash and transient AST/ALT elevation.
2. ATP-mimetic, competitive tyrosine kinase inhibitor which inhibits the activation of IGF-1R homodimer, IR homodimer and IGF-1R/IR heterdimers through IGF-1, IGF-2 and insulin. OSI-906, BMS-754807 and XL-288 are currently in phase I clinical development. To date, no clinical studies in soft tissue sarcomas have been reported.
3. Antibody binds to IGF-1 and IGF-2 leading to inactivation of IGF-1R and hybrid IR/IGF-1R, while sparing the binding of insulin to IR-B, resulting in the absence of hyperglycemia. Recently, a phase I study of MEDI-573 was reported and no hyperglycemia was observed and no response was observed.[53]

Preclinical studies suggested the level of IGF-1R expression may be a biomarker for clinically efficacy for these antibodies, clinical confirmation remains to be reported. Thus far, there has been no biomarker for response to small molecule reported. Anti-tumour activity in soft tissue sarcoma by targeting the IGF-1R/IR pathway through IGF-1R antibody has been modest. This is possibly related to the fact that most soft tissue sarcoma subtypes have upregulation of IGF-2, which signals through the IGF-1R/IR-A hybrid receptor and is not blocked by IGF-1R antibody.[33,34,36,41] Furthermore, some of the soft tissue sarcoma subtypes have pTEN loss, increase in PI3K/Akt mRNA level or activation of IRS-2, circumventing the blockade by the antibody upstream.[36,41-44] Last but not least, there has been no direct comparison in clinical efficacy amongst these three therapeutic approaches.

PI3K/Akt/mTOR pathway

Growth factor receptor tyrosine kinases activation will lead to recruitment and activation of PI3K to the cytoplasmic side of the cell membrane, which in turn phosphyorylates phosphatidylinositol-4,5-phosphate to phosphatidylinositol-3,4,5-phosphate (PIP3). PIP3 is dephosphorylated and inactivated by pTEN, and activates Akt through recruitment to the cell membrane, which in turn activates mTOR-1 directly and indirectly through inhibition of negative regulator of mTOR-1, tubuerus sclerosis complex 2. In mammalian cells, there are 2 mTOR complexes, mTOR-1, which is rapalogue sensitive, and mTOR-2, which is rapalogue insensitive. Recently, mTOR-2 is found to activate Akt, leading to mTOR-1 activation.[54,55]

The PI3K/Akt/mTOR pathway is an ideal anti-cancer target, including soft tissue sarcomas, as it is activated by all the growth factor receptor tyrosine kinases, such as IGF-1R, VEGFR, PDGFR, or by the loss of pTEN or upregulation of PI3K/Akt.[41,43,44] In turn, the pathway will lead to cell survival and anti-apoptosis through Akt and to cell growth, proliferation, metastasis and angiogenesis through activation of S6-kinase and p70. Preclinical study by Friedrichs et al. reported activation of PI3K/Akt/mTOR in synovial sarcoma cell lines and inhibition of mTOR or PI3K led to tumour regression.[56] Similarly, inhibition of mTOR by rapamycin led to p53-dependent apoptosis of rhabdomyosarcoma cell lines.[57] Wan et al. found that this is due to inhibition of the mTOR/HIF-1α/VEGF pathway via S6 kinase.[58]

Sapi et al. reported a differential activation of mTOR-1 among 108 cases with GIST with c-KIT, PDGFR-α and WT mutations (38.4% versus 83.3% versus 73.9%, respectively).[59] In imatinib-resistant GIST cell lines, despite treatment with imatinib, there is continual hyperactivation of c-KIT with no increase in total c-KIT exprerssion. Either PI3 kinase, MEK or mTOR inhibition leads to decrease in growth, but only PI3 kinase inhibition led to apoptosis.[60] Similarly, prolonged treatment with sunitinib leads to silencing of pTEN expression through methylation, which in turn leads to activation of the PI3K/AKT pathway.[61] Ikezoe et al. demonstrated synergism of suntinib with PI3K or mTOR in imatinib-resistant GIST.[62]

There are currently 3 rapamycin-analogues targeting mTOR-1, temsirolimus, everolimus and ridaforolimus, being developed in the clinics. Only temsirolimus (CCI-779) and ridoforolimus (AP 23573) have been tested in soft tissue sarcomas. Okuno et al.[63] reported a phase II study of temsirolimus in metastatic soft tissue sarcoma patients and 22% had prior chemotherapy. Two out of 40 evaluable patients attained a partial response for 3 and 17 months, respectively. But disappointingly, the median time-to-progression (TTP) was only 2 months or 6-month progression-free rate (PFR) was only 14%, which is deemed to be inactive according to the EORTC criteria.[64] The median survival was 7.6 months.

A phase II study of ridaforolimus in osteosarcoma, leiomyosarcoma, liposarcoma and other soft tissue sarcomas was reported in abstract form. 93% of patients had prior chemotherapy. The primary endpoint was clinical benefit rate at 16 weeks, which were 30% (4 partial response), 33%, 30% and 23%, respectively and were deemed active by the authors. The corresponding 6-month PFR were 23%, 22%, 25% and 23%. The median overall survival of the entire population was 40.1 weeks (range 37.9-44.1 weeks).[65]

In 2011, the phase III study of ridaforolimus versus placebo as a maintenance therapy after first to third-line therapy in the metastatic settings for soft tissue and bone sarcomas was reported with progression free survival (PFS) as the primary endpoint and overall survival (OS) as the main secondary endpoint. In the overall population, the PFS and OS was improved from 14.6 weeks to 17.7 weeks in the ridaforolimus treated patients (HR=0.72, p<0.0001) and from 19.2 months to 21.4 months (HR=0.88, p=0.22) after first analysis. Subgroup analysis including histology, number of prior lines of therapy, etc is pending.[66]

A combined phase I/II study combining everolimus and imatinib in pretreated metastatic GIST patients was reported. The recommended phase II dose of the combination was 2.5 mg daily of everolimus in combination with 600 mg daily of imatinib, denoting pharmacokinetic interaction. Two strata were enrolled: stratum 1 failed imatinib alone and stratum 2 failed imatinib and other therapies. A 37% progression free rate was observed in stratum 2 with a corresponding PFS and OS at 3.5 and 10.7 months, respectively.[67] This combination was suggested by the authors to take forward for further development. The biological activity seen may be related to the silencing of pTEN as reported by Yang and colleagues after treatment with sunitinib.[61] Unfortunately, no biopsy samples were available in this trial to further elucidate the biology underlying this combination in this heavily-pretreated GIST population.

Toxicities of rapalogues are considered as tolerable with <10% patients experienced grade 3 or 4 toxicities. Common toxicities include stomatitis, hyperglycemia, hyperlipidemia, fatigue and thrombocytopenia.

In summary, the clinical efficacy of rapalogues in sarcomas has been modest, which may be explained by the following resistance mechanisms. Wan et al. reported inhibition of mTOR by rapalogues led to the loss of the negative feedback of S6 kinase on IRS-1, leading to activation of pAKT.[68] Cao et al.[69] found that after initial inhibition of IGF-1R and Akt phosphorylation by IGF-1R antibody, at 72 hours such inhibition was lost through mechanisms independent to pTEN loss or activation of epidermal growth factor. The activation of the Ras/Raf/MEK/Erk pathway led to inhibition of mTOR leading to loss of addiction to the IGF pathway.[70,71]

To circumvent these resistance mechanisms, phase I/II studies of combined PI3K/mTOR inhibitors such as BEZ235, IGF-1R-mTOR and Akt-MEK (MK-2206 and AZD 6244) combinations in solid tumours are currently being performed. The improvements in clinical efficacy in soft tissue sarcomas remain to be reported.

Complicating the development of rapalogues is the lack of biomarkers. Despite pTEN loss leads to constitutional activation of mTOR, pTEN status did not predict clinical benefit.[72] Similarly, inhibition of S6 kinase and p70 activation did not predict clinical benefits.

Targeting Akt or PI3K upstream from mTOR may offer an alternative strategy in the treatment of soft tissue sarcomas. Barrentina et al.[73] reported 18% of mxyoid/round cell liposarcoma had PIK3CA mutation leading to Akt activation, which is associated with poor survival. Zhu et al.[74] found activation of PI3K and Akt in all the soft tissue sarcoma cell lines. Inhibition of PI3K or Akt led to inhibition of downstream pathway, leading to cycle cell arrest at G2 phase through upregulation of GADD45α. Activation of Akt and mTOR was observed in 61% and 66% of the 140 sarcoma samples, particularly in malignant nerve sheath tumours, rhabdomyosarcoma and synovial sarcoma, independent from EGFR activation. Phosphorylation of Akt was associated with metastatic disease.[75]

Inhibition of both PI3K and mTOR by BEZ235 leads to G1 phase cell cycle arrest without apoptosis in both *in vitro* and *in vivo* sarcoma models including Ewing's and rhabdomyosarcoma. As a single agent, no apoptosis was observed. But synergistic anti-tumour effect was observed when BEZ235 is combined with classical active chemotherapeutic agents in sarcoma, including doxorubicin, when chemotherapy is given first. Simultaneous targeting with IGF-1R showed synergistic activity probably due to decrease in IC50 for PI3K inhibition by BEZ235.[76] Therefore, clinical studies of PI3K inhibitor in mxyoid/round cell liposarcoma and of PI3K or Akt inhibitors in malignant nerve sheath tumour, rhabdomyosarcoma and synovial sarcoma may be of value.

As mentioned previously, PI3K inhibition with concurrent imatinib not only leads to growth inhibition but also apoptosis in imatinib-resistant GIST cell lines as compared to mTOR inhibition. Therefore, clinical investigation of PI3K inhibitor in combination with imatinib in imatinib failure GIST patients may be of value. Similarly, the activation of PI3K/AKT/mTOR due to methylation of pTEN from prolonged sunitinib treatment can be exploited as a novel therapeutic option for sunitinib failure.

3. Vascular endothelial growth factors, fibroblast growth factors and receptors

Angiogenesis is a complex biological process involved in the formation of new blood vessels in normal and pathological tissues, including cancer.[77,78] A battery of proangiogenic and antiangiogenic factors is involved in angiogenesis, which is tightly controlled in normal tissues, but not in pathological processes including cancer.[77,78] In cancer, angiogenesis is a result from the interaction of various proangiogenic and antiangiogenic factors and their receptor produced or present in tumour cells, endothelial cells, extracellular matrix and inflammatory cells.[79]

A number of proangiogenic and antiangiogenic factors have been identified (Table 3). The most important proangiogenic factor is vascular endothelial factor (VEGF) which is present in six isoforms, VEGF A to E and placental growth factor (PIGF).[80] Furthermore, VEGFA exists as 6 proangiogenic isoforms (VEGF 121, 145, 148, 165, 183, 189 and 206) and 6 corresponding antiangiogenic isoforms, generated through alternative splicing of exons 6, 7 and 9 of VEGFA gene.[79,81]

There are a total of 4 VEGFR, namely VEGFR-1, VEGFR-2, VEGFR-3 and VEGFR-4. Interaction of VEGFR-2 and its ligands, VEGFA and PIGF, represents the most important angiogenic pathway. Whereas, VEGFA, VEGF-B and PIGF bind to VEGFR-1 for angiogenesis and VEGF-C and D bind to VEGFR-3 for lymphogenesis.[80]

Increasing level of angiogenesis or elevation of VEGF expression in soft tissue sarcoma samples has been reported to be associated with high grade, increase risk of metastases and poor prognosis.[82-84] Serum VEGF expression is elevated in all soft tissue sarcomas[85-87] especially epithelial subtypes including epithelioid sarcoma and alveolar soft part sarcoma (ASPS),[88] and high grade fibrosarcoma of no specific subtype (previously known as malignant fibrous histiocytoma) and leiomyosarcoma.[89] In addition, VEGF A, B and C and their corresponding VEGFR-1, -2 and -3 are overexpressed in angiosarcoma, demonstrating an autocrine or paracrine growth pathway, with corresponding activation of the PI3K/Akt/mTOR pathway.[90-92] Antonescu et al. also demonstrated overexpression of TIE-2, VEGFR-1 and -2 in angiosarcoma, and 10% of the samples demonstrated mutations in either exon 15 in the extracellular domain and exon 16 in the transmembrane domain.[93]

Thus, targeting VEGFs and their receptors is an attractive strategy for the treatment of soft tissue sarcomas, especially angiosarcoma, and ASPS.

Targeting VEGF can be achieved through

1. Monoclonal antibody to VEGF-A by Bevacizumab: A phase II study combining 7.5 mg/kg of bevacizumab with standard dose doxorubicin at 75 mg/m^2 every 3 weeks in patients with metastatic soft tissue sarcomas was reported D'Adamo et al. 17 patients were treated and only 2 PRs were observed with a median time-to-progression and median overall survival of 8 and 16 months, respectively. Despite dexrazoxane, 6 patients experienced at least grade 2 congestive heart failure, making it too toxic for further development of the combination.[94] Bevacizumab at 15 mg/kg every 3 weeks was tested in a phase II study of patients with metastatic angiosarcoma and epithelioid hemagioendothelioma. 29 patients were enrolled and out of 26 evaluable patients, 3 PRs were observed. Currently, the development of bevacizumab is unclear despite this level of activity in angiosarcoma.[95] Common toxicities include hypertension, macular or papular erythematous rash, diarrhea, mucosal bleeding (most common as epitaxis) and proteinuria. Other rare toxicities are hemorrhage, hypertensive emergency and reversible posterior leukoencephalopathy syndrome, arterial thromoembolism (especially in patients over 65 years), bowel perforation and fistulae.
2. Aflibercept is a decoy recombinant protein of the second Ig domain of VEGFR-1 and third Ig domain of VEGFR-2 fused to the Tc domain of human IgG1, with pM affinity to VEGF-A, -B and PIGF. In vivo rhbadomyosarcoma model treated with aflibercept at 2.5 mg/kg twice weekly demonstrated significant anti-tumour activity.[96,97] Late stage clinical development in metastatic non-small cell lung cancer, colorectal cancer and other solid tumours are either ongoing or reported. But no development plan in soft tissue sarcoma has been made. Toxicities are consistent with other anti-VEGF/VEGFR agents, such as hypertension, headache, proteinuria, fatigue, dysphonia, bleeding (epistaxis and hemoptysis), anorexia, abdominal pain, nausea, diarrhea or constipation, and arthalgia.
3. Small molecules ATP-mimetic receptor tyrosine kinase inhibitors: VEGFR is a member of the split kinase class III receptor which shares structural homology in the ATP binding domain with platelet derived growth factor (PDGFR), FLT-3, c-kit, and Tie-2. Although in preclinical models, co-inhibition of PDGFR and VEGFR may yield synergistic anti-tumour activity through targeting of the endothelial cells and pericytes in the tumour vasculature, resepctively and delay in tumour resistance,[98-102] additional toxicities are expected. Additional receptor tyrosine kinases are inhibited by some of these small molecules at clinically relevant plasma concentration, such as RET in motesanib, vandatinib, FGFR-1, 2 or 3 in BIBF 1120 and brivanib[103,104] and c-met in foretinib, cabozantinib and MGCD265,[105] leading to possible synergistic anti-tumour activity.

The early phase development of sunitinib,[106,107] sorafenib[108-111] and pazopanib[112] in various types of soft tissue sarcomas is summarized in Table 4. With the observed progression-free survival benefit in the phase II trial of pazopanib across all soft tissue sarcoma subtypes, a phase III trial comparing pazopanib and placebo in metastatic soft tissue sarcoma was reported in the 2011 annual meeting of the American Society of Clinical Oncology with progression-free survival as the primary endpoint. Patients had prior anthracyclin but had no more than 4 prior lines of therapy, and performance status of 0-1. With a median follow-up of 15 months, and 19% of patients still on study, the median progression-free survival in the pazopanib treated patients was improved from 1.5 to 4.6 months ($p<0.0001$). The interim median overall survival was 11.9 versus 10.4 months ($p>0.05$), favouring the pazopanib arm.[113]

Based on the success of sunitinib as second-line therapy for metastatic GIST, other antiangioenic compounds have been in clinical development in pretreated GIST. Campbell et al. reported a phase II study of sorefenib in imatinib- and sunitinib-pretreated metastatic GIST patients. An impressive 13% response rate was observed with median PFS at 5.2 months and OS at 11.6 months which were compared to that of sunitinib.[114] In the annual meeting of the American Society of Clinical Oncology Meeting in 2011, the final result of a phase II study of regorafenib in pretreated GIST was reported. Regorafenib is a multi-targeted tyrosine kinase inhibitor targeting VEGFR 1-3, TIE2, PDGFR-β, FGFR-1, as well as B-RAF, C-RAF and p38 MAPK at nanomolar concentration. Three PRs and a median PFS of 10 months were observed for the entire population. Due to the small patient numbers, median PFS were 10, 6 and 8 months for those harboured exon 11, 9 and WT c-KIT mutation respectively. Interesting, one patient was found to have B-RAF mutation in exon 15.[115] Agaram et al. reported up to 7% of WT GIST had V600E mutation in B-RAF.[116] In preclinical models, sorafenib has superior inhibitory activity in secondary mutations in the activation loop, such as D816H, D820A/G, V822K, and Y823D, of c-KIT as that of sunitinib, and similar activity towards ATP pocket secondary mutations, such as V654A and T670I, and exon 9 c-kit mutations.[117] Sorafenib, most likely regorafenib, inhibits cell proliferation, induces apoptosis and decreases angiogenesis through the inhibition of Ras/Raf/MEK/ERK pathway as well as induction of p15 and p27 and decrease in p21, cyclin A and B1 as well as cdc-2.[118] Based on these biological rationales, sorafenib and regorafenib will expect to have substantial clinical activity in GIST. A phase III study of regorafenib in the imatinib- and sunitinib-pretreated metastatic GIST patients has just finished enrollment.

The VEGF and FGF pathways are associated with growth and poor prognosis in soft tissue sarcomas.[119] Upregulation of other proangiogenic pathways, such as the FGF pathway, has been conferred as resistance mechanism for anti-VEGF strategies.[120] Tumour growth suppression has been observed in preclinical soft tissue sarcoma xenografts by FGF inhibition.[121] Therefore, combined FGFR and VEGFR tyrosine kinase inhibitors may have improved anti-tumour activity and duration of response in soft tissue sarcomas. In a retrospective analysis of 43 solid tumour samples through a phase I study of brivanib, expression of FGF-2 was associated with longer progression-free survival and higher disease control rate.[122] Schwartz et al. reported the preliminary result of a randomized discontinuation study of brivanib in metastatic soft tissue sarcomas to detect an HR of 0.5 in progression free survival in the FGF-2 positive patients. 251 patinets were enrolled with a median age of 54, and all patients were ECOG 0-1 and 80% had prior systemic therapy with a median of 2 regimens. During the first 12 weeks of open label brivanib, 130 patients had PD and 35 patients were taken off study due to reasons other than PD. Seven patients had a PR, and 3 were either angiosarcoma or hemangiopericytoma. Out of the 78 patients who had SD and underwent randomization to brivanib or placebo, 53 patients had FGF-2 positive tumours, and the median progression-free survival was 2.8 months in the brivanib arm as compared to 1.4 months in the placebo arm ($HR=0.58$, $p=0.08$). The progression-free rate at 12 weeks in the overall population was 31% and no difference was observed across all histological subtypes. In the FGF-2 negative tumours, the corresponding progression-free survival was 2.6 and 1.4 months ($HR=0.8$). The median progression-free survival was 4.1

months in those in the placebo arm who crossed over to brivanib at progression. Brivanib was considered as well tolerated. All grade 3 or higher toxicities occurred in less than 5% except for fatigue (10%) and hypertension (15%).[123]

Clinical benefit with tyrosine kinase inhibitors observed in angiosarcoma is particularly of interests as clinical response with classical chemotherapy, such as doxorubicin, liposomal doxorubicin and paclitaxel, is usually short-lived.[108-110] Various reports have demonstrated overexpression of VEGFR-2 and VEGFR-3 and their corresponding ligands, VEGF-A, VEGF-C, in pulmonary and cutaneous angiosarcomas, denoting the paracrine and/or autocrine role in their development and proliferation.[90,124,125]

Alveolar soft part sarcoma (ASPS) is known to be chemotherapy resistant and therefore development of novel agents is essential. Stacchioti et al.[126] reported a series of 10 patients. Five patients had prolonged PR and 3 other had prolonged stable disease, with a median duration of response of more than 9 months. Similar impressive clinical benefit of 4 out of 7 patients had a PR and 3 patients with SD by RECISTS were reported for cediranib.[127] The investigators in the National Cancer Institute reported the preliminary results of a phase II study of cediranib with 14 PRs in 33 untreated or second-line metastatic ASPS patients. Biopsies for gene expression profile alterations were performed before and after treatment and VEGFR-1, VEGFR-2 and angiopoietin-2 expression were downregulated whereas CXCR7, CCL-2 and transgelin were upregulated.[128] Currently, a cross-over phase II trials comparing cedarinib and sunitinib is being planned. The transcription factor activity of the ASPACR1-TFE3 chromosomal translocation leads to overexpression of growth factor receptors, including VEGFR-2, PDGFR, c-Met, RET and EGFR, and transcription factor, HIF-1α. The activation of these pathways leads to activation of both the PI3K/Akt/mTOR and ERK pathway.[126,129-131]

4. Monoclonal antibody to the extracellular domain of VEGFRs or PDGFR: IMC1121B (ramucirumab) and IMC18F-1, targeting the VEGFR-2 and VEGFR-1 extracellular domain respectively, are currently under clinical development as a single agent or in combination with chemotherapy in other solid tumours. IMC-3G3, a monoclonal antibody against the extracellular domain of PDGFR, is currently in clinical development including in PDGFR mutated metastatic GIST.

The preliminary phase II and III trial result in antiangiogenic compounds look promising in all soft tissue sarcomas, especially for angiosarcoma, hemangiopericytoma, ASPS, which devoid of effective systemic therapy. Further development of this class of agent in these uncommon subtypes is definitely worthwhile. Given the activation of multiple growth factor pathways, like VEGFR, PDGFR, Tie-2, the use of tyrosine kinase inhibitor may be more likely to provide clinical benefit, unlike that in other solid tumours. With the activation of downsteam pathways, including the PI3K/Akt/mTOR or MEK/ERK pathway, combination with antiangiogenic strategy, especially for tyrosine kinase inhibitors, may be at least additive. Furthermore, combinations with doxorubicin and other cytotoxic chemotherapy will be reported in the next couple of years, which have the potential of improving their anti-tumour activity. Like the identification of FGF-2 expression as a potential biomarker for efficacy for brivanib, further exploration for biomarker for antiangiogenic therapeutics is important which allows us to identify the corresponding patient subgroups and to improve the understand of the biology of angiogenesis and thus the mechanisms of resistance and corresponding therapeutic strategies.

4. Epigenetic modification and histone deactylase inhibitors

Histones and histone deactylase

There are 5 members of the histone family, H1, H2A, H2B, H3 and H4 in eukaryotic cells. Tetramer of H3 and H4 and dimmers of H2A and H2B make up nucelosomes, around which DNA winds. H1 makes this complex more compact. The amino terminal of histones undergoes post-translational modification by acetylation, phsophorylation and methylation, leading to change in the structure and function of the histones. Acetylation and deacetylation are the most studied processes. The lysine residues in histones, particularly H3 and H4, undergo acetylation by histone acetyltransferase (HAT) and deacetylation by histone deacetylation (HDAC) which determine the fate of gene expression.[132] Acetylation leads to neutralization of the positive charges in the lysine residues of H3, decrease in the affinity to DNA, and thus generating an open or euchromatin structure which allows the binding of transcription factors. Conversely, deacetylation leads to tight interaction between the histones and DNA, generating a closed or heterochromatin structure which prevents gene transcription. [132,133]

There are 4 classes of HDAC: Class I includes HDAC 1, 2, 3, and 8 and is ubiquitously present in the nucleus; Class II includes Class IIa (HDAC 4, 5, 6 and 7) and Class IIb (9 and 10), which shuttles between the cytoplasm and nucleus and is tissue specific, Class III includes SIRT 1-7 and is NAD+ dependent for its activity and Class IV includes HDAC 11 and properties of Classes I and II.[134-136] Classes I, II and IV are homologous in their structure with a zinc-containing catalytic domain.

Recently, HDAC Classes II is found to modulate acetylation status of proteins, such as heat short protein 90 (Hsp 90). Acetylation of Hsp 90 leads to release of oncoproteins, such as Her-2, Akt, c-kit, bcr-Abl, and subsequently subject to proteosome-mediated degradation.[135] This process is believed to account for at least a good portion of the anti-tumour activity of HDAC inhibitors. Specifically, inhibition of HDAC 6 and 10 leads to downregulation of VEGFR1 and 2 expression through acetylation of Hsp90.[137] Other members of Class II HDAC are involved in either cell proliferation and survival or cell migration, which is crucial for angiogenesis.[138,139]

Histone deacetylase and sarcoma

Overexpression of one or more members of Class I and II HDAC has been well reported in breast, prostate and colorectal cancer,[135] which has not been reported in soft tissue sarcoma.

Preclinical studies of HDAC inhibitors demonstrated not only tumour growth suppression but also tumour regression and differentiation in human synovial sarcoma xenografts.[140,141] Synovial sarcoma is characterized by the expression of oncoprotein, STY-SSX, which co-localizes with the Polycomb repressor complex leading to HDAC-mediated chromatin condensation.[142-144] In particular, the interaction among the Polycomb protein, the SS18 component of the oncoprotein and a transcriptional corepressor protein called TLE was observed.[145] One of the repression targets of this complex is the tumor suppressor gene EGR1.[146] HDAC inhibitor will reverse the repression by the Polycomb protein, leading to de-repression of EGR1 and followed by apoptosis.

Similar preclinical anti-tumour effect has been observed in Ewing sarcoma,[147-149] clear cell sarcoma,[150] endometrial stromal sarcoma,[151] mxyoid chondrosarcoma[152] and alveolar rhabdomyosarcoma.[149] Treatment of HDAC inhibitor leads to increase in expression of p21 and G2/S arrest and decrease in mTOR expression and activity, leading to apoptosis and autophagy.[151]

In addition, Lopez et al. reported G2/M arrest and S phase depletion of fibrosarcoma, leiomyosarcoma and rhabdomyosarcoma cell lines with PCI-24781, a novel HDAC inhibitor, followed by decrease in RAD51 and apoptosis.[153] Synergistic anti-tumour activity has been observed when combining doxorubicin with HDAC inhibitor, when modest anti-tumour activity was observed after treatment with doxorubicin or HDAC alone.[153,154]

Based on these promising preclinical data, clinical development of HDAC inhibitor in translocation associated sarcoma is definitive of interest. Combination with doxorubicin will be of interests in both translocation associated sarcomas and in soft tissue sarcomas with complex karyotypes. Inhibition of HDACs can lead to at least partial decrease of VEGFR-1 and -2 and significant clinical efficacy has been observed with VEGFR tyrosine kinase inhibitors in patients with ASPS, angiosarcoma, etc, so clinical development of these combination will likely provide improved clinical efficacy, with caution about the possibility of increase toxicity. Other combinations that may be of interests include HDAC inhibitor with therapeutics targeting the PI3K/Akt/mTOR pathway and PARP inhibition.

Double strand DNA damage due to radiation leads to activation of ATM which subsequently activates other downstream DNA repair proteins, including p53, CHK-2, BRCA-1, leading to cell cycle delay or apoptosis.[155] HDAC1 interacts with ATM which leads to its activation and DNA repair.[156] HDAC inhibitor is a radiosensitizer through suppression of DNA repair by decreasing the expression of DNA repair proteins such as DNA protein kinase.[157] Therefore, combination of HDAC inhibitor and radiation in the management of localized limb or retroperitoneal sarcomas will be worth studying.

HDAC inhibitors in clinical development

There are four classes of HDAC inhibitor, short fatty acid, hydroxamic acid, cyclic tetrapeptide, and benzamide. Except for the first class, all the others are in clinical development. Focus will be placed on the hydroxamic acid and benzamide class of HDAC inhibitors.

Hydroxamic acid analogues

Vorinostate or suberoylanilide hydroxamic acid (SAHA) is the first orally administered HDAC inhibitor in clinical development, which targets Class I, IIa and IIb HDAC. A dose of 300 mg twice daily 3 days every week or 400 mg daily or 200 mg twice daily.[158] It is currently licensed for the treatment of cutaneous T-cell lymphoma. The result of vorinostat as a second-line therapy in malignant pleural mesothelioma is anticipated in later part of 2011. Clinical development in combination with chemotherapy in various solid tumours has been slow due to toxicity compared to chemotherapy alone. Marked production of reactive oxygen species was observed in preclinical model was treated with the combination of bortezomib and HDAC inhibitor through suppression by bortezomib on NF-κB production induced by HDAC inhibitor, which in turn leads to reactive oxygen species production.[159,160]

A phase II study of vorinostat in combination with bortezomib in second-line soft tissue sarcoma reported with no response in 16 evaluable patients.[161]

Panobinostat (LBH-589) is another Class I, IIa, and IIb HADC inhibitor in clinical development with both oral and intravenous formulation. Dose-limiting toxicity is prolonged QTc, thrombocytopenia, neutropenia and hypophosphatemia and diarrhea, fatigue and thrombocytopenia for intravenous[162] and oral panobinostat,[163,164] respectively.

Early phase studies of either as a single agent or in combination with chemotherapy and novel agents to Hsp 90, Her-2, EGFR, VEGFR, etc are ongoing.
Belinostat (PDX-101) is again a Class I, IIa, and IIb HDAC inhibitor. An intravenous formulation entered clinical development as a daily for 5 day every 3 week schedule. 1000 mg/m^2/day was determined to be the phase II dose. Histone H4 hyperacetylation lasted for 4-24 hours after each infusion. Best response was SD, and amongst which 2 soft tissue sarcoma patients lasted for 7 and 14 months, respectively.[165] A preliminary report of 14 patients using various schedules, daily, twice or three times daily, at doses ranging from 900-1000 mg/m^2/dose and for one day to for 5 days every 21 days.[166] Clinical development plan of both single agent in various solid tumours and haematological malignancies and combination with chemotherapy and demethylating compounds are ongoing including a phase I/II trial in combination with doxorubicin in soft tissue sarcoma.
Other hydroxamic acid analogues are in clinical development including PCI-24781, a Class I, IIa and IIb HDAC inhibitor with high potency against HDAC 1 and 3, which is being developed in haematological malignancies and solid tumours.[167] Based on the synergistic anti-tumour effect in combination with doxorubicin, possibly through hyperacetylation of topo-II, a phase I/II study is currently recruiting patients.

Benzamide analogues

MS-275 was initially developed at the US NCI using various schedules, daily for 4 out of 6 weeks, once every 2 weeks and weekly for 4 out 6 weeks.[168,169] Due to excess toxicity and prolonged half-life, only the latter 2 schedules are being developed mostly in combination with other protein targets of HDAC class IV.
MGCD0103 is HDAC 1, 2, 3 and 11 specific HDAC inhibitor. Siu et al.[170] reported the phase I study using a three times a week schedule with 45 mg/m^2/day as the phase II dose. Acetylation at H4 increased in a dose-dependent fashion and significantly acetylation in white cells was observed at doses above 45 mg/m^2/day. No objective response was observed except SD in 5 patients for 4 or more months. Currently, development of MGCD0103 in concentrated in lymphoma and other haematological malignancies.[171]
SB939, a HDAC Class I, II, and IV, has been tested in weekly 3 out 4 weeks and daily for 5 day every 2 weeks schedules with improved intra-tumour accumulation and transit time, HDAC inhibition as well as half-life.[172] 60 mg a day was determined to be the dose for either schedule.[173,174] Only SDs for a median of 5 months, as best response, were observed. Proof of concept phase II study in translocation associated soft tissue sarcomas led by the NCIC-CTG is accruing patients.
Fatigue, nausea, vomiting, diarrhea and anorexia are common to all classes of HDAC inhibitors in oral or intravenous formulations. In the absence of comparative trials, cardiac toxicity, such as arrhythmia and prolongation of QTc, seems to be occur more frequently in the intravenous formulation, which is probably related to the peak concentration of HDAC inhibitor is approached the inhibitory concentration of cardiac ion channels. This observation may favour the development of oral formulation but careful cardiac monitoring will be essential when combined with therapeutics that have been associated with cardiac toxicities including HER-2, VEGF/VEGFR. Thrombocytopenia is the only observed haematological toxicities, though mostly grade 1 and 2. The mechanism is still being investigated.

HDAC inhibition in peripheral blood mononuclear cells as a pharmacodynamic marker for anti-tumour activity and drug exposure has not been consistent. Identification of such a marker is still essential.

The mechanisms of action of HDAC inhibitor are likely multi-fold and inhibition of different classes of HDAC may have different anti-tumour effects.[135] Thus clinical activity may be different and whether cross-resistance will occur. Fantin et al. reviewed the potential mechanisms of resistance for HDAC inhibitors such as increase in DNA hypermethylation, upregulation of protection against oxidative stress, and overexpression of anti-apoptotic proteins, such as Bcl-2 and Bcl-XL.[175]

5. DNA repair by poly (ADP-ribose) polymerases (PARP)

Poly (ADP-ribose) polymerases (PARP)

DNA damage leads to the activation of PARP, which consists of 17 members[176,177] that have a conserved catalytic domain.[178] PARP1 is the most well characterized nuclear protein with three functional domains: the zinc finger containing DNA binding domain, which is responsible for the detection of DNA breaks and localization to the nuclei; the auto-modification domain which includes the breast cancer gene-1 (BRCA-1) C-terminal domain; and the C-terminal catalytic domain.[179,180] Any single strand DNA break detected by the DNA binding domain of PARP1 leads to ADP-ribose polymerization with base excision repair proteins, such as XRCC-1, DNA polymerase-β and DNA ligase III, histones and PARP1, by the catalytic domain, which is NAD-dependent.[181,182] In turn, this complex process affect DNA replication, transcription, differentiation, gene regulation, protein degradation and mitotic spindle maintenance. Only in the absence of PARP-1, which accounts for 90% of PARP activity, PARP2 will be involved in DNA repair.[183]

Relevance of PARP and soft tissue sarcomas

Farmers et al.[184] demonstrated homozygous deletion of BRCA-1 or BRCA-2 led to sensitivity to PARP1 inhibition, resulting in apoptosis. Apoptosis is postulated to be the loss of homologous recombination repair after single strand DNA breaks as a result of both PARP1 inhibition and loss of BRCA-1 or -2. To date no BRCA-1 or -2 germline loss has been documented in soft tissue sarcomas. But Xing et al. reported 29% of uterine leiomyosarcoma had decrease or absent BRAC-1 protein expression, which is postulated to be due to methylation of BRCA-1 gene promoter.[185] Schoffski et al.[186] reported decrease in BRCA-1 in 50% of the soft tissue sarcoma samples.

In addition, members of the Fanconi family proteins are involved in double strand DNA repair through activation of ATM and ATR and formation of a nuclear complex of 5 Fanconi family proteins. This complex subsequently co-localizes with BRCA1 and -2 for DNA repair.[187] Loss of function or expression of any of these protein or "BRCA-ness" confers sensitivity to PARP1 inhibition.[188] [189] ATM is a serine/threonine kinase that activates checkpoint kinase -2 (Chk-2) in the presence of DNA damage and sequentially, leads to increase in RAD51 and BRCA1 and -2 activity.[155] A study of leiomyosarcoma and gastrointestinal stromal sarcoma samples showed frequent 13q21-q32 amplification, which corresponds to BRCA-2 and RB1 gene location, and 11q22-q24 loss, which contains the ATM gene, in high grade and >5 cm leiomyosarcoma. 83% of the samples had either absence or weak ATM expression by immunohistochemistry and out of which 50% had 11q loss.[190]

Similarly, loss of ATM was reported in 41% of alveolar rhabdomyosarcoma.[191] Concurrent ATR loss and K-ras G12D mutation in p53 heterogyous mice developed lung adenocarcinoma and sarcomas.[192] Germline Chk-2 loss has not been reported in sarcoma except in osteosarcoma[193], and a variant of Li-Fraumeni syndrome-related malignancies

RAD51 is transcriptionally controlled by pTEN. Loss of pTEN[43] and rarely pTEN mutation[194,195] has been documented in leiomyosarcoma and uterine leiomyosarcoma, respectively and 12% of various soft tissue sarcomas had hypermethylation of the pTEN gene.[196] Interestingly, only truncated pTEN but not point mutation confers sensitivity to PARP1 inhibition.[197] Whereas increase in RAD51 expression in soft tissue sarcoma leads to resistance to doxorubicin due to S/G2 phase arrest. In the presence of wild type p53 through activator protein 2, RAD51 expression was downregulated through decrease in promotor activity.[198]

PARP inhibitor potentiates chemotherapy and radiation

Potentiation of preclinical anti-tumour efficacy was observed when combining PARP inhibitor with methylating agents (DTIC, temozolamide), alkylating agent (cyclophosphamide, ifosfamide), doxorubicin, topoisomerase I inhibitors and platinum agents, which are of relevance in soft tissue sarcomas.[199-202] Soft tissue sarcomas that have low BRCA1 expression had statistically significantly higher response rate, PFR at 6 months, and OS to trabectadin, thus, one may suspect that the combination of PARP inhibition with trabectadin may confer additive or synergistic anti-tumour activity.

Radiation is commonly being given pre-operatively or post-operative for localized soft tissue sarcomas of the limbs and retroperitonium. Single strand and sometimes double strand DNA breaks occur after radiation lead to PARP1 activation followed by DNA repair. Similar potentiation of radiation induced anti-tumour efficacy has been observed when given with PARP1 inhibitor.[199-202]

Thus PARP1 inhibitors either as a single agent or in combination with DNA damaging agents and radiation will be worthwhile to explore in soft tissue sarcomas. One may predict that single agent activity will be observed only in those soft tissue sarcomas that have a low BRCA1 protein expression resulting from promoter methylation or other post-translational mechanisms. To select this selected population, immunohistochemistry of BRCA1 and BRCA2 will suffice. When use in combination with DNA damaging agents and radiation, PARP1 inhibitor will act as a potentiating agent. But one may still expect those tumours with a low BRCA1 protein level will have a better response.

PARP inhibitor in clinical development

Olaparib (AZD2281; KU-0059436) is a phthalazione class PARP1 and 2 inhibitor. A phase I study of 60 solid tumour patients were treated at doses from 100 mg to 600 mg twice daily on either a 2 weeks on 1 week off or continuous schedules. Grade 1 or 2 drug-related anemia, lymphopenia, fatigue, vomiting dyguesia and anorexia were reported. Dose-limiting toxicity included grade 3 mood alteration, grade 3 fatigue, grade 3 somnolence and grade 4 throbocytopenia were observed in 1 and 2 patients, respectively in the continuous schedule at 400 and 600 mg twice daily. As predicted by preclinical data, responses were observed in BRCA 2 mutation positive ovarian and breast cancer. One BRCA2 mutation positive prostate cancer had 50% reduction of PSA and resolution of bone metastases.[203] Forty percent of BRCA1/2 mutation positive BRCA1/2 mutation positive ovarian cancer had a PR or reduction of CA125 for a median of 28 weeks.[204]

AG014699 (PF-01367338) is a PARP1 and 2 inhibitor administered intravenously. Based on synergistic preclinical anti-tumour activity with temozolomide, a phase I study was reported. The addition of PF-01367338 did not increase temozolomide related toxicity, allowing administration of full dose temozolomide at 200 mg/m^2/day for 5 days. Increase in single strand DNA break was observed only when PF-01367338 was administered concurrently with temozolomide. A PR was observed in one melanoma, one pretreated desmoids tumour. Stable disease for more than 6 months was observed in 4 patients, including one leiomyosarcoma.[205]

Adoption of the novel phase 0 design, Kummar et al. found a good correlation of PARP inhibition in tumour and peripheral blood mononuclear cells by ABT 888. A minimum of 50% reduction of PARP activity was observed with 25-50 mg of ABT 888 daily. Due to an average 70% of ABT 888 is excreted in urine unchanged during the 24 hours at 50 mg or higher daily, continuous dosing will be necessary.[206]

BSI-201 was initially thought to be an intravenously administered irreversible PARP1 inhibitor, but due to recent preclinical and clinical data showed that PARP1 is not inhibited at clinically relevant concentration. Thus no further discussion will be presented in this book chapter.

MK-4827 is an orally administered PARP1 and 2 inhibitor. Sandhu et al. reported a phase I study of MK-4827 given daily at doses 30-210 mg. Dose-limiting toxicity included grade 3 fatigue, pneumonitis and anorexia. Common toxicities were all grade 1-2 such as nausea and myelosuppression. At doses of 110 mg daily, sustained PARP inhibition was observed in peripheral blood mononuclear cells. Responses and SD for more than 16 weeks were observed in sporadic and BRCA-related breast or ovarian cancer. One heavily-pretreated non-small cell lung cancer patient had SD for more than 42 weeks.[207]

A number of other PARP inhibitors are in phase I clinical development, including E7016 (PARP1 and 2 inhibitor) and CEP-8983 and its prodrug, CEP-9722 (PARP1 and 2 inhibitor).

Based on the preclinical and translational research information, PARP inhibitor in combination with DNA damaging agents (anthracyclin, ifosfamide, DTIC and trabectedin) and radiation will be of interest. As reported by Plummer et al., enhanced DNA breaks is observed only when PARP inhibitor is administered concurrently with chemotherapy. Thus careful preclinical and clinical study of the schedule of these combination should be performed not only to enhance anti-tumour activity, but also to reduce unnecessary toxicities.

Development as a single agent may only be applicable to those with low BRCA1 protein expression, low ATM expression such as gastrointestinal stromal tumour, leiomyosarcoma and alveolar rhabdomyosarcoma and low RAD51 expressing sarcomas.

Development of resistance is the rule rather than exception for PARP inhibitor. Reversal of loss of nonsense mutation in BRCA2 due to a second mutation has been reported.[208] Pre- and post-treatment biopsies in the setting of localized disease or metastatic disease may proven to be valuable in further our understanding of the predictive biomarker for response, the biological effect of PAPR inhibitors alone and/or in combination with other agents and more importantly, the mechanisms of resistance. For example, the activation of PARP 1 by Ras/Raf/Erk pathway has been observed.[209] Thus, such combination may be of clinical relevance. PARP activity is at least in part responsible for HIF-1α expression.[208] Building on the clinical benefit of anti-VEGFR TKI in soft tissue sarcoma, the combinations with PARP inhibitor have been initiated.

Protective effects of PARP inhibition on doxorubicin related cardiac toxicities[210], platinum- and taxane related neurotoxicities[211] and cisplatin-related nephrotoxicities[212] without compromising anti-tumour activities have been reported in preclinical models. Careful study of the incidence of toxicity will be fruitful during clinical debelopment such as randomized phase II studies with toxicities as one of the main endpoints will be worthwhile.

Apoptosis pathways

Apoptosis, otherwise known as programmed cell death, is a critical process required for maintaining tissue homeostasis. Furthermore, it prevents tumorigenesis by eliminating damaged cells. Apoptosis occurs through two major pathways. The extrinsic or death receptor pathway is turned on in response to extracellular signals resulting in activation of plasma membrane receptors. This ultimately leads to processes that trigger initiator caspases which in turn activate executioner caspases.[213] The intrinsic or mitochondrial pathway is turned on in response to a diverse set apoptotic signals which include DNA damage, growth factor withdrawal and viral infection. Mitochondria release co-factors from their intermembrane space which promote and amplify the apoptotic cascade including the formation and activation of apoptosomes.[214] Although these pathways have their own distinct regulatory processes, there is also significant cross-talk in many situations.[215] Defects in apoptosis can lead to oncogenic transformation and contribute to therapeutic resistance.[216]

Bcl-2 family

The members of the Bcl-2 family of proteins are the key regulators of mitochondrial response to apoptotic signals and are divided into three subfamilies based on function and structure. The anti-apoptotic members include Bcl-2, Bcl-X_L, Mcl-1, Bcl-w, and A1/Bfl1. The pro-apoptotic members include Bax and Bak. The third subfamily is the BH3-only group which is largely responsible for sensing apoptotic signals and transmitting them to the other Bcl-2 family members.[217] Members of this subfamily include Bid, Bad, PUMA, and Noxa.[214] A network of interactions between these subfamilies decides the apoptotic fate of the cell and an imbalance within this network leads to a variety of disease states.

The Bcl-2 family of proteins is a common target for deregulation in cancers. Anti-apoptotic members may be overexpressed or pro-apoptotic members may be mutated or silenced. These abnormalities have been demonstrated in soft tissue sarcomas. Bcl-2 overexpression has been demonstrated in synovial sarcoma, Kaposi's sarcoma, solitary fibrous tumor and gastrointestinal stromal tumor (GIST).[218,219] Focal positivity has been observed in both benign and malignant peripheral nerve sheath tumors. Sarcomas of fibroblastic type, including low-grade myxofibrosarcoma, malignant fibrous histiocytoma and fibrosarcoma showed variable expression of Bcl-2.[218] The bcl-2 overexpression in synovial sarcoma include immunohistochemical expression of bcl-2, bax, bcl-x, and bac. Furthermore, this has been correlated with poor prognosis.[220,221]

Oblimersen sodium (G3139, Genasense), the first agent targeting Bcl-2 to enter clinical trials, is a phosporothioate Bcl-2 antisense oligodeoxynucleotide that targets Bcl-2 mRNA. The cell death mechanisms of Bcl-2 antisense can be classified in two categories exerting either an apoptotic or a nonapoptotic effect based on their involvement in cell death pathways. Pre-clinical data in combination with doxorubicin in the FU-SY-1 synovial sarcoma cell line enhanced doxorubicin-induced cell killin.[222] Clinical development of oblimersen is unknown.

Similarly ABT 737 (A-779024, Abbott Laboratories), a small molecule that targets anti-apoptotic Bcl-2 family proteins (Bcl-2, Bcl-X_L, and Bcl-w), in combination with imatinib in GIST cell lines inhibits the proliferation and induces apoptosis in all GIST cell lines. Strong synergistic drug interactions at clinically relevant in vitro combinations were reported.[223] Clinical development of ABT-263 is ongoing in various solid tumours and chronic lymphocytic leukemia and in combination with other chemotherapeutic and targeted agents. ABT-263 is administered orally and thrombocytopenia is the dose-limiting and most common toxicity, which occurs on day 15 followed by a rebound by days 21-28 and due to mechanistic inhibition of Bcl-XL in mature platelets.[224] Impressive anti-tumour activity has been observed in commonly Bcl-2 amplified chronic lymphocytic leukemia.[225] SDs and a few PRs have been observed in solid tumours, including small-cell lung cancer which has overexpression of Bcl-2.[224,226]

Many additional agents have been identified or designed to target the Bcl-2 family at the mRNA or protein level and pre-clinical data suggests these agents should be developed further in the subtypes of soft tissue sarcomas demonstrating Bcl-2 overexpression.

Stem cell pathways

The developmental pathways important to normal stem cells are also important to cancer stem cells (CSC). Like normal stem cells, CSC are thought to possess the capacity for unlimited self renewal through symmetric division, the ability to give rise to progeny cells through assymetric division, and an innate resistance to cytotoxic therapies.[227,228] However where the process of differentiation initiated by the normal stem cell results in a specialized progeny that has no proliferative potential, te CSC gives rise to progeny that do not undergo terminal differentiation but instead exhibit uncontrolled proliferation.[229]

Due to similarities to normal stem cells, CSCs are predicted to rely on the same pathways that govern development, self-renewal and cell fate. In embryonic stem cells, the Notch, Wnt, and Hedgehog (HH) pathways largely regulate these processes.[230] These pathways are frequently dysregulated in many types of cancers, and specifically within subpopulations of these cancers that possess stem cell like properties (Li et al, 2010; Barker et al, 2006; Haegebarth et al, 2009; Wang et al, 2010).[231-233]

Hedgehog (HH) pathway[234]

Under normal conditions, HH signaling plays important roles in embryonic development tissue regeneration in adults (Ingham PW et al, 2001; Vajosalo M et al, 2008). HH signaling is comprised of multiple ligands that regulate receptor activity. HH signaling is initiated when one of three HH ligands (Sonic, Indian and Desert) bind the receptor Patched (Ptch1). The ligand/receptor interactions may be autocrine or paracrine. Receptor engagement results in activation of the transmembrane Smoothened (Smo), which is inactive state in the absence of a ligand. Subsequently, Smo activation regulates transcription of genes involved in HH signaling such as Gli1, Gli2 adn Gli3. Gli1/2/3 regulate the transcription of genes involved in HH signaling such as Gli1 and Ptch1 as well as genes involved in epithelial-mesenchymal transitin (EMT), such as SNAIL1.[235]

Dysregulation of nearly every step of the HH signaling pathway has been linked to cancer development and progression. In rhabdomyosarcoma (RMS), the most common soft tissue sarcoma in children, HH signaling is preferentially activated in specific subgroups of RMS.[236-239] Ptch1, Gli1, and Gli3 are expressed at significant higher levels in embryonal RMS

than in fusion-gene negative alveolar RMS than in fusion-gene positive alveolar RMS. High expression of Ptch1 significantly correlated with reduced cumulative survival.[238]
Betullinic acid possesses anti-tumoral acivity and overcomes resistance by inducing apoptosis in a variety of human cancers.[240] In preclinical study using RMS-13 cells, which is known to display an activate HH pathway caused by DNA amplification of the Gli1 locus, betullinic acid effectively suppressed HH target gene expression.[238]
Early phase clinical trials are underway which include patients with soft tissue sarcomas with agents such as GDC 0449 (Genetech),[241-244] LDE225 (Novartis Pharmaceuticals)[245] and BMS-833923[246] which both selectively inhibit Smo. Preliminary anti-tumour activity in consistently in basal cell carcinoma and medulloblastoma and in sporadiac cases of non-small cell lung cancer. All are orally administered on a daily schedule. Only IPI-926 is a cyclopamine analogue that is administered intravenously.[247] Toxicity includes gastrointestinal (nausea, vomiting), anorexia, muscle spasm/cramps, fatigue and dysguesia. Due to the long half-life of days, various alternative dosing schedules are being tested to optimize toxicity and anti-tumour activity. Combination with various chemotherapy and targeted agents are ongoing, such as PI3K inhibitor.

Notch signaling pathway

The Notch pathway is a highly conserved regulatory signaling network with the basic molecular players in the pathway including 5 ligands (Dll 1, 3, 4 and Jagged 1, 2), Notch receptors (Notch 1 to Notch 4) and the transcription factors. A complex signaling pathway is initiated when a ligand expressed on one cell engages a receptor expressed on another cell. Upon ligand/receptor interaction a cleavage event removes the Notch/ligand complex from the membrane bound portion of Notch. The cytoplasmic region of Notch then undergoes a proteolytic cleavage mediated by ϒ-secretase, releasing an intracellular domain peptide which translocates to the nucleus and drives transcription of Notch target genes.[230] The physiologic functions of Notch signaling are multifaceted and include maintenance of stem cells, specification of cell fate, and regulation of differentiation in development as well as oncogenesis.[248,249]
ϒ-secretase inhibitors are a promising therapeutic approach as they act downstream of the ligand/receptor interactions and therefore should not be affected by the diversity of ligands, receptors and combinations thereof. Currently several ϒ-secretase inhibitors are being evaluated in early Phase human studies.
Aberrant Notch signaling has been reported in rhabdomyosarcoma and Kaposi sarcoma cell lines.[250,251] A striking increase in Notch 2 expression was observed. In addition a slight upregulation of Notch 3 was also noted. However, Notch 1 and 4 were not significantly increased. Increased expression of two downstream effectors, Hes1 and Hey1, correlated with invasiveness of the cell lines. The addition of ϒ-secretase inhibitors significantly decreased the Hes1 and Hey1 expression. Furthermore, with addition of ϒ-secretase inhibitors, a significant reduction in cell mobility was observed suggesting the Notch pathway may play a role in the invasiveness of the cell lines.[250] In pre-clinical studies, a ϒ-secretase inhibitor also blocked Notch activation and induces apoptosis in Kaposi's sarcoma tumor cells.[251] These findings show that the Notch pathway is important in regulating these subtypes of soft tissue sarcoma and may ϒ-secretase inhibitors be useful therapeutic agents.

Wnt pathway

Wnts are secreted glycoproteins that bind to cell surface receptors initiating signaling cascades which are important in many physiologic settings including embryogenesis, development, cell polarization, differentiation and proliferation .[252-256] The Wnt signaling pathways fall into two categories: canonical and non-canonical, characterized by their dependence on β-catenin. Canonical Wnt will be the focus of this section as it is better characterized in mammalian systems. Canonical Wnt signaling is initiated when a Wnt ligand engages co-receptors of the Frizzled (Fzd) and low-density lipoprotein receptor-related protein (LRP) families, leading to β-catenin stabilization, nuclear translocation and activation of target genes.[230,257]

The relevance of Wnt signaling in human cancers is highlighted by the frequency of which this pathway is aberrantly activated across a vast range of malignancies. There are numerous mechanisms that drive aberrant Wnt/β-catenin signaling than nearly always occur in a mutually exclusive manner. In one study, 50% of human sarcomas and 65% of sarcoma cell lines of diverse histological subtypes exhibit upregulated autocrine canonical Wnt signaling. Furthermore, in Wnt autocrine cell lines, alterations included overexpression or gene amplification of Wnt ligands and/or LRP5/6 coreceptors and epigenetic silencing of different cell surface Wnt antagonists.[258] High level of nuclear expression of β-catenin has reported in solitary fibrous tumor, endometrial stromal sarcoma, synovial sarcoma, dedifferentiated liposarcoma, and malignant fibrous histiocytoma.[259-262]

There are three major areas of targeting the Wnt pathway which include receptor/ligand interactions, cytosolic signaling components, and nuclear signaling components. In pre-clinical studies, monoclonal antibodies against Wnt1 induced apoptosis in a number of cell lines including sarcoma.[263,264] *In vitro* results are encouraging and warrant further development. An alternate approach to inhibiting ligand/receptor interactions would be to target the Wnt co-receptors. The LRP family is comprised of 2 highly homologous members, LRP5 and LRP6 which are long single- pass transmembrane receptors which could be targeted through antibodies.[265] The Fzd family of transmembrane receptors also shares a high degree of homology in their cysteine rich domain which could be targeted through an antibody to block Wnt signaling.[266]

Targeting the cytosolic signaling components of the Wnt pathway are in preclinical or phase I early development. No clinical information is currently available. The small molecules in development include those targeting Dvl, Tankyrase1 and 2, Axin, Porcupine, and β-catenin.[230] Similarly nuclear signaling small molecules which would interrupt the β-catenin interaction with TCF/LEF are also in early development.

6. Conclusions

With decades of research into the biology of each target, its interaction with other pathways or targets, and the relevance in sarcoma, it is an exciting time in drug development in soft tissue sarcomas. But the academia and industry must remember that soft tissue sarcoma is a collective term for a florid of many different diseases, though some share similar characteristics, such as the translocation associated sarcomas and their fusion proteins with transcription factor activity, each target may only be relevant to a small number of subtypes. A lot of investment and time will be needed in order to bring these agents to the market with a small return.

During the development of these agents, it is important to understand the biology of these targets and their effects on the sarcoma cells, cytostatic or cytotoxic, as it will influence the clinical endpoints, progression-free survival or progression-free rate versus response rate, respectively, in proof of concept phase II studies. This approach will lessen our chance of failure in the phase III setting.

Furthermore, how can a target, expression/overexpression, amplification, mutation, or translocation, be considered to be of clinical relevance for clinical therapeutics? There seems to be a different answer for different cancer. Therefore, detail preclinical modeling and translational research using archival tumour samples will be important. It is important to collect tumour (fresh biopsies before and after therapy and archival samples), blood or even urine samples during proof of concept studies in order to validate the target identify and to evaluate novel predictive markers for clinical benefit.

Resistance is universal for any cancer therapeutics. Preclinical, translational and clinical research should be done to elucidate these escape mechanisms. Such information can help us not only to develop combinatorial therapeutics to delay or prevent resistance and thus more prolonged clinical benefits, but also to understand the biology of sarcomas and thus new therapeutic options when resistance emerges.

With the constant quest of the sarcoma community to understand and to develop new agents for this vastly diverse cancer, it is the hope that more effective and less toxic agents will be available for the treatment of this disease.

7. References

[1] O'Sullivan B, Davis AM, Turcotte R, et al: Preoperative versus postoperative radiotherapy in soft-tissue sarcoma of the limbs: a randomised trial. Lancet 359:2235-41, 2002

[2] Figueredo A, Bramwell VH, Bell R, et al: Adjuvant chemotherapy following complete resection of soft tissue sarcoma in adults: a clinical practice guideline. Sarcoma 6:5-18, 2002

[3] Woll PJ, van Glabbeke, M, Hohenberger, P, et al.: Adjuvant chemotherapy with doxorubicin and ifosfamide in resected soft tissue sarcoma (STS): interim analysis of a randomised phase III trial Proceedings Am Soc Clin Oncol, J Clin Oncol, 2007, pp A10008

[4] Bramwell VH, Anderson D, Charette ML: Doxorubicin-based chemotherapy for the palliative treatment of adult patients with locally advanced or metastatic soft tissue sarcoma. Cochrane Database Syst Rev:CD003293, 2003

[5] Kindblom LG, Remotti HE, Aldenborg F, et al: Gastrointestinal pacemaker cell tumor (GIPACT): gastrointestinal stromal tumors show phenotypic characteristics of the interstitial cells of Cajal. Am J Pathol 152:1259-69, 1998

[6] Sircar K, Hewlett BR, Huizinga JD, et al: Interstitial cells of Cajal as precursors of gastrointestinal stromal tumors. Am J Surg Pathol 23:377-89, 1999

[7] Corless CL, McGreevey L, Haley A, et al: KIT mutations are common in incidental gastrointestinal stromal tumors one centimeter or less in size. Am J Pathol 160:1567-72, 2002

[8] Heinrich MC, Corless CL, Duensing A, et al: PDGFRA activating mutations in gastrointestinal stromal tumors. Science 299:708-10, 2003

[9] Hirota S, Isozaki K, Moriyama Y, et al: Gain-of-function mutations of c-kit in human gastrointestinal stromal tumors. Science 279:577-80, 1998

[10] Rubin BP, Singer S, Tsao C, et al: KIT activation is a ubiquitous feature of gastrointestinal stromal tumors. Cancer Res 61:8118-21, 2001
[11] Tarn C, Merkel E, Canutescu AA, et al: Analysis of KIT mutations in sporadic and familial gastrointestinal stromal tumors: therapeutic implications through protein modeling. Clin Cancer Res 11:3668-77, 2005
[12] Corless CL, Fletcher JA, Heinrich MC: Biology of gastrointestinal stromal tumors. J Clin Oncol 22:3813-25, 2004
[13] Blanke CD, Rankin C, Demetri GD, et al: Phase III randomized, intergroup trial assessing imatinib mesylate at two dose levels in patients with unresectable or metastatic gastrointestinal stromal tumors expressing the kit receptor tyrosine kinase: S0033. J Clin Oncol 26:626-32, 2008
[14] Blanke CD, Demetri GD, von Mehren M, et al: Long-term results from a randomized phase II trial of standard- versus higher-dose imatinib mesylate for patients with unresectable or metastatic gastrointestinal stromal tumors expressing KIT. J Clin Oncol 26:620-5, 2008
[15] Verweij J, Casali PG, Zalcberg J, et al: Progression-free survival in gastrointestinal stromal tumours with high-dose imatinib: randomised trial. Lancet 364:1127-34, 2004
[16] Verweij J, van Oosterom A, Blay JY, et al: Imatinib mesylate (STI-571 Glivec, Gleevec) is an active agent for gastrointestinal stromal tumours, but does not yield responses in other soft-tissue sarcomas that are unselected for a molecular target. Results from an EORTC Soft Tissue and Bone Sarcoma Group phase II study. Eur J Cancer 39:2006-11, 2003
[17] Dematteo RP, Ballman KV, Antonescu CR, et al: Adjuvant imatinib mesylate after resection of localised, primary gastrointestinal stromal tumour: a randomised, double-blind, placebo-controlled trial. Lancet 373:1097-104, 2009
[18] Joensuu H, Eriksson M, Hatrmann J, et al: Twelve versus 36 months of adjuvant imatinib (IM) as treatment of operable GIST with a high risk of recurrence: Final results of a randomized trial (SSGXVIII/AIO). J Clin Oncol 29:A:LBA 1, 2011
[19] Demetri GD, van Oosterom AT, Garrett CR, et al: Efficacy and safety of sunitinib in patients with advanced gastrointestinal stromal tumour after failure of imatinib: a randomised controlled trial. Lancet 368:1329-38, 2006
[20] Osuna D, de Alava E: Molecular pathology of sarcomas. Rev Recent Clin Trials 4:12-26, 2009
[21] Todd R, Lunec J: Molecular pathology and potential therapeutic targets in soft-tissue sarcoma. Expert Rev Anticancer Ther 8:939-48, 2008
[22] Lazar A, Abruzzo LV, Pollock RE, et al: Molecular diagnosis of sarcomas: chromosomal translocations in sarcomas. Arch Pathol Lab Med 130:1199-207, 2006
[23] Borden EC, Baker LH, Bell RS, et al: Soft tissue sarcomas of adults: state of the translational science. Clin Cancer Res 9:1941-56, 2003
[24] Maleddu A, Pantaleo MA, Nannini M, et al: Mechanisms of secondary resistance to tyrosine kinase inhibitors in gastrointestinal stromal tumours (Review). Oncol Rep 21:1359-66, 2009
[25] Pollak MN: Insulin-like growth factors and neoplasia. Novartis Found Symp 262:84-98; discussion 98-107, 265-8, 2004

[26] Rodon J, DeSantos V, Ferry RJ, Jr., et al: Early drug development of inhibitors of the insulin-like growth factor-I receptor pathway: lessons from the first clinical trials. Mol Cancer Ther 7:2575-88, 2008

[27] Samani AA, Yakar S, LeRoith D, et al: The role of the IGF system in cancer growth and metastasis: overview and recent insights. Endocr Rev 28:20-47, 2007

[28] Pollak MN, Schernhammer ES, Hankinson SE: Insulin-like growth factors and neoplasia. Nat Rev Cancer 4:505-18, 2004

[29] Frasca F, Pandini G, Scalia P, et al: Insulin receptor isoform A, a newly recognized, high-affinity insulin-like growth factor II receptor in fetal and cancer cells. Mol Cell Biol 19:3278-88, 1999

[30] Sciacca L, Costantino A, Pandini G, et al: Insulin receptor activation by IGF-II in breast cancers: evidence for a new autocrine/paracrine mechanism. Oncogene 18:2471-9, 1999

[31] Sciacca L, Mineo R, Pandini G, et al: In IGF-I receptor-deficient leiomyosarcoma cells autocrine IGF-II induces cell invasion and protection from apoptosis via the insulin receptor isoform A. Oncogene 21:8240-50, 2002

[32] Pavelic K, Bukovic D, Pavelic J: The role of insulin-like growth factor 2 and its receptors in human tumors. Mol Med 8:771-80, 2002

[33] Zhang L, Zhan S, Navid F, et al: AP-2 may contribute to IGF-II overexpression in rhabdomyosarcoma. Oncogene 17:1261-70, 1998

[34] Zhan S, Shapiro DN, Helman LJ: Activation of an imprinted allele of the insulin-like growth factor II gene implicated in rhabdomyosarcoma. J Clin Invest 94:445-8, 1994

[35] Sun Y, Gao D, Liu Y, et al: IGF2 is critical for tumorigenesis by synovial sarcoma oncoprotein SYT-SSX1. Oncogene 25:1042-52, 2006

[36] Steigen SE, Schaeffer DF, West RB, et al: Expression of insulin-like growth factor 2 in mesenchymal neoplasms. Mod Pathol 22:914-21, 2009

[37] Ayalon D, Glaser T, Werner H: Transcriptional regulation of IGF-I receptor gene expression by the PAX3-FKHR oncoprotein. Growth Horm IGF Res 11:289-97, 2001

[38] Werner H, Idelman G, Rubinstein M, et al: A novel EWS-WT1 gene fusion product in desmoplastic small round cell tumor is a potent transactivator of the insulin-like growth factor-I receptor (IGF-IR) gene. Cancer Lett 247:84-90, 2007

[39] Karnieli E, Werner H, Rauscher FJ, 3rd, et al: The IGF-I receptor gene promoter is a molecular target for the Ewing's sarcoma-Wilms' tumor 1 fusion protein. J Biol Chem 271:19304-9, 1996

[40] Xie Y, Skytting B, Nilsson G, et al: Expression of insulin-like growth factor-1 receptor in synovial sarcoma: association with an aggressive phenotype. Cancer Res 59:3588-91, 1999

[41] Gloudemans T, Prinsen I, Van Unnik JA, et al: Insulin-like growth factor gene expression in human smooth muscle tumors. Cancer Res 50:6689-95, 1990

[42] Tricoli JV, Rall LB, Karakousis CP, et al: Enhanced levels of insulin-like growth factor messenger RNA in human colon carcinomas and liposarcomas. Cancer Res 46:6169-73, 1986

[43] Hernando E, Charytonowicz E, Dudas ME, et al: The AKT-mTOR pathway plays a critical role in the development of leiomyosarcomas. Nat Med 13:748-53, 2007

[44] Chang Q, Li Y, White MF, et al: Constitutive activation of insulin receptor substrate 1 is a frequent event in human tumors: therapeutic implications. Cancer Res 62:6035-8, 2002

[45] Agaram NP, Laquaglia MP, Ustun B, et al: Molecular characterization of pediatric gastrointestinal stromal tumors. Clin Cancer Res 14:3204-15, 2008

[46] Janeway KA, Zhu MJ, Barretina J, et al: Strong expression of IGF1R in pediatric gastrointestinal stromal tumors without IGF1R genomic amplification. Int J Cancer 127:2718-22, 2010

[47] Pantaleo MA, Nannini M, Di Battista M, et al: Combined treatment strategies in gastrointestinal stromal tumors (GISTs) after imatinib and sunitinib therapy. Cancer Treat Rev 36:63-8, 2010

[48] Tarn C, Rink L, Merkel E, et al: Insulin-like growth factor 1 receptor is a potential therapeutic target for gastrointestinal stromal tumors. Proc Natl Acad Sci U S A 105:8387-92, 2008

[49] Braconi C, Bracci R, Bearzi I, et al: KIT and PDGFRalpha mutations in 104 patients with gastrointestinal stromal tumors (GISTs): a population-based study. Ann Oncol 19:706-10, 2008

[50] Hailey J, Maxwell E, Koukouras K, et al: Neutralizing anti-insulin-like growth factor receptor 1 antibodies inhibit receptor function and induce receptor degradation in tumor cells. Mol Cancer Ther 1:1349-53, 2002

[51] Pappos AS, Patel S, Crowley J, et al: Activity of R1507, a monoclonal antibody to the insulin-like growth factor-1 receptor (IGF1R), in patients (pts) with recurrent or refractory Ewing's sarcoma family of tumors (ESFT): Results of a phase II SARC study., Proc Am Soc Clin Oncol, 2010, pp A10000

[52] Tap WD, Demetri GD, Barnette P, et al: AMG 479 in relapsed or refractory Ewing's family tumors (EFT) or desmoplastic small round cell tumors (DSRCT): Phase II results., Proc Am Soc Clin Oncol, 2010, pp A10001

[53] Menefee M, LoRusso P, Viner J, et al: MEDI-573, a dual IGF-1/-2 neutralizing antibody blocks IGF-1R and IR-A signaling and maintains glucose hemostasis in a Phase I study for advanced solid tumors. 22nd EORTC-NCI-AACR Symposiumon Molecular Targets and Cancer Therapeutics, 2010

[54] Jiang BH, Liu LZ: Role of mTOR in anticancer drug resistance: perspectives for improved drug treatment. Drug Resist Updat 11:63-76, 2008

[55] Wan X, Helman LJ: The biology behind mTOR inhibition in sarcoma. Oncologist 12:1007-18, 2007

[56] Friedrichs N, Trautmann M, Endl E, et al: Phosphatidylinositol-3'-kinase/AKT signalling is essential in synovial sarcoma. Int J Cancer, 2010

[57] Hosoi H, Dilling MB, Shikata T, et al: Rapamycin causes poorly reversible inhibition of mTOR and induces p53-independent apoptosis in human rhabdomyosarcoma cells. Cancer Res 59:886-94, 1999

[58] Wan X, Shen N, Mendoza A, et al: CCI-779 inhibits rhabdomyosarcoma xenograft growth by an antiangiogenic mechanism linked to the targeting of mTOR/Hif-1alpha/VEGF signaling. Neoplasia 8:394-401, 2006

[59] Sapi Z, Fule T, Hajdu M, et al: The activated targets of mTOR signaling pathway are characteristic for PDGFRA mutant and wild-type rather than KIT mutant GISTs. Diagn Mol Pathol 20:22-33, 2011
[60] Bauer S, Duensing A, Demetri GD, et al: KIT oncogenic signaling mechanisms in imatinib-resistant gastrointestinal stromal tumor: PI3-kinase/AKT is a crucial survival pathway. Oncogene 26:7560-8, 2007
[61] Yang J, Ikezoe T, Nishioka C, et al: Long-term exposure of gastrointestinal stromal tumor cells to sunitinib induces epigenetic silencing of the PTEN gene. Int J Cancer, 2011
[62] Ikezoe T, Yang Y, Nishioka C, et al: Effect of SU11248 on gastrointestinal stromal tumor-T1 cells: enhancement of growth inhibition via inhibition of 3-kinase/Akt/mammalian target of rapamycin signaling. Cancer Sci 97:945-51, 2006
[63] Okuno SH, Bailey H, Mahoney MR, et al: A Phase II study of temsirolimus (CCI-779) in patients with soft tissue sarcoma. A srydt of the Mayo Phase II Consortium. Cancer, 2011
[64] Van Glabbeke M, Verweij J, Judson I, et al: Progression-free rate as the principal end-point for phase II trials in soft-tissue sarcomas. Eur J Cancer 38:543-9, 2002
[65] Chawla SP, Tolcher AW, Staddon AP, et al: Survival results with AP23573, a novel mTOR inhibitor, in patients (pts) with advanced soft tissue or bone sarcomas: Update of phase II trial. Proc Am Soc Clin Oncol 25, 2007
[66] Chawla SP, Blay JY, Ray-Coquard IL, et al: Results of the phase III, placebo-controlled trial (SUCCEED) evaluating the mTOR inhibitor ridaforolimus (R) as maintenance therapy in advanced sarcoma patients (pts) following clinical benefit from prior standard cytotoxic chemotherapy (CT). J Clin Oncol 29:A10005, 2011
[67] Schoffski P, Reichardt P, Blay JY, et al: A phase I-II study of everolimus (RAD001) in combination with imatinib in patients with imatinib-resistant gastrointestinal stromal tumors. Ann Oncol 21:1990-8, 2010
[68] Wan X, Harkavy B, Shen N, et al: Rapamycin induces feedback activation of Akt signaling through an IGF-1R-dependent mechanism. Oncogene 26:1932-40, 2007
[69] Cao L, Yu Y, Darko I, et al: Addiction to elevated insulin-like growth factor I receptor and initial modulation of the AKT pathway define the responsiveness of rhabdomyosarcoma to the targeting antibody. Cancer Res 68:8039-48, 2008
[70] Silvany RE, Eliazer S, Wolff NC, et al: Interference with the constitutive activation of ERK1 and ERK2 impairs EWS/FLI-1-dependent transformation. Oncogene 19:4523-30, 2000
[71] Benini S, Manara MC, Cerisano V, et al: Contribution of MEK/MAPK and PI3-K signaling pathway to the malignant behavior of Ewing's sarcoma cells: therapeutic prospects. Int J Cancer 108:358-66, 2004
[72] Italiano A, Kind M, Stoeckle E, et al: Temsirolimus in advanced leiomyosarcomas: patterns of response and correlation with the activation of the mammalian target of rapamycin pathway. Anticancer Drugs 22:463-7, 2011
[73] Barretina J, Taylor BS, Banerji S, et al: Subtype-specific genomic alterations define new targets for soft-tissue sarcoma therapy. Nat Genet 42:715-21, 2010

[74] Zhu QS, Ren W, Korchin B, et al: Soft tissue sarcoma cells are highly sensitive to AKT blockade: a role for p53-independent up-regulation of GADD45 alpha. Cancer Res 68:2895-903, 2008

[75] Dobashi Y, Suzuki S, Sato E, et al: EGFR-dependent and independent activation of Akt/mTOR cascade in bone and soft tissue tumors. Mod Pathol 22:1328-40, 2009

[76] Manara MC, Nicoletti G, Zambelli D, et al: NVP-BEZ235 as a new therapeutic option for sarcomas. Clin Cancer Res 16:530-40, 2010

[77] Hyder SM, Stancel GM: Regulation of angiogenic growth factors in the female reproductive tract by estrogens and progestins. Mol Endocrinol 13:806-11, 1999

[78] Folkman J: Angiogenesis in cancer, vascular, rheumatoid and other disease. Nat Med 1:27-31, 1995

[79] Ferrara N: Vascular endothelial growth factor as a target for anticancer therapy. Oncologist 9 Suppl 1:2-10, 2004

[80] Veikkola T, Alitalo K: VEGFs, receptors and angiogenesis. Semin Cancer Biol 9:211-20, 1999

[81] Harper SJ, Bates DO: VEGF-A splicing: the key to anti-angiogenic therapeutics? Nat Rev Cancer 8:880-7, 2008

[82] Pakos EE, Goussia AC, Tsekeris PG, et al: Expression of vascular endothelial growth factor and its receptor, KDR/Flk-1, in soft tissue sarcomas. Anticancer Res 25:3591-6, 2005

[83] Chao C, Al-Saleem T, Brooks JJ, et al: Vascular endothelial growth factor and soft tissue sarcomas: tumor expression correlates with grade. Ann Surg Oncol 8:260-7, 2001

[84] Yudoh K, Kanamori M, Ohmori K, et al: Concentration of vascular endothelial growth factor in the tumour tissue as a prognostic factor of soft tissue sarcomas. Br J Cancer 84:1610-5, 2001

[85] Graeven U, Andre N, Achilles E, et al: Serum levels of vascular endothelial growth factor and basic fibroblast growth factor in patients with soft-tissue sarcoma. J Cancer Res Clin Oncol 125:577-81, 1999

[86] Hayes AJ, Mostyn-Jones A, Koban MU, et al: Serum vascular endothelial growth factor as a tumour marker in soft tissue sarcoma. Br J Surg 91:242-7, 2004

[87] Yoon SS, Segal NH, Park PJ, et al: Angiogenic profile of soft tissue sarcomas based on analysis of circulating factors and microarray gene expression. J Surg Res 135:282-90, 2006

[88] Kuhnen C, Lehnhardt M, Tolnay E, et al: Patterns of expression and secretion of vascular endothelial growth factor in malignant soft-tissue tumours. J Cancer Res Clin Oncol 126:219-25, 2000

[89] Potti A, Ganti AK, Tendulkar K, et al: Determination of vascular endothelial growth factor (VEGF) overexpression in soft tissue sarcomas and the role of overexpression in leiomyosarcoma. J Cancer Res Clin Oncol 130:52-6, 2004

[90] Tokuyama W, Mikami T, Masuzawa M, et al: Autocrine and paracrine roles of VEGF/VEGFR-2 and VEGF-C/VEGFR-3 signaling in angiosarcomas of the scalp and face. Hum Pathol 41:407-14, 2010

[91] Yonemori K, Tsuta K, Ando M, et al: Contrasting Prognostic Implications of Platelet-Derived Growth Factor Receptor-beta and Vascular Endothelial Growth Factor Receptor-2 in Patients with Angiosarcoma. Ann Surg Oncol, 2011

[92] Lahat G, Dhuka AR, Hallevi H, et al: Angiosarcoma: clinical and molecular insights. Ann Surg 251:1098-106, 2010

[93] Antonescu CR, Yoshida A, Guo T, et al: KDR activating mutations in human angiosarcomas are sensitive to specific kinase inhibitors. Cancer Res 69:7175-9, 2009

[94] D'Adamo DR, Anderson SE, Albritton K, et al: Phase II study of doxorubicin and bevacizumab for patients with metastatic soft-tissue sarcomas. J Clin Oncol 23:7135-42, 2005

[95] Agulnik M, Okuno S, Von Mehren M, et al: An open-label multicenter phase II study of bevacizumab for the treatment of angiosarcoma. J Clin Oncol 27:A10522, 2009

[96] Holash J, Davis S, Papadopoulos N, et al: VEGF-Trap: a VEGF blocker with potent antitumor effects. Proc Natl Acad Sci U S A 99:11393-8, 2002

[97] Cursiefen C, Chen L, Borges LP, et al: VEGF-A stimulates lymphangiogenesis and hemangiogenesis in inflammatory neovascularization via macrophage recruitment. J Clin Invest 113:1040-50, 2004

[98] Bran B, Bran G, Hormann K, et al: The platelet-derived growth factor receptor as a target for vascular endothelial growth factor-mediated anti-angiogenetic therapy in head and neck cancer. Int J Oncol 34:255-61, 2009

[99] Erber R, Thurnher A, Katsen AD, et al: Combined inhibition of VEGF and PDGF signaling enforces tumor vessel regression by interfering with pericyte-mediated endothelial cell survival mechanisms. FASEB J 18:338-40, 2004

[100] Shen J, Vil MD, Zhang H, et al: An antibody directed against PDGF receptor beta enhances the antitumor and the anti-angiogenic activities of an anti-VEGF receptor 2 antibody. Biochem Biophys Res Commun 357:1142-7, 2007

[101] Timke C, Zieher H, Roth A, et al: Combination of vascular endothelial growth factor receptor/platelet-derived growth factor receptor inhibition markedly improves radiation tumor therapy. Clin Cancer Res 14:2210-9, 2008

[102] Kuhnert F, Tam BY, Sennino B, et al: Soluble receptor-mediated selective inhibition of VEGFR and PDGFRbeta signaling during physiologic and tumor angiogenesis. Proc Natl Acad Sci U S A 105:10185-90, 2008

[103] Auguste P, Gursel DB, Lemiere S, et al: Inhibition of fibroblast growth factor/fibroblast growth factor receptor activity in glioma cells impedes tumor growth by both angiogenesis-dependent and -independent mechanisms. Cancer Res 61:1717-26, 2001

[104] Huang X, Yu C, Jin C, et al: Ectopic activity of fibroblast growth factor receptor 1 in hepatocytes accelerates hepatocarcinogenesis by driving proliferation and vascular endothelial growth factor-induced angiogenesis. Cancer Res 66:1481-90, 2006

[105] You WK, Sennino B, Williamson CW, et al: VEGF and c-Met Blockade Amplify Angiogenesis Inhibition in Pancreatic Islet Cancer. Cancer Res 71:4758-68, 2011

[106] George S, Merriam P, Maki RG, et al: Multicenter phase II trial of sunitinib in the treatment of nongastrointestinal stromal tumor sarcomas. J Clin Oncol 27:3154-60, 2009

[107] Vigil CE, Chiappori AA, Williams CA, et al: Phase II study of sunitinib malate in subjects with metastatic and/or surgically unresctable non-GIST soft tissue sarcomas. J Clin Oncol 26:A10535, 2008

[108] Maki RG, D'Adamo DR, Keohan ML, et al: Phase II study of sorafenib in patients with metastatic or recurrent sarcomas. J Clin Oncol 27:3133-40, 2009

[109] von Mehren M, Rankin C, Goldblum JR, et al: Phase 2 Southwest Oncology Group-directed intergroup trial (S0505) of sorafenib in advanced soft tissue sarcomas. Cancer, 2011

[110] Penel N, Ray-Coquard I, Cioffi A, et al: A stratified phase II trial investigating sorafenib in patients with metastatic or locally advanced angiosarcoma. J Clin Oncol 28:A 10026, 2010

[111] Bertuzzi A, Stroppa EM, Secondino S, et al: Efficacy and toxicity of sorafenib monotherapy in patients with advanced soft tissue sarcoma failing anthracycline-based chemotherapy. J Clin Oncol 28:A10025, 2010

[112] Sleijfer S, Ray-Coquard I, Papai Z, et al: Pazopanib, a multikinase angiogenesis inhibitor, in patients with relapsed or refractory advanced soft tissue sarcoma: a phase II study from the European organisation for research and treatment of cancer-soft tissue and bone sarcoma group (EORTC study 62043). J Clin Oncol 27:3126-32, 2009

[113] Van Der Graaf WT, Blay JY, Chawla SP, et al: PALETTE: A randomized, double-blind, phase III trial of pazopanib versus placebo in patients (pts) with soft-tissue sarcoma (STS) whose disease has progressed during or following prior chemotherapy—An EORTC STBSG Global Network Study (EORTC 62072). J Clin Oncol 29:LBA10002, 2011

[114] Campbell N, Wroblewski K, Maki R, et al: Final results of a Unoversity of Chicago phase II consortium trial of sorafenib (SOR) in patients, (pts) with imatinib (IM)-and sunitinib (SU)-resistant (RES) gastrointestinal stromal tumors (GIST). J Clin Oncol 29:A4, 2011

[115] George S, Von Mehren M, Heinrich MC, et al: A multicenter phase II study of regorafenib in patients (pts) with advanced gastrointestinal stromal tumor(GIST), after therapy with imatinib (IM) and sunitinib (SU). J Clin Oncol 29:A10007., 2011

[116] Agaram NP, Wong GC, Guo T, et al: Novel V600E BRAF mutations in imatinib-naive and imatinib-resistant gastrointestinal stromal tumors. Genes Chromosomes Cancer 47:853-9, 2008

[117] Heinrich M, Carden R, Griffith D, et al: In vitro activity of sorafenib againist imatinib-and sunitinib resistant kinase mutations associated with drug resistant GI stromal tumors. J Clin Oncol 27:A10500., 2009

[118] Huynh H, Lee JW, Chow PK, et al: Sorafenib induces growth suppression in mouse models of gastrointestinal stromal tumor. Mol Cancer Ther 8:152-9, 2009

[119] Schmitt T, Kasper B: New medical treatment options and strategies to assess clinical outcome in soft-tissue sarcoma. Expert Rev Anticancer Ther 9:1159-67, 2009

[120] Bergers G, Hanahan D: Modes of resistance to anti-angiogenic therapy. Nat Rev Cancer 8:592-603, 2008

[121] Ishibe T, Nakayama T, Okamoto T, et al: Disruption of fibroblast growth factor signal pathway inhibits the growth of synovial sarcomas: potential application of signal inhibitors to molecular target therapy. Clin Cancer Res 11:2702-12, 2005

[122] Plateros S, Mokliatchouk O, Jayson GC, et al: Correlation of FGF2 tumor expression with tumor response, PFS, and changes in plasma pharmacodynamic (PD) markers

following treatment with brivanib alaninate, an oral dual inhibitor of VEGFR and FGFR tyrosine kinases. . J Clin Oncol 26:A3506, 2008
[123] Schwartz GK, Maki RG, Ratain MJ, et al: Brivanib (BMS-582664) in advanced soft tissue sarcoma (STS): biomarker and subset results of a phase II randomized discontinuation trial. J Clin Oncol 29:A10000, 2011
[124] Itakura E, Yamamoto H, Oda Y, et al: Detection and characterization of vascular endothelial growth factors and their receptors in a series of angiosarcomas. J Surg Oncol 97:74-81, 2008
[125] Stacher E, Gruber-Mosenbacher U, Halbwedl I, et al: The VEGF-system in primary pulmonary angiosarcomas and haemangioendotheliomas: new potential therapeutic targets? Lung Cancer 65:49-55, 2009
[126] Stacchiotti S, Tamborini E, Marrari A, et al: Response to sunitinib malate in advanced alveolar soft part sarcoma. Clin Cancer Res 15:1096-104, 2009
[127] Gardner KH, Judson I, Leahy M, et al: Activity of cediranib, a highly potent and selective VEGF signaling inhibitor, in alveolar soft part sarcoma. J Clin Oncol 27:A10523, 2009
[128] Kummar A, Strassberger A, MMonks A, et al: An evaluation of cediranib as a new agent for alveolar soft part sarcoma (ASPS). J Clin Oncol 29:A10001, 2011
[129] Lazar AJ, Das P, Tuvin D, et al: Angiogenesis-promoting gene patterns in alveolar soft part sarcoma. Clin Cancer Res 13:7314-21, 2007
[130] Wang J, Coltrera MD, Gown AM: Cell proliferation in human soft tissue tumors correlates with platelet-derived growth factor B chain expression: an immunohistochemical and in situ hybridization study. Cancer Res 54:560-4, 1994
[131] Vistica DT, Hollingshead M, Borgel SD, et al: Therapeutic vulnerability of an in vivo model of alveolar soft part sarcoma (ASPS) to antiangiogenic therapy. J Pediatr Hematol Oncol 31:561-70, 2009
[132] Grunstein M: Nucleosomes: regulators of transcription. Trends Genet 6:395-400, 1990
[133] Strahl BD, Allis CD: The language of covalent histone modifications. Nature 403:41-5, 2000
[134] Gray SG, Ekstrom TJ: The human histone deacetylase family. Exp Cell Res 262:75-83, 2001
[135] Bolden JE, Peart MJ, Johnstone RW: Anticancer activities of histone deacetylase inhibitors. Nat Rev Drug Discov 5:769-84, 2006
[136] Glozak MA, Seto E: Histone deacetylases and cancer. Oncogene 26:5420-32, 2007
[137] Park JH, Kim SH, Choi MC, et al: Class II histone deacetylases play pivotal roles in heat shock protein 90-mediated proteasomal degradation of vascular endothelial growth factor receptors. Biochem Biophys Res Commun 368:318-22, 2008
[138] Wilson AJ, Byun DS, Nasser S, et al: HDAC4 promotes growth of colon cancer cells via repression of p21. Mol Biol Cell 19:4062-75, 2008
[139] Mottet D, Bellahcene A, Pirotte S, et al: Histone deacetylase 7 silencing alters endothelial cell migration, a key step in angiogenesis. Circ Res 101:1237-46, 2007
[140] Ito T, Ouchida M, Morimoto Y, et al: Significant growth suppression of synovial sarcomas by the histone deacetylase inhibitor FK228 in vitro and in vivo. Cancer Lett 224:311-9, 2005

[141] Kwan W, Terry T, Siu S, et al: Effect of depsipeptide (NSC 630176), a histone deacetylase inhibitor, on human synovial sarcoma in vitro. J Clin Oncol 23:A9039, 2006

[142] Soulez M, Saurin AJ, Freemont PS, et al: SSX and the synovial-sarcoma-specific chimaeric protein SYT-SSX co-localize with the human Polycomb group complex. Oncogene 18:2739-46, 1999

[143] van der Vlag J, Otte AP: Transcriptional repression mediated by the human polycomb-group protein EED involves histone deacetylation. Nat Genet 23:474-8, 1999

[144] Furuyama T, Banerjee R, Breen TR, et al: SIR2 is required for polycomb silencing and is associated with an E(Z) histone methyltransferase complex. Curr Biol 14:1812-21, 2004

[145] Yochum GS, Ayer DE: Pf1, a novel PHD zinc finger protein that links the TLE corepressor to the mSin3A-histone deacetylase complex. Mol Cell Biol 21:4110-8, 2001

[146] Lubieniecka JM, de Bruijn DR, Su L, et al: Histone deacetylase inhibitors reverse SS18-SSX-mediated polycomb silencing of the tumor suppressor early growth response 1 in synovial sarcoma. Cancer Res 68:4303-10, 2008

[147] Sakimura R, Tanaka K, Nakatani F, et al: Antitumor effects of histone deacetylase inhibitor on Ewing's family tumors. Int J Cancer 116:784-92, 2005

[148] Sonnemann J, Dreyer L, Hartwig M, et al: Histone deacetylase inhibitors induce cell death and enhance the apoptosis-inducing activity of TRAIL in Ewing's sarcoma cells. J Cancer Res Clin Oncol 133:847-58, 2007

[149] Jaboin J, Wild J, Hamidi H, et al: MS-27-275, an inhibitor of histone deacetylase, has marked in vitro and in vivo antitumor activity against pediatric solid tumors. Cancer Res 62:6108-15, 2002

[150] Liu S, Cheng H, Kwan W, et al: Histone deacetylase inhibitors induce growth arrest, apoptosis, and differentiation in clear cell sarcoma models. Mol Cancer Ther 7:1751-61, 2008

[151] Hrzenjak A, Kremser ML, Strohmeier B, et al: SAHA induces caspase-independent, autophagic cell death of endometrial stromal sarcoma cells by influencing the mTOR pathway. J Pathol 216:495-504, 2008

[152] Sakimura R, Tanaka K, Yamamoto S, et al: The effects of histone deacetylase inhibitors on the induction of differentiation in chondrosarcoma cells. Clin Cancer Res 13:275-82, 2007

[153] Lopez G, Liu J, Ren W, et al: Combining PCI-24781, a novel histone deacetylase inhibitor, with chemotherapy for the treatment of soft tissue sarcoma. Clin Cancer Res 15:3472-83, 2009

[154] Sampson ER, Amin V, Schwarz EM, et al: The histone deacetylase inhibitor vorinostat selectively sensitizes fibrosarcoma cells to chemotherapy. J Orthop Res 29:623-32, 2011

[155] Shiloh Y: The ATM-mediated DNA-damage response: taking shape. Trends Biochem Sci 31:402-10, 2006

[156] Bakkenist CJ, Kastan MB: DNA damage activates ATM through intermolecular autophosphorylation and dimer dissociation. Nature 421:499-506, 2003

[157] Munshi A, Kurland JF, Nishikawa T, et al: Histone deacetylase inhibitors radiosensitize human melanoma cells by suppressing DNA repair activity. Clin Cancer Res 11:4912-22, 2005

[158] Kelly WK, O'Connor OA, Krug LM, et al: Phase I study of an oral histone deacetylase inhibitor, suberoylanilide hydroxamic acid, in patients with advanced cancer. J Clin Oncol 23:3923-31, 2005

[159] Yu C, Rahmani M, Conrad D, et al: The proteasome inhibitor bortezomib interacts synergistically with histone deacetylase inhibitors to induce apoptosis in Bcr/Abl+ cells sensitive and resistant to STI571. Blood 102:3765-74, 2003

[160] Pei XY, Dai Y, Grant S: Synergistic induction of oxidative injury and apoptosis in human multiple myeloma cells by the proteasome inhibitor bortezomib and histone deacetylase inhibitors. Clin Cancer Res 10:3839-52, 2004

[161] Attia S, Mahoney MR, Okuno S, et al: A phase II consortium trial of vorinostat and bortezomib for advanced soft tissue sarcomas. J Clin Oncol 29:A10079, 2011

[162] Sharma S, Vogelzang NJ, Beck Y, et al: Phase I pharmacokinetic (PK) and pharmacodynamic (PD) study of LBH589, a novel deacetylase (DAC) inhibitor given intravenously on a new once weekly schedule. J Clin Oncol 25:A14019, 2007

[163] Prince HM, George D, Patnaik A, et al: Phase I study of oral LBH589, a novel deacetylase (DAC) inhibitor in advanced solid tumors and non-hodgkin's lymphoma. 2007 25:A3500, 2007

[164] Fukutomi A, Hatake K, Matsui K, et al: A phase I study of oral panobinostat (LBH589) in Japanese patients with advanced solid tumors. Invest New Drugs, 2011

[165] Steele NL, Plumb JA, Vidal L, et al: A phase 1 pharmacokinetic and pharmacodynamic study of the histone deacetylase inhibitor belinostat in patients with advanced solid tumors. Clin Cancer Res 14:804-10, 2008

[166] Steele NL, Plumb JA, Vidal L, et al: Pharmacokinetic and pharmacodynamic properties of an oral formulation of the histone deacetylase inhibitor Belinostat (PXD101). Cancer Chemother Pharmacol 67:1273-9, 2011

[167] Rivera-Del Valle N, Gao S, Miller CP, et al: PCI-24781, a Novel Hydroxamic Acid HDAC Inhibitor, Exerts Cytotoxicity and Histone Alterations via Caspase-8 and FADD in Leukemia Cells. Int J Cell Biol 2010:207420, 2010

[168] Ryan QC, Headlee D, Acharya M, et al: Phase I and pharmacokinetic study of MS-275, a histone deacetylase inhibitor, in patients with advanced and refractory solid tumors or lymphoma. J Clin Oncol 23:3912-22, 2005

[169] Kummar S, Gutierrez M, Gardner ER, et al: Phase I trial of MS-275, a histone deacetylase inhibitor, administered weekly in refractory solid tumors and lymphoid malignancies. Clin Cancer Res 13:5411-7, 2007

[170] Siu LL, Pili R, Duran I, et al: Phase I study of MGCD0103 given as a three-times-per-week oral dose in patients with advanced solid tumors. J Clin Oncol 26:1940-7, 2008

[171] Bonfils C, Kalita A, Dubay M, et al: Evaluation of the pharmacodynamic effects of MGCD0103 from preclinical models to human using a novel HDAC enzyme assay. Clin Cancer Res 14:3441-9, 2008

[172] Novotny-Diermayr V, Sangthongpitag K, Hu CY, et al: SB939, a novel potent and orally active histone deacetylase inhibitor with high tumor exposure and efficacy in mouse models of colorectal cancer. Mol Cancer Ther 9:642-52, 2010

[173] Razak AR, Hotte SJ, Siu LL, et al: Phase I clinical, pharmacokinetic and pharmacodynamic study of SB939, an oral histone deacetylase (HDAC) inhibitor, in patients with advanced solid tumours. Br J Cancer 104:756-62, 2011

[174] Yong W, Gob B, Toh H, et al: Phase I study of SB939 three times weekly for 3 weeks every 4 weeks in patients with advanced solid malignancies. J Clin Oncol 27:A2560, 2009

[175] Fantin VR, Richon VM: Mechanisms of resistance to histone deacetylase inhibitors and their therapeutic implications. Clin Cancer Res 13:7237-42, 2007

[176] Otto H, Reche PA, Bazan F, et al: In silico characterization of the family of PARP-like poly(ADP-ribosyl)transferases (pARTs). BMC Genomics 6:139, 2005

[177] Gagne JP, Hendzel MJ, Droit A, et al: The expanding role of poly(ADP-ribose) metabolism: current challenges and new perspectives. Curr Opin Cell Biol 18:145-51, 2006

[178] Yelamos J, Schreiber V, Dantzer F: Toward specific functions of poly(ADP-ribose) polymerase-2. Trends Mol Med 14:169-78, 2008

[179] de Murcia G, Schreiber V, Molinete M, et al: Structure and function of poly(ADP-ribose) polymerase. Mol Cell Biochem 138:15-24, 1994

[180] de Murcia G, Menissier de Murcia J: Poly(ADP-ribose) polymerase: a molecular nick-sensor. Trends Biochem Sci 19:172-6, 1994

[181] Dantzer F, Ame JC, Schreiber V, et al: Poly(ADP-ribose) polymerase-1 activation during DNA damage and repair. Methods Enzymol 409:493-510, 2006

[182] Schreiber V, Dantzer F, Ame JC, et al: Poly(ADP-ribose): novel functions for an old molecule. Nat Rev Mol Cell Biol 7:517-28, 2006

[183] Menissier de Murcia J, Ricoul M, Tartier L, et al: Functional interaction between PARP-1 and PARP-2 in chromosome stability and embryonic development in mouse. EMBO J 22:2255-63, 2003

[184] Farmer H, McCabe N, Lord CJ, et al: Targeting the DNA repair defect in BRCA mutant cells as a therapeutic strategy. Nature 434:917-21, 2005

[185] Xing D, Scangas G, Nitta M, et al: A role for BRCA1 in uterine leiomyosarcoma. Cancer Res 69:8231-5, 2009

[186] Schoffski P, Taron M, Jimeno J, et al: Predictive impact of DNA repair functionality on clinical outcome of advanced sarcoma patients treated with trabectedin: a retrospective multicentric study. Eur J Cancer 47:1006-12, 2011

[187] Turner N, Tutt A, Ashworth A: Hallmarks of 'BRCAness' in sporadic cancers. Nat Rev Cancer 4:814-9, 2004

[188] McCabe N, Turner NC, Lord CJ, et al: Deficiency in the repair of DNA damage by homologous recombination and sensitivity to poly(ADP-ribose) polymerase inhibition. Cancer Res 66:8109-15, 2006

[189] Williamson CT, Muzik H, Turhan AG, et al: ATM deficiency sensitizes mantle cell lymphoma cells to poly(ADP-ribose) polymerase-1 inhibitors. Mol Cancer Ther 9:347-57, 2010

[190] Ul-Hassan A, Sisley K, Hughes D, et al: Common genetic changes in leiomyosarcoma and gastrointestinal stromal tumour: implication for ataxia telangiectasia mutated involvement. Int J Exp Pathol 90:549-57, 2009

[191] Zhang P, Bhakta KS, Puri PL, et al: Association of ataxia telangiectasia mutated (ATM) gene mutation/deletion with rhabdomyosarcoma. Cancer Biol Ther 2:87-91, 2003
[192] Gilad O, Nabet BY, Ragland RL, et al: Combining ATR suppression with oncogenic Ras synergistically increases genomic instability, causing synthetic lethality or tumorigenesis in a dosage-dependent manner. Cancer Res 70:9693-702, 2010
[193] Miller CW, Ikezoe T, Krug U, et al: Mutations of the CHK2 gene are found in some osteosarcomas, but are rare in breast, lung, and ovarian tumors. Genes Chromosomes Cancer 33:17-21, 2002
[194] Amant F, de la Rey M, Dorfling CM, et al: PTEN mutations in uterine sarcomas. Gynecol Oncol 85:165-9, 2002
[195] Lancaster JM, Risinger JI, Carney ME, et al: Mutational analysis of the PTEN gene in human uterine sarcomas. Am J Obstet Gynecol 184:1051-3, 2001
[196] Kawaguchi K, Oda Y, Saito T, et al: DNA hypermethylation status of multiple genes in soft tissue sarcomas. Mod Pathol 19:106-14, 2006
[197] Mendes-Pereira AM, Martin SA, Brough R, et al: Synthetic lethal targeting of PTEN mutant cells with PARP inhibitors. EMBO Mol Med 1:315-22, 2009
[198] Hannay JA, Liu J, Zhu QS, et al: Rad51 overexpression contributes to chemoresistance in human soft tissue sarcoma cells: a role for p53/activator protein 2 transcriptional regulation. Mol Cancer Ther 6:1650-60, 2007
[199] Tentori L, Graziani G: Chemopotentiation by PARP inhibitors in cancer therapy. Pharmacol Res 52:25-33, 2005
[200] Tentori L, Leonetti C, Scarsella M, et al: Inhibition of poly(ADP-ribose) polymerase prevents irinotecan-induced intestinal damage and enhances irinotecan/temozolomide efficacy against colon carcinoma. FASEB J 20:1709-11, 2006
[201] Bernges F, Zeller WJ: Combination effects of poly(ADP-ribose) polymerase inhibitors and DNA-damaging agents in ovarian tumor cell lines--with special reference to cisplatin. J Cancer Res Clin Oncol 122:665-70, 1996
[202] Donawho CK, Luo Y, Penning TD, et al: ABT-888, an orally active poly(ADP-ribose) polymerase inhibitor that potentiates DNA-damaging agents in preclinical tumor models. Clin Cancer Res 13:2728-37, 2007
[203] Fong PC, Boss DS, Yap TA, et al: Inhibition of poly(ADP-ribose) polymerase in tumors from BRCA mutation carriers. N Engl J Med 361:123-34, 2009
[204] Fong PC, Yap TA, Boss DS, et al: Poly(ADP)-ribose polymerase inhibition: frequent durable responses in BRCA carrier ovarian cancer correlating with platinum-free interval. J Clin Oncol 28:2512-9, 2010
[205] Plummer R, Jones C, Middleton M, et al: Phase I study of the poly(ADP-ribose) polymerase inhibitor, AG014699, in combination with temozolomide in patients with advanced solid tumors. Clin Cancer Res 14:7917-23, 2008
[206] Kummar S, Kinders R, Gutierrez ME, et al: Phase 0 clinical trial of the poly (ADP-ribose) polymerase inhibitor ABT-888 in patients with advanced malignancies. J Clin Oncol 27:2705-11, 2009
[207] Sandhu SK, WenHam RM, Wilding G, et al: First-in-human trial of a poly(ADP-ribose) polymerase (PARP) inhibitor MK-4827 in advanced cancer patients (pts) with

antitumor activity in BRCA-deficient and sporadic ovarian cancers. J Clin Oncol 28:A3001, 2010

[208] Lord CJ, Ashworth A: Targeted therapy for cancer using PARP inhibitors. Curr Opin Pharmacol 8:363-9, 2008

[209] Cohen-Armon M, Visochek L, Rozensal D, et al: DNA-independent PARP-1 activation by phosphorylated ERK2 increases Elk1 activity: a link to histone acetylation. Mol Cell 25:297-308, 2007

[210] Pacher P, Liaudet L, Bai P, et al: Activation of poly(ADP-ribose) polymerase contributes to development of doxorubicin-induced heart failure. J Pharmacol Exp Ther 300:862-7, 2002

[211] Bardos G, Moricz K, Jaszlits L, et al: BGP-15, a hydroximic acid derivative, protects against cisplatin- or taxol-induced peripheral neuropathy in rats. Toxicol Appl Pharmacol 190:9-16, 2003

[212] Racz I, Tory K, Gallyas F, Jr., et al: BGP-15 - a novel poly(ADP-ribose) polymerase inhibitor - protects against nephrotoxicity of cisplatin without compromising its antitumor activity. Biochem Pharmacol 63:1099-111, 2002

[213] Dejean LM, Ryu SY, Martinez-Caballero S, et al: MAC and Bcl-2 family proteins conspire in a deadly plot. Biochim Biophys Acta 1797:1231-8, 2010

[214] Kang MH, Reynolds CP: Bcl-2 inhibitors: targeting mitochondrial apoptotic pathways in cancer therapy. Clin Cancer Res 15:1126-32, 2009

[215] Li H, Zhu H, Xu CJ, et al: Cleavage of BID by caspase 8 mediates the mitochondrial damage in the Fas pathway of apoptosis. Cell 94:491-501, 1998

[216] Johnstone RW, Ruefli AA, Lowe SW: Apoptosis: a link between cancer genetics and chemotherapy. Cell 108:153-64, 2002

[217] Leibowitz B, Yu J: Mitochondrial signaling in cell death via the Bcl-2 family. Cancer Biol Ther 9:417-22, 2010

[218] Suster S, Fisher C, Moran CA: Expression of bcl-2 oncoprotein in benign and malignant spindle cell tumors of soft tissue, skin, serosal surfaces, and gastrointestinal tract. Am J Surg Pathol 22:863-72, 1998

[219] Hirakawa N, Naka T, Yamamoto I, et al: Overexpression of bcl-2 protein in synovial sarcoma: a comparative study of other soft tissue spindle cell sarcomas and an additional analysis by fluorescence in situ hybridization. Hum Pathol 27:1060-5, 1996

[220] Kawauchi S, Fukuda T, Oda Y, et al: Prognostic significance of apoptosis in synovial sarcoma: correlation with clinicopathologic parameters, cell proliferative activity, and expression of apoptosis-related proteins. Mod Pathol 13:755-65, 2000

[221] Oda Y, Sakamoto A, Satio T, et al: Molecular abnormalities of p53, MDM2, and H-ras in synovial sarcoma. Mod Pathol 13:994-1004, 2000

[222] Joyner DE, Albritton KH, Bastar JD, et al: G3139 antisense oligonucleotide directed against antiapoptotic Bcl-2 enhances doxorubicin cytotoxicity in the FU-SY-1 synovial sarcoma cell line. J Orthop Res 24:474-80, 2006

[223] Reynoso D, Nolden LK, Yang D, et al: Synergistic induction of apoptosis by the Bcl-2 inhibitor ABT-737 and imatinib mesylate in gastrointestinal stromal tumor cells. Mol Oncol 5:93-104, 2011

[224] Gandhi L, Camidge DR, Ribeiro de Oliveira M, et al: Phase I study of Navitoclax (ABT-263), a novel Bcl-2 family inhibitor, in patients with small-cell lung cancer and other solid tumors. J Clin Oncol 29:909-16, 2011

[225] Wilson W, O'Connor OO, Roberts AW, et al: ABT-263 activity and safety in patients with relapsed or refractory lymphoid malignancies in particular chronic lymphocytic leukemia (CLL)/small lymphocytic lymphoma (SLL). J Clin Oncol 27:A8574, 2009

[226] Rudin CM, Oliveria MR, Garon EB, et al: A phase IIa study of ABT-263 in patients with relapsed small-cell lung cancer (SCLC). J Clin Oncol 28:A7046, 2010

[227] Reya T, Morrison SJ, Clarke MF, et al: Stem cells, cancer, and cancer stem cells. Nature 414:105-11, 2001

[228] Visvader JE, Lindeman GJ: Cancer stem cells in solid tumours: accumulating evidence and unresolved questions. Nat Rev Cancer 8:755-68, 2008

[229] Shackleton M, Quintana E, Fearon ER, et al: Heterogeneity in cancer: cancer stem cells versus clonal evolution. Cell 138:822-9, 2009

[230] Curtin JC, Lorenzi MV: Drug discovery approaches to target Wnt signaling in cancer stem cells. Oncotarget 1:563-77, 2010

[231] Wang Z, Li Y, Banerjee S, et al: Emerging role of Notch in stem cells and cancer. Cancer Lett 279:8-12, 2009

[232] Barker N, Clevers H: Mining the Wnt pathway for cancer therapeutics. Nat Rev Drug Discov 5:997-1014, 2006

[233] Haegebarth A, Clevers H: Wnt signaling, lgr5, and stem cells in the intestine and skin. Am J Pathol 174:715-21, 2009

[234] Willert K, Brown JD, Danenberg E, et al: Wnt proteins are lipid-modified and can act as stem cell growth factors. Nature 423:448-52, 2003

[235] Ingham PW: Hedgehog signaling: a tale of two lipids. Science 294:1879-81, 2001

[236] Tostar U, Malm CJ, Meis-Kindblom JM, et al: Deregulation of the hedgehog signalling pathway: a possible role for the PTCH and SUFU genes in human rhabdomyoma and rhabdomyosarcoma development. J Pathol 208:17-25, 2006

[237] Oue T, Yoneda A, Uehara S, et al: Increased expression of the hedgehog signaling pathway in pediatric solid malignancies. J Pediatr Surg 45:387-92, 2010

[238] Zibat A, Missiaglia E, Rosenberger A, et al: Activation of the hedgehog pathway confers a poor prognosis in embryonal and fusion gene-negative alveolar rhabdomyosarcoma. Oncogene 29:6323-30, 2010

[239] Pressey JG, Anderson JR, Crossman DK, et al: Hedgehog pathway activity in pediatric embryonal rhabdomyosarcoma and undifferentiated sarcoma: A report from the Children's Oncology Group. Pediatr Blood Cancer, 2011

[240] Alakurtti S, Makela T, Koskimies S, et al: Pharmacological properties of the ubiquitous natural product betulin. Eur J Pharm Sci 29:1-13, 2006

[241] Lorusso PM, Jimeno A, Dy GK, et al: Pharmacokinetic dose-scheduling study of hedgehog pathway inhibitor vismodegib (GDC-0449) in patients with locally-advanced or metastatic solid tumors. Clin Cancer Res, 2011

[242] LoRusso PM, Rudin CM, Reddy JC, et al: Phase I trial of hedgehog pathway inhibitor vismodegib (GDC-0449) in patients with refractory, locally advanced or metastatic solid tumors. Clin Cancer Res 17:2502-11, 2011

[243] Von Hoff DD, LoRusso PM, Rudin CM, et al: Inhibition of the hedgehog pathway in advanced basal-cell carcinoma. N Engl J Med 361:1164-72, 2009

[244] Rudin CM, Hann CL, Laterra J, et al: Treatment of medulloblastoma with hedgehog pathway inhibitor GDC-0449. N Engl J Med 361:1173-8, 2009

[245] Rodon Ahnert J, Basalga J, Tawbi HA, et al: A phase I dose-escalation study of LDE225, a smoothened (Smo) antagonist, in patients with advanced solid tumors. J Clin Oncol 28:A2500, 2010

[246] Siu LL, Papdopoulos K, Alberta SR, et al: A first-in-human, phase I study of an oral hedgehog (HH) pathway antagonist, BMS-833923 (XL139), in subjects with advanced or metastatic solid tumors. J Clin Oncol 28:A2501, 2010

[247] Rudin CM, Jimeno A, Miller WH, et al: A phase I study of IPI-926, a novel hedgehog pathway inhibitor, in patients (pts) with advanced or metastatic solid tumors. J Clin Oncol 29:A3014, 2011

[248] Artavanis-Tsakonas S, Rand MD, Lake RJ: Notch signaling: cell fate control and signal integration in development. Science 284:770-6, 1999

[249] Greenwald I: LIN-12/Notch signaling: lessons from worms and flies. Genes Dev 12:1751-62, 1998

[250] Roma J, Masia A, Reventos J, et al: Notch pathway inhibition significantly reduces rhabdomyosarcoma invasiveness and mobility in vitro. Clin Cancer Res 17:505-13, 2011

[251] Curry CL, Reed LL, Golde TE, et al: Gamma secretase inhibitor blocks Notch activation and induces apoptosis in Kaposi's sarcoma tumor cells. Oncogene 24:6333-44, 2005

[252] Nusse R, Varmus HE: Wnt genes. Cell 69:1073-87, 1992

[253] Cadigan KM, Nusse R: Wnt signaling: a common theme in animal development. Genes Dev 11:3286-305, 1997

[254] Van der Flier LG, Sabates-Bellver J, Oving I, et al: The Intestinal Wnt/TCF Signature. Gastroenterology 132:628-32, 2007

[255] Clevers H, Batlle E: EphB/EphrinB receptors and Wnt signaling in colorectal cancer. Cancer Res 66:2-5, 2006

[256] Clevers H: Wnt/beta-catenin signaling in development and disease. Cell 127:469-80, 2006

[257] Rao TP, Kuhl M: An updated overview on Wnt signaling pathways: a prelude for more. Circ Res 106:1798-806, 2010

[258] Vijayakumar S, Liu G, Rus IA, et al: High-frequency canonical Wnt activation in multiple sarcoma subtypes drives proliferation through a TCF/beta-catenin target gene, CDC25A. Cancer Cell 19:601-12, 2011

[259] Ng TL, Gown AM, Barry TS, et al: Nuclear beta-catenin in mesenchymal tumors. Mod Pathol 18:68-74, 2005

[260] Hasegawa T, Yokoyama R, Matsuno Y, et al: Prognostic significance of histologic grade and nuclear expression of beta-catenin in synovial sarcoma. Hum Pathol 32:257-63, 2001

[261] Saito T, Oda Y, Sakamoto A, et al: APC mutations in synovial sarcoma. J Pathol 196:445-9, 2002

[262] Sakamoto A, Oda Y, Adachi T, et al: Beta-catenin accumulation and gene mutation in exon 3 in dedifferentiated liposarcoma and malignant fibrous histiocytoma. Arch Pathol Lab Med 126:1071-8, 2002

[263] He B, You L, Uematsu K, et al: A monoclonal antibody against Wnt-1 induces apoptosis in human cancer cells. Neoplasia 6:7-14, 2004

[264] Mikami I, You L, He B, et al: Efficacy of Wnt-1 monoclonal antibody in sarcoma cells. BMC Cancer 5:53, 2005

[265] Bafico A, Liu G, Yaniv A, et al: Novel mechanism of Wnt signalling inhibition mediated by Dickkopf-1 interaction with LRP6/Arrow. Nat Cell Biol 3:683-6, 2001

[266] Dann CE, Hsieh JC, Rattner A, et al: Insights into Wnt binding and signalling from the structures of two Frizzled cysteine-rich domains. Nature 412:86-90, 2001

Part 5

Prognosis of Soft Tissue Tumors

13

Prognostic Factors in Soft Tissue Sarcoma

Luiz Eduardo Moreira Teixeira,
Jose Carlos Vilela and Ivana Duval De Araujo
Federal University of Minas Gerais
Brazil

1. Introduction

Soft tissue sarcoma (STS) represents a heterogeneous group of mesenchymal malignant tumors with variable natural history. This term was first introduced to describe a circumscribed neoplasm consisting of malignant fat cell occurring principally in the trunk (Abernethy, 1817). Nowadays, more than 30 types of STS have been described, and many of these present innumerable subtypes. Despite this wide range of entities, they represent less than 1% of all types of cancer, but still one of the most therapeutically challenging group of tumor (Choong & Rudiger, 2008). Surgery is the keystone of treatment, associated or not to adjuvant method, and the two aims are avoid metastatic spread and local relapse.

Despite advances in local control of the sarcomas, the metastatic disease, which is the cause of death for most patients, presents little recent advances. In fact, 10% of patients have metastasis at the diagnosis and 25% with localized disease will develop distant spread (Delaney et al, 1991). The systemic disease occurs primarily by hematogenic spread, and the lungs are the most common distant organs involved by the distant metastasis. Some subtypes demonstrated predilection for lymphatic route of dissemination such as synovial sarcoma and epithelioid sarcoma while the alveolar sarcoma targets the brain involvement.

In contrast to bone sarcomas, soft tissue malignancies do not respond well to chemotherapies schemes. This may be explained by the diversities of subgroups or by different factors that affect the prognosis. Therefore, the difficult in treating soft tissue sarcomas is determinate which patients will need the adjuvant chemotherapy or radiation therapy. The indication of these methods is guided by factors that predict the risk of metastatic disease or local recurrence. These factors are called prognostic factors and the purpose of this chapter is to define the different prognostic factors of soft tissue sarcoma.

As a heterogeneous group, the behavior and natural evolution of this tumor are variable, but, in general aspects the metastatic spreading is observed in about one third of the patients, local relapse is seen in 10% to 30% and the global 5-year survival is 60%. Different factors are reported in the literature such as tumor grade, size, location, vascular invasion, histological necrosis and presence of cytogenetic markers. However, the importance of each factor is unclear. In this chapter we will discuss each prognostic factor including: age, sex, location, size, subtype, histological aspects, grade, surgical manipulation, recurrence, imunohistochemical pattern, genetic and gene markers.

In this chapter the prognostic factors can be separated into three categories: patient factors, tumor factors and treatment factors.

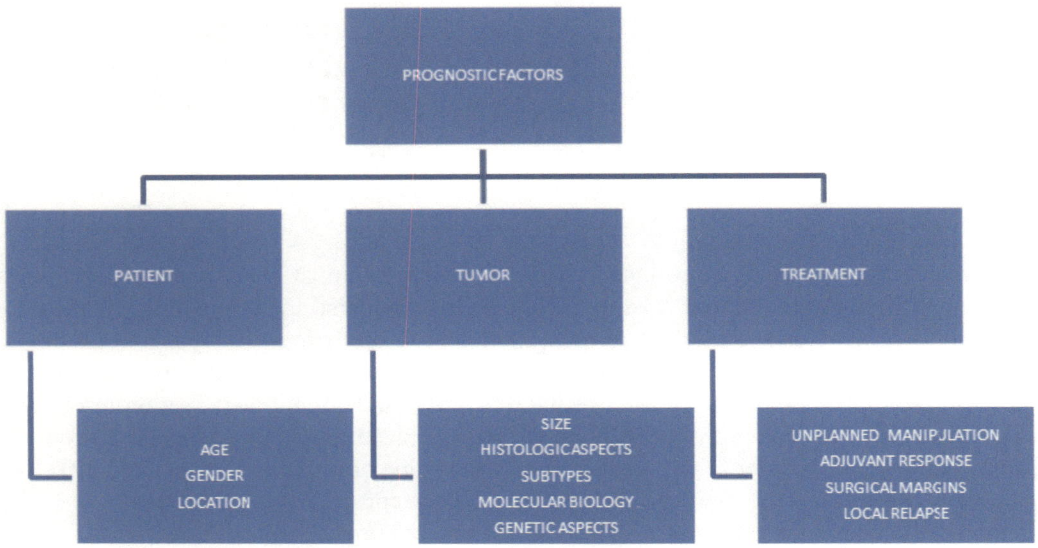

Fig. 1. Resume of prognostic factor of soft tissue Sarcoma

2. Prognostic factors

2.1 Patient factors

The factors in the literature related to patients are: age, gender and tumor localization. In some studies, patients older than 50 years and male are associated with a bad prognostic (Gustafson et al. , 1994). Nevertheless, these factors have not been proven of value in predicting the risk for local recurrence and metastasis. Although the shorter survival observed in the elderly, this seems to be related to tumor size and aggressiveness in this age group 35, 36. Even if gender and age had some importance, this seems to be a minor one. (Teixeira et al., 2009)

Localization has also been evaluated as a prognostic factor, according to the segment involved, depth or the site related to the anatomical compartments. The depth in relation to the muscle fascia is considered a relevant factor for the prognosis, being included in some prognostic systems as the AJCC/UICC. However, some studies doubt the validity of depth as an isolated factor of worse prognosis, they have found the same survival rate when the tumors are adjusted by the histological malignancy and size (Rydholm & Gustafson, 2003).

The extra compartmental localization also seems to be associated with a bad prognostic. The tumors considered extra compartmental usually present more difficult surgical treatment and thinner margins, provided that they are in close contact to neurovascular structures. Both, the difficult to obtain proper margins and the fact that they are situated in areas with rich vascularization and lymphatic drainage help to systemic disseminate and local recur, which may explain the results obtained by some studies. (Teixeira et al., 2009)
More proximal tumors, situated in the scapular or pelvic girdle, in general present delayed diagnosis and a bigger size, thus a worse prognosis. On the other side, more distal tumors present longer survival rate, but many times they require amputations in order to achieve the desired surgical margin. Some studies pointed out a survival rate of 47%, with a local recurrence of 35% in tumors of the gluteus area, while tumors in hands and feet present a survival rate between 80% and 82% in five years and a local recurrence rate between 17% and 21% (Behranwala et al., 2004). Despite the disparity in the survival and local recurrence rates, the risk does not seem to be associated with the localization but with the size of the tumor in the moment of the diagnostic, as long as distal tumors tend to present earlier and smaller.

2.2 Tumor's factors

The factors associated with tumors seem to be the most important ones to determine the prognostic of systemic spread. Among them, we call special attention for size, histological and genetic aspects and the histological subtypes.

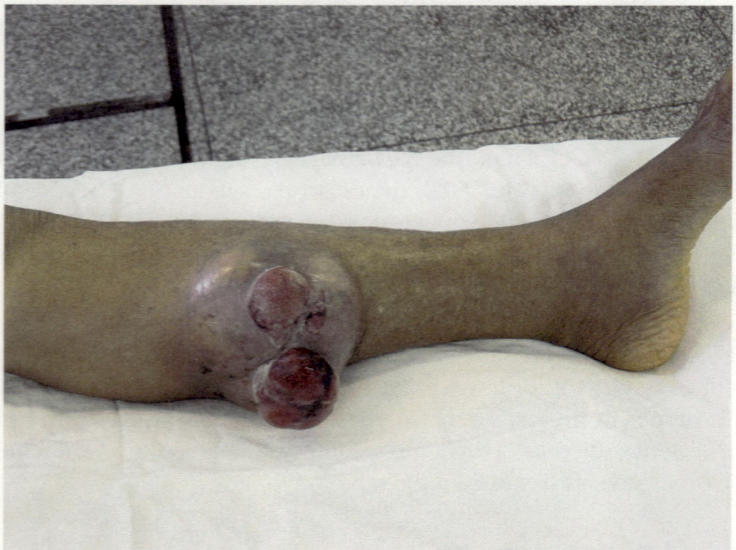

Fig. 2. Large tumors representing an adverse effect in survival

The size of the tumor is implicated as an important factor for systemic disease and local recurrence. However, there is no consensus determining the cutoff for groups at high risk. Some clinical trials use 5cm, 8cm or 10cm as the cutoff. In general, the growth of 5cm in the tumor size increases the risk for metastasis 1.5 times (Trovik et al., 1994). Provided that, the tumors bigger than 5 cm should been considered as possessing a worse prognostic.

The histologic grading is a method for stratifying STS into groups of different prognosis based on histological aspects such as cellularity, atypia, mitotic index, necrosis, pleomorphism and histotype. Most of studies show that high grade of malignancy possess a strong influence in developing metastasis and local recurrence, being one of the most important independent factors related to the aggressiveness of the STS. However, the lack of universal classification, the inaccuracy of each histological component, the examiner subjectivity and the different grades of aggressiveness of each histological subtypes reduce the reproducibility. The combination of these factors creates several grading systems and prognostic models. Some schemes, such as that of the American Joint Committee on Cancer (AJCC), have also included nodal involvement. The most widely used grading systems include those proposed by the *French Federation Nationale des Centres de Lutte Contre le Cancer* (FNCLCC) and the National Cancer Institute (NCI), the staging system established by the AJCC, and a sarcoma-specific mortality nomogram developed at the Memorial Sloan-Kettering Cancer Center (MSKCC). Despite of this, the high-grade histologic aspect of the tumor must be considered one of most determinant factor in overall survival.

Among the specific histologic aspects, vascular invasion and necrosis seem the most important one as an isolated prognostic factor. Vascular invasion represents a well-established prognostic factor in several tumor types, including malignant melanoma, papillary thyroid cancer, endometrial cancer, and testicular cancer. In STS, vascular invasion has repeatedly shown prognostic value, but it is generally not applied systematically in pathological evaluations. Vascular invasion has been identified with variable prevalence in different studies, which may hamper its clinical application. Tumor necrosis has repeatedly been established as a negative prognostic factor in STS.23,30-34 It also represents an important factor in the FNCLCC and the NCI grading systems, which apply cutoff values of 15% (microscopic evaluation) and 50% (macroscopic evaluation), respectively. A more recent histologic find used in the STS grading is the pattern of growth. Growth pattern was classified as pushing or infiltrative, irrespective of the extent of infiltration. Soft tissue tumors with microscopically infiltrative pattern of growing have a significantly higher risk for local and systemic recurrence compared with a "pushing" growth pattern.

The histologic subtypes was previously not considered a important factor in the prognosis of patients with STS, but the differences in response to adjuvant treatments improve the value of the histotypes in predicting metastatic spreading. Some subtypes have a high risk to develop distant disease such as synovial sarcoma, epithelioid sarcoma, rhabdomyosarcoma and soft tissue Ewing`s sarcoma

2.2.1 Genetics and molecular aspects

Prognostication for adults with STS is primarily based on tumor size, histologic grade, depth, location, histologic subtype, and the presence or absence of distant metastasis. However, recent studies suggest that proliferation markers may improve the prognostic value of standard clinical-pathologic markers. These studies evaluated the DNA activity, antigen markers and oncogenes. The first studies have shown that tumor cell proliferative activity and/or DNA content are related to the outcome of patients with STS. Several methods have been used to assess cell proliferation, including enumeration of mitotic figures, thymidine labeling indices, DNA-flow cytometric analysis, and immunohistochemical analysis of proteins associated with proliferation. Furthermore, multivariate analysis revealed that DNA content was an independent prognostic indicator. The widespread availability of DNA analysis by flow cytometry and image analysis, as well as the magnitude of the difference in predicting survival, suggest that DNA analysis may be useful clinically, for example in selecting candidates for adjuvant systemic therapy. However, such statement will require further study (Levine, 1999). .

The second aspect is histological markers. The most studied is Ki-67, an antigen described in 1983 as a human nuclear antigen associated with cellular proliferation. Ki-67 expression has been found related to other proliferation markers and to p53 mutations. To date, the threshold value of immunohistochemical staining for Ki-67 expression that defines a high-risk lesion for Ki-67 expression is unclear, but is observed in 40% as a "positive" level of expression. Although his prognostic significance is unclear, it has been associated with prognosis (Ueda *et al.* 1989).

The third aspect is the effect of oncogenes. The oncogenes most studied are p53, ras gene family, myc, and the RB1.

The p53 gene, located on human chromosome 17p13, encodes a nuclear phosphoprotein involved in transcriptional regulation, translational control, DNA repair, cell cycle control, cell differentiation, and apoptosis. The p53 gene is the most commonly mutated gene in human solid tumors (Bartek *et al.*, 1991), its mutant expression is observed in about 61% of patients with STS (Wadayama *et al.*, 1993) and is associated with poor prognosis for distant spread, disease free-survival and drug resistance. Although its clinical validity is unclear.

The ras gene family consists of three genes located on chromosomes 1,11, and 12. Several small series of STS have shown low incidence of ras mutations in the range of 3% to 35%. Although ras mutations are demonstrable in some types of STS, it is doubtful that this represents the original stimulation for malignant transformation or a clinically useful prognostic marker.

The myc oncogene encodes the production of a nuclear phosphoprotein, which binds to DNA and can transform cells both in vitro and in vivo [50]. This gene is normally a single copy on chromosome 2. Amplification myc has been shown to be a poor prognostic indicator for children with neuroblastoma. Several reports have been published of myc expression in STS (Dias *et al.*, 1990). In a study of rhabdomyosarcomas, another report suggested that myc amplification is limited to the alveolar subtype. A study of 23 STS cases found myc amplification in 30% and suggested it was correlated with higher grade and poorer survival [54]. Although the data for myc expression/ amplification suggest a putative relationship between myc with progression and survival, confirmatory studies are needed before validating myc as a prognostic factor in routine clinical practice (Barrios *et al.*, 1994).

The c-erbB2 is located on human chromosome17 and encodes a transmembrane protein (p185) which has remarkable homology with the epidermal growth factor receptor (EGFR).

Few reports have analyzed c-erbB2 amplifications or overexpression in STS. Amplification in STS seems to be unusual, occurring in only six of 105 cases in one report (. No studies have attached clinical significance to c-erbB2 amplification and/or overexpression. Furthermore, the low rates of c-erbB2 alterations do not suggest a role in the initiation or progression of STS.

The human retinoblastoma gene, RB1, located on chromosome 13, is another tumor suppressor gene involved in the genesis of STS. Germline's mutations of RB1 result in the hereditary form of retinoblastoma. In addition, somatic mutations of this gene and/or absent p110RB protein expression have been observed in various human tumors and tumor cell lines. Alterations in RB1 or p110RB protein expression have been observed in up to 70% of the STS studied, but do not appear to consistently have clinical prognostic value (Karpeh *et al.*,1995).

2.3 Treatment factor

Although STSs do not have a good response as for bone sarcomas, some subtypes can be treated with chemotherapy schemes. Systemic chemotherapy is considered the only therapeutic option for patients presenting with widely metastatic disease or with locally advanced disease not amenable to surgery or radiotherapy. For the majority of these patients, cytotoxic chemotherapy should be regarded as palliative, although in a small subset of patients long-term survival may be achieved. The standard chemotherapy is doxorubicin-based therapy, but others subtypes have a good response to ifosfamide like synovial sarcoma. Rhabdomyosarcoma, soft tissue Ewing`s sarcoma and others round cell soft tissue tumors have good response to this adjuvant treatment. So the response to the treatment can be used as a prognostic factor, but the clinical use is still unclear.

Other question concerning the influence of the treatment in the prognosis is the previous manipulation of the tumor by an unplanned resection. Many times patient and the assistant physician came across a diagnosis of an unsuspected sarcoma after a lump resection. This manipulation can spread cell tumor. We consider that the clinical problems following an unplanned resection of a sarcoma are more dependent of the technical difficulties concerning the oncological surgery principles when reoperating the patient than the malignance of the tumor itself. If the salvage treatment could be performed appropriately, the oncological outcomes may not be influenced.

Another topic is the effects of a local recurrence in the survival and metastatic disease. There is little doubt in the literature that local relapse is associated with a worse prognosis. The unsolved issue is whether local relapse is causative. The occurrence of local relapse per se might favor the systemic spread of disease and, therefore, directly affect survival, or it might simply be a marker of biological tumor aggressiveness. Theoretically, the two mechanisms may coexist and possibly interact, with both contributing to the outcome. Some patients had a local relapse after surgery performed at nonreferral centers, with unplanned resections with marginal or intralesional margins. Others, relapse even with wide margins and planned procedure. In the last cases, the recurrence suggests an aggressive sarcoma and probably is associated with worse prognosis. If tumor aggressiveness could be objectively assessed initially, a different surgical policy might be justified from the very beginning (Gronchi et al., 2007).

3. Conclusion

Soft tissue sarcomas have many factors that can influence the overall survival of the patients. These factors are related to the patients, tumor and treatment. To achieve the best possible result, the physician must take all of them in consideration and try to control the factors that have influence in the outcome and are possible to be handled to minimize the effects of the others witch he can´t modify.

4. References

Albernethy J. Surgical Aberrations. J Surgical Aberrations 1817, 2, 17 - 30.

Barrios C, Castresana JS, Kriecbergs A: Clinicopathologic correlations and short-term prognosis in musculoskeletal sarcoma with cmyc oncogene amplification. Am J Clin Oncol 1994;17:273–276.

Bartek J, Bartkova J, Vojtesek B, et al: Aberrant expression of the p53 oncoprotein is a common feature of a wide spectrum of human malignancies. Oncogene 1991;6:1699–1703.

Behranwala KA, A´Hern R, Omar A, Thomas M. Prognosis of lymph node metastasis in soft tissue sarcoma. Ann Surg Oncol 2004, 11(7): 714 - 719.

Choong PFM, Rudiguer HA. Prognostic fator in soft tissue sarcoma: what have we learned? Expert Rev Anticancer Ther, 8(2): 139-146, 2008.

Delaney T, Yang J, Glatstein E. Adjuvant Therapies for adult patients with soft tissue sarcoma. Oncology 5, 105-118, 1991.

Dias P, Kumar P, Marsden HB, et al: N-myc gene is amplified in alveolar rhabdomyosarcomas (RMS) but not in embryonal RMS. Int J Cancer 1990;45:593–596.

Gustafson P, Dreinhofer K, Ryldhom A. Soft tissue sarcoma should be treated at a tumor center. A comparison of quality of surgery in 375 patients. Acta Orthop Scand. 1994; 65: 47-50.

Karpeh MS, Brennan MF, Cance WG, et al: Altered patterns of retinoblastoma gene product expression in adult soft-tissue sarcomas. Br J Cancer 1995;72:986–991.

Levine EA. Prognostic Factors in Soft Tissue Sarcoma. Semin. Surg. Oncol. 17:23–32, 1999.

Rydholm A and Gustafson P. Should tumor depth be included in prognostication of soft tissue sarcoma? BMC Cancer 2003, 3:17 (http: //www.biomedcentral.com/1471-2407/3/17).

Teixeira LE, Araújo ID, de Andrade MA, Gomes RA, Salles PG, Ghedini DF. Local recurrence in soft tissue sarcoma: prognostic factors. Rev Col Bras Cir 2009, 36(5):377-81.

Trovik CS, Bauer HC Local recurrence of soft tissue sarcoma a risk factor for late metastases. 379 patients followed for 0.5 - 20 years. Acta Orthop Scand 1994, 65: 553 -558.

Uda RB, Cundiff D, August CZ, et al: Growth factor receptor andrelated oncogene determination in mesenchymal tumors. Cancer1993;71:3526–3530.

Ueda T, Aozasa K, Tsujimoto M, et al: Prognostic significance of Ki-67 reactivity in soft tissue sarcomas. Cancer 1989;63:1607–1611.

Wadayama B, Toguchida J, Yamaguchi T, et al: p53 expression and its relationship to DNA alterations in bone and soft tissue sarcomas. Br J Cancer 1993;68:1134–1139.

14

Metastatis of Soft Tissue Sarcomas

Fethi Derbel et al.*
Department of Surgery, University Hospital Sahloul, Sousse
Tunisia

1. Introduction

Although soft-tissue sarcomas account for <1% of all malignancies, they represent a high percentage of cancer-related deaths worldwide [1]. These tumors may arise in virtually any anatomic site, but most originate in an extremity (59%), the trunk (19%), the retroperitoneum (15%), or the head and neck (9%) [2]. Currently, more than 50 histologic types of soft tissue sarcoma have been identified, but the most common are malignant fibrous histiocytoma (28%), leiomyosarcoma (12%), liposarcoma (15%), synovial sarcoma (10%), and malignant peripheral nerve sheath tumors (6%) [3]. Rhabdomyosarcoma is the most common soft tissue sarcoma of childhood.

2. The role of the pathology

As part of the evaluation by a specialist multidisciplinary team, accurate histological characterisation is essential before initiating treatment. The mainstay of diagnosis is histological interpretation±immunohistochemistry, although cytogenetic and molecular genetics investigations and, occasionally, electron microscopy are useful ancillary tools. Cytological analysis of fine-needle aspirates has a limited role in primary diagnosis, but can be used to confirm recurrent disease, or nodal metastases.

The histopathology report is an interpretation based on tumour morphology and immunoprofile in the available sampled tissue, and clinicopathological correlation is mandatory.

Diagnosis is most frequently made on needle core biopsy material, and tumour subtype and grade can be determined in about 80% of core biopsies [4], although pathologists experienced in examining soft tissue tumours have a diagnostic accuracy of 95-99% [4,5]. The amount of tissue can be a limitation, as the biopsy may not represent the entire, frequently heterogeneous tumour, or may miss the tumour. For this reason, correlation

* Sonia Ziadi[1], Medi Ben Hadj Hamida[2], Jaafar Mazhoud[2], Mohamed Ben Mabrouk[2], Abdallah Mtimet[2], Sabri Youssef[2], Ajmi Chaouch[3], Ali Ben Ali[2], Ibtissam Hasni[4], Mrad Dali Kaouthar[4], Jemni Hela[4], Moncef Mokni[1] and Ridha Ben Hadj Hamida[2]

[1]*Department of Pathology, University Hospital Farhat Hached, Sousse, Tunisia*
[2]*Department of Surgery, University Hospital Sahloul, Sousse, Tunisia*
[3]*Department of Anesthesiology and Intensive Care, University Hospital Sahloul, Sousse, Tunisia*
[4]*Department of Medical Imaging, University Hospital Sahloul Sousse, Tunisia*

between the clinicoradiological features and the histopathology report is essential, and rebiopsy considered if there is any discrepancy.

The mitotic count, amount of necrosis and degree of cellular atypia can be underrepresented in biopsies, and a significant proportion of tumours are upgraded after subsequent resection.

The limitations of histology should be appreciated. There is notable morphological overlap between different groups of malignant tumours, with different clinical behaviours and therapeutic responses.

Some tumours are resected after neoadjuvant chemotherapy, or post-adjuvant chemotherapy or radiation. Post-treatment changes include stromal fibrosis and tumoral infarct, the latter difficult to distinguish from necrosis, making grading difficult. Radiation can cause reactive atypia of stromal fibroblasts, obscuring distinction between tumour and stromal tissue.

The clinical behavior of most soft tissue sarcomas is similar and, as defined by the staging system, is determined by the anatomic location (depth), grade, and size of the tumor. The histologic grade of a soft tissue sarcoma remains the most important prognostic factor.

The features that define the grade are the degree of cellularity, differentiation, pleomorphism, and necrosis as well as the number of mitoses. Certain tumors have an assigned grade based on the histologic diagnosis (eg, Grade 1 for well-differentiated liposarcomas; Grade 3 for rhabdomyosarcoma).

3. Metastasis of sarcomas

The current American Joint Committee on Cancer (AJCC) staging criteria for soft tissue sarcomas rely on the histologic grade, the tumor size and depth, and the presence of distant or nodal metastases [6]. In the 2002 AJCC staging system, four tumor grades are designated: well differentiated (G1), moderately differentiated (G2), poorly differentiated (G3), and undifferentiated (G4). In this four-tiered system, Grades 1 and 2 are considered low grade and Grades 3 and 4 are considered high grade [6]. Some recommend using other grading systems based on necrosis [7]or mitoses and necrosis [8].

The metastatic potentials for soft tissue sarcomas by grade are as follows: 5% to 10% for low-grade lesions, 25% to 30% for intermediate grade lesions, and 50% to 60% for high-grade tumors [9].

Superficial sarcomas are generally less aggressive than their deeper counterparts; for example, atypical fatty tumours in the subcutis do not metastasise or dedifferentiate and rarely recur, unlike similar intramuscular or retroperitoneal tumours [10].

The dominant pattern of metastasis is hematogenous. Lymph node metastasis of soft tissue sarcomas is rare; less than 5% show nodal spread. A few histologic subtypes, including rhabdomyosarcoma, epithelioid sarcoma, synovial sarcoma, angiosarcoma, clear cell sarcoma, and malignant fibrous histiocytoma, show a higher incidence of nodal involvement (10% to 20%) [11]. Alveolar rhabdomyosarcoma can present with widespread nodal as well as bone marrow metastases. Myxoid liposarcoma is known for metastasizing to other soft tissue sites [10].

Distant metastases occur most often to the lung. Of patients with extremity sarcoma, approximately 20% will have isolated pulmonary metastatic disease at some point in the course of their disease [12]. Although pulmonary metastases most commonly arise from

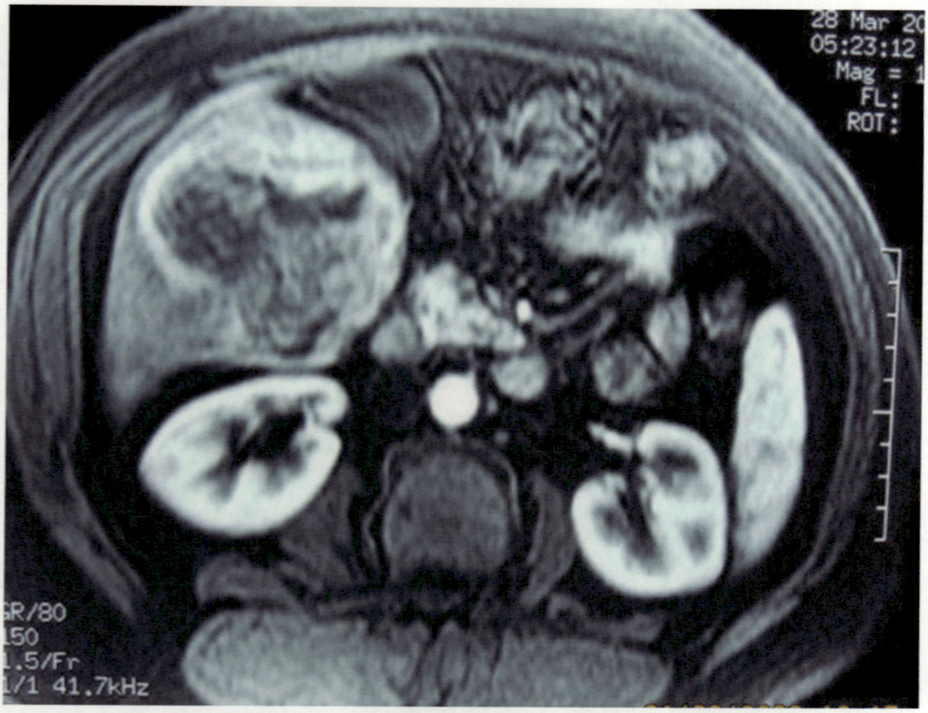

Fig. 1. Abdominal magnetic resonance imaging showing a 5-cm hepatic mass of segment V [26].

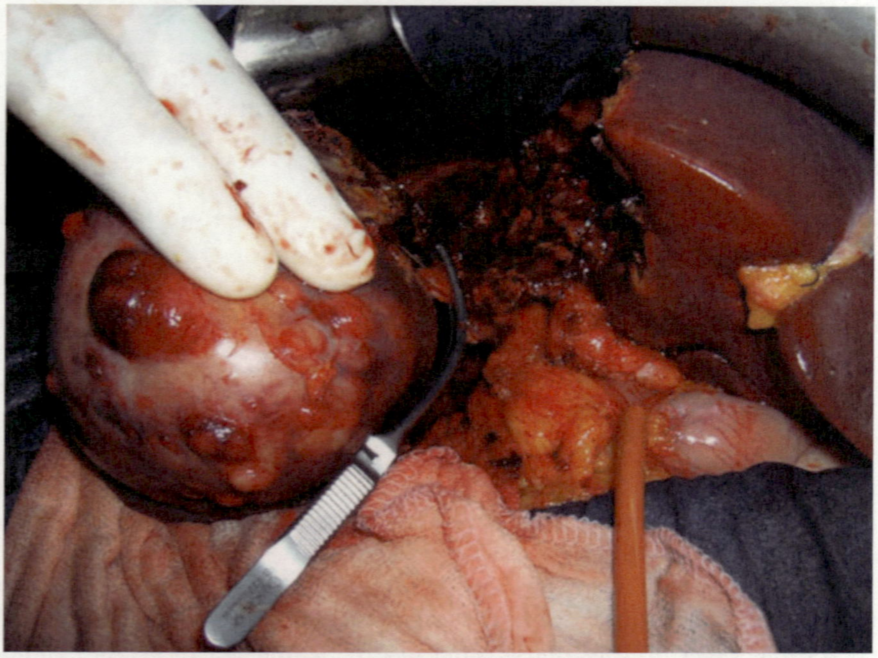

Fig. 2. Operative view showing a large firm mass in segments V and VI of the liver [26].

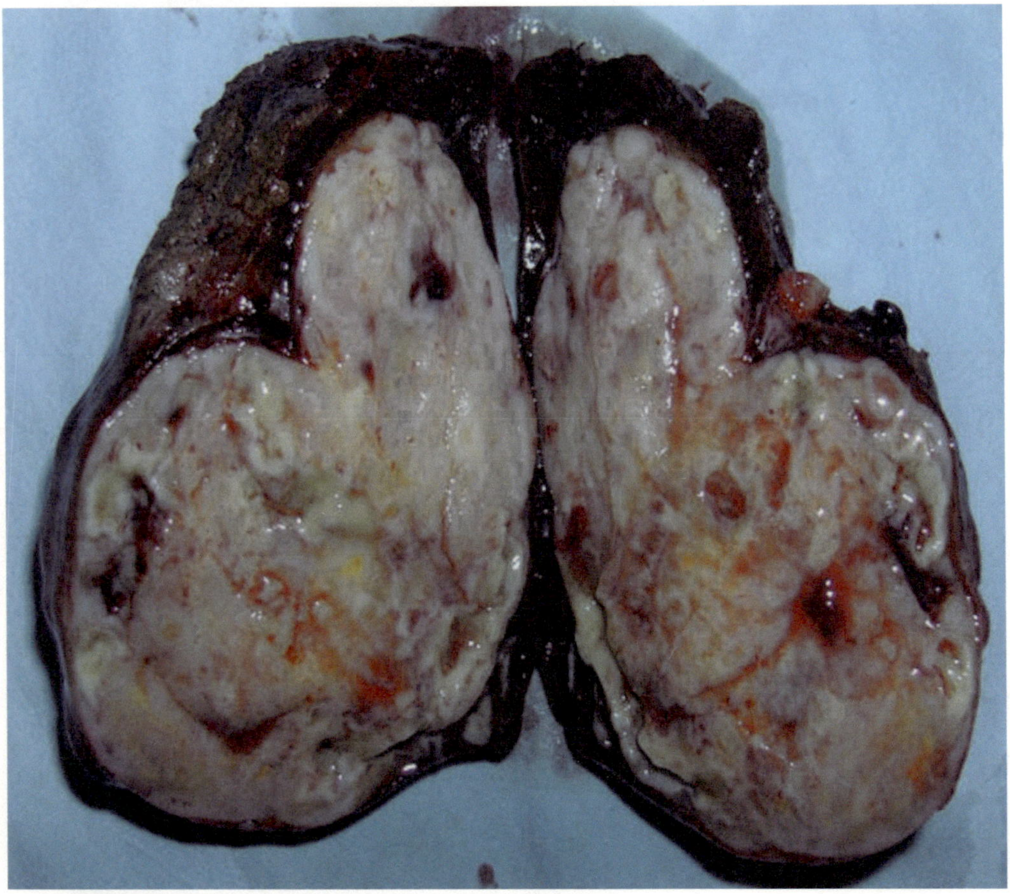

Fig. 3. Section in the mass in segments V and VI [26].

primary tumors in the extremities, they may arise from almost any histologic variant or primary site [13]. Extrapulmonary metastases usually appear after lung metastasis and represent disseminated disease [14]. Initial metastases to other sites such as the liver, brain, and soft tissue distant from the primary tumor are rare [15, 16]. In our study, we report one case of liver metastases of malignant fibrous histiocytoma[fig 1-4]. Pezzi et al. reported that most metastases of MFH occurred in the lungs (90%), followed by bone (8%). However, liver metastases of this tumour are very rare (1%) [24] [26].

Liposarcoma has a documented tendency for spread to distant extrapulmonary sites other than regional lymph nodes [17, 18, 19]. Cheng et al [17] reported on 60 patients with extremity liposarcoma, of which 22 developed metastases. Of these 22 liposarcoma patients, 13 had exclusively extrapulmonary disease on recurrence.

Distant soft tissue was the most common location of unusual initial spread reported by Cheng et al, including the brain and abdomen [17]. Many investigators have noted an increased prevalence of myxoid liposarcoma to exhibit unusual metastases compared to other subtypes of liposarcoma [19].

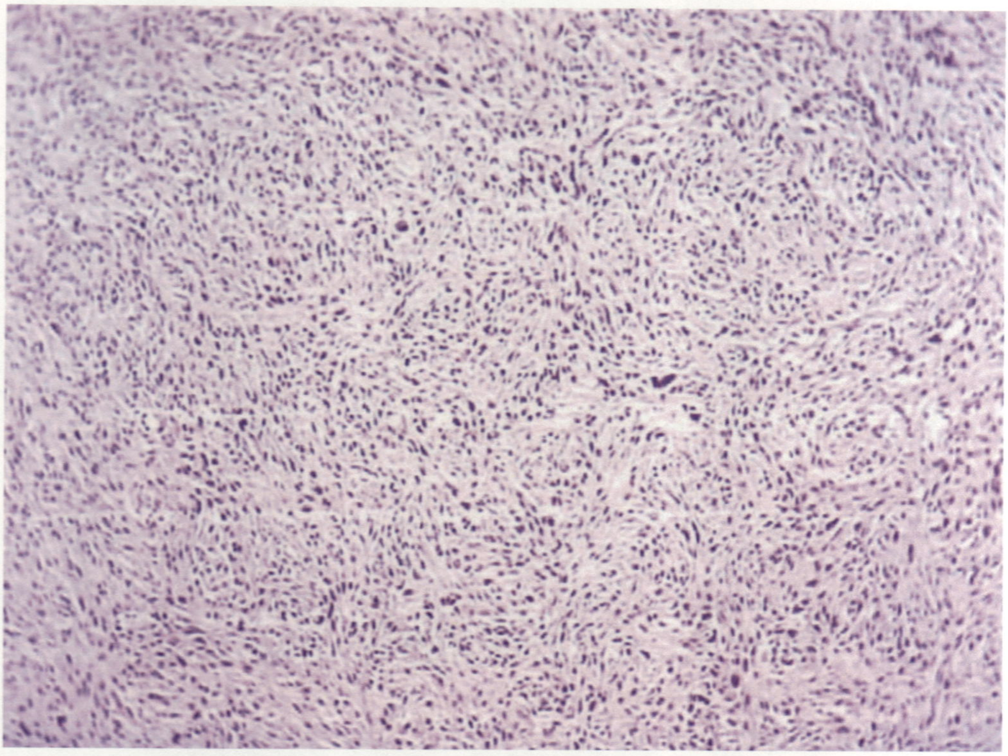

Fig. 4. Histological examination showing spindle-shaped and pleomorphic malignant cells intermingled with bizarre giant cells and inflammatory cells with a storiform pattern [26].

Other large series including all histologic types of high-grade sarcoma have reported unusual metastatic patterns. Potter et al found 15 distant extrapulmonary metastases in their series of 563 patients (2.7%) [20]. Vezeridis et al [21] also documented extrapulmonary distant metastases, but both of these studies were failing to demonstrate a consistent pattern in terms of anatomic location of the initial unusual metastatic site.

In our experience, over a period of 10 years (1998-2007), 13,737 cases of cancer are registered in the central region of Tunisia. 357 (2.6%) cases are soft tissue sarcomas, and 40 (11.2%) of them were diagnosed with metastatic disease.

Histological types who give most metastases are synovial sarcoma, stromal tumor and undifferentiated sarcoma (Table No. I). The lung was the most common site of metastatic sarcomas.

Postulating that soft-tissue sarcomas metastasize via the venous system may account for the predominance of distant recurrence in the lungs. The mechanism of extrapulmonary metastasis is less clear. In 1946, Tedeschi [22] proposed the concept of pluricentric anlage, referring to systemically altered lipid metabolism causing stimulation of undifferentiated mesenchymal cells to explain patients he observed with fatty tumors in multiple soft-tissue locations. While this concept has been used to explain the development of multiple subcutaneous nodules in patients with neurofibromatosis, it seems to be a less robust explanation for the usual clinical course of sarcoma [23]. The mechanism of unusual distant metastasis remains obscure.

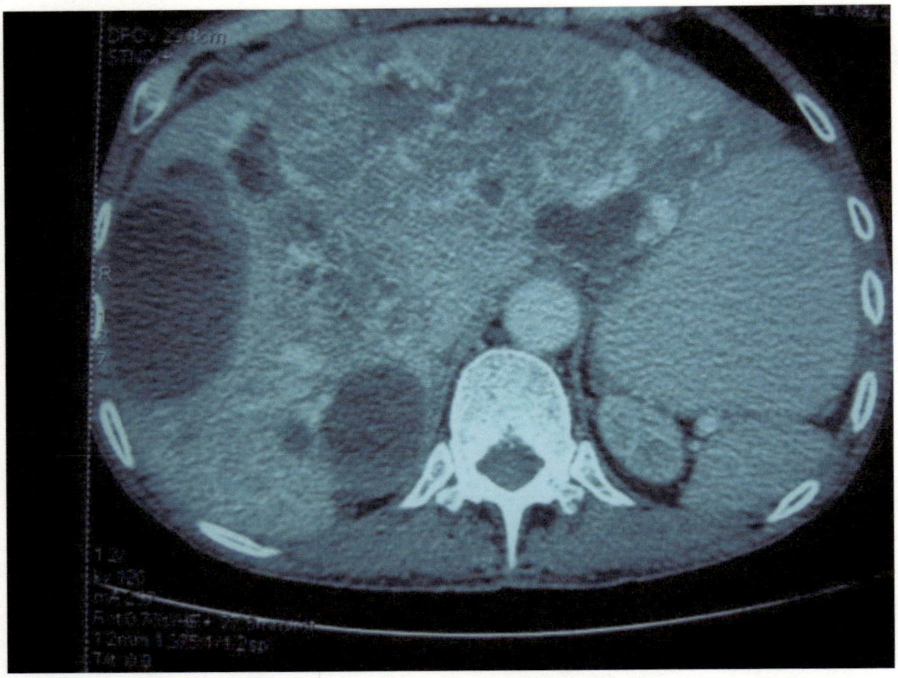

Fig. 5. Abdominal CT scan showing multiple cystic metastasis of a GIST with intracystic enhancing nodules

Histologic type	All of cases	Sarcomas Stage IV	Metastatic site
Undifferentiated sarcoma	**82**	**11** (13,41%)	Lung (6), liver (5), bone (1), lymph node (1)
stromal tumor (GIST)	**33**	**7** (21.21%)	liver (6), peritonium (1)
Synovialosarcoma	**21**	**6** (28.57%)	Lung (6), bone (2)
Leiomyosarcoma	**26**	**5** (19.23%)	Lung (6), bone (2), lymph node (1)
Ewing sarcoma	**7**	**3** (42.85%)	Lung (3), brain (1)
Rhabdomyosarcoma	**23**	**3** (13%)	Lung (1), peritonium (2)
Malignant fibrous histiocytoma	**25**	**2** (8%)	peritonium (1), lymph node (1)
Desmoplastic Intrabdominal round cell tumor	**8**	**2** (25%)	Rectum (1), bladder (1)
Fibrosarcoma	**14**	**1** (7.14%)	Liver (1)
Other sarcomas	**118**	**0**	
Total	**357**	**40** (11.2%)	

Table 1. Histological type of sarcoma stage IV and metastatic sites (1998-2007: The Central region of Tunisia)

Liver metastasis of GIST are frequent. It mainly occurs after incomplete resection of the primitive lesion. Surgical resection is the preferred treatment, but there is a high rate of recurrence. Imatinib is the treatment of choice for these cases. With effective treatment, GIST becomes entirely cystic. Upon reactivation, the cysts develop intracystic enhancing nodules [25]

We report a case of liver metastasis of GIST that occurred three years after the incomplete resection of the intestinal tumor treated with Imatinib. The CT scan showed the development of intracystic enhancing nodules within Six months of Imatinib.

4. References

[1] Rosenthal TC, Kraybill W. Soft tissue sarcomas: integrating primary care recognition with tertiary care center treatment. *Am Fam Physician*. 1999; 60(2):567-572.

[2] DeVita VT Jr, Hellman S, Rosenberg SA, eds. Cancer: Principles and Practice of Oncology. 6th ed. Philadelphia, PA: Lippincott Williams & Wilkins, 2001:1841–1891.

[3] Coindre JM, Terrier P, Guillou L, et al. Predictive value of grade for metastasis development in the main histologic types of adult soft tissue sarcomas: a study of 1240 patients from the French Federation of Cancer Centers Sarcoma Group. Cancer 2001;91:1914–1926.

[4] Hoeber I, Spillane AJ, Fisher C, Thomas JM. Accuracy of biopsy techniques for limb and limb girdle soft tissue tumors. Ann Surg Oncol 2001;8:80e87.

[5] Heslin MJ, Lewis JJ, Woodruff JM, Brennan MF. Core needle biopsy for diagnosis of extremity soft tissue sarcoma. Ann Surg Oncol 1997;4:425e431.

[6] Greene FL, Page DL, Fleming FD, et al. (eds). American Joint Committee on Cancer: Cancer Staging Manual. 6th ed. New York, NY: Springer; 2002:221–226.

[7] Costa J, Wesley RA, Glatstein E, Rosenberg SA. The grading of soft tissue sarcomas. Results of a clinicohistopathologic correlation in a series of 163 cases. Cancer 1984;53:530–541.

[8] Guillou L, Coindre JM, Bonichon F, et al. Comparative study of the National Cancer Institute and French Federation of Cancer Centers Sarcoma Group grading systems in a population of 410 adult patients with soft tissue sarcoma. J Clin Oncol 1997;15:350–362.

[9] Coindre JM, Terrier P, Bui NB, et al. Prognostic factors in adult patients with locally controlled soft tissue sarcoma. A study of 546 patients from the French Federation of Cancer Centers Sarcoma Group. J Clin Oncol 1996;14:869–877.

[10] Thway K. Pathology of soft tissue sarcomas. Clin Oncol (R Coll Radiol). 2009 Nov;21(9):695-705. Epub 2009 Sep 6.

[11] Fong Y, Coit DG, Woodruff JM, Brennan MF. Lymph node metastasis from soft tissue sarcoma in adults. Analysis of data from a prospective database of 1772 sarcoma patients. Ann Surg 1993;217:72–77.

[12] Gadd MA, Casper ES, Woodruff JM, et al. Development and treatment of pulmonary metastases in adult patients with extremity soft tissue sarcoma. Ann Surg 1993; 218(6):705–712.

[13] Lewis JJ, Brennan MF. Soft tissue sarcomas. Curr Probl Surg 1996; 33(10):817- 872.

[14] Lewis JJ, Brennan MF. Soft tissue sarcomas. *Curr Probl Surg*. 1996; 33(10):817-872.

[15] Potter DA, Glenn J, Kinsella T, et al. Patterns of recurrence in patients with high-grade soft-tissue sarcomas. *J Clin Oncol*. 1985; 3(3):353-366.

[16] Fong Y, Coit DG, Woodruff JM, Brennan MF. Lymph node metastasis from soft tissue sarcoma in adults: analysis of data from a prospective database of 1772 sarcoma patients. *Ann Surg*. 1993; 217(1):72-77.

[17] Cheng EY, Springfield DS, Mankin HJ. Frequent incidence of extrapulmonary sites of initial metastasis in patients with liposarcoma. Cancer. 1995; 75(5):1120-1127.

[18] Pearlstone DB, Pisters PW, Bold RJ, et al. Patterns of recurrence in extremity liposarcoma: implications for staging and follow-up. Cancer. 1999; 85(1):85-92.

[19] Vassilopoulos PP, Voros DN, Kelessis NG, Katsilieris JN, Apostolikas NG. Unusual spread of liposarcoma. Anticancer Res. 2001; 21(2B):1419-1422.

[20] Potter DA, Glenn J, Kinsella T, et al. Patterns of recurrence in patients with high-grade soft-tissue sarcomas. J Clin Oncol. 1985; 3(3):353-366.

[21] Vezeridis MP, Moore R, Karakousis CP. Metastatic patterns in soft tissue sarcomas. Arch Surg. 1983. 118(8):915-918.

[22] Tedeschi CG. Systemic multicentric lipoblastosis. Arch Pathol. 1946; 42:320-337.

[23] Enzinger FM, Winslow DJ. Liposarcoma: a study of 103 cases. Virchows Arch Pathol Anat Physiol Klin Med. 1962; 335:367-388.

[24] Pezzi CM, Rawlings Jr MS, Esgro JJ, et al. Prognostic factors in 227 patients with malignant fibrous histiocytoma. Cancer 1992;69(8):2098–103

[25] Burkill G, et al. Malignant Gastrointestinal Stromal Tumor: Distribution, Imaging Features, and Pattern of Metastatic Spread. *Radiology* 2003; 226: 527-532.

[26] Fethi Derbel, Hassene Hajji, Abdallah Mtimet, Mehdi Ben Hadj Hamida, Jaafar Mazhoud, Sabri Youssef, Ali Ben Ali, Habib Khochtali, Ajmi Chaoucha, Moncef Mokni, Hela Jemni, Ridha Ben Hadj Hamida. Liver metastasis of malignant fibrous histiocytoma: A case report Arab Journal of Gastroenterology June 2010 (Vol. 11, Issue 2, Pages 113-115)